AYURVEDA
FOR OBESITY AND
GUT HEALTH

"Dr. L. Eduardo Cardona-Sanclemente's new book, following his previous title *Ayurveda for Depression*, is a major contribution to the interface between ayurveda and modern medicine. It is a detailed guide to understanding the mind-body relationship according to ayurveda, empowering the reader to take practical steps toward healthy weight management, especially after years of unsuccessful self-management. This guide is a must-read and a timely work for physicians to integrate with their patients when addressing obesity, being overweight, and gut health."

DR. JAISRI M. LAMBERT, AYURVEDA PHYSICIAN (NAMA) AND
FOUNDER OF THE CANADA AYURVEDA RESEARCH
& EDUCATION FOUNDATION (CARE)

"This book on ayurveda for obesity and gut health is a seminal piece of work, particularly now that we are truly in a 'global obesity and gut health pandemic.' The gut microbiome—the gut-brain axis—is at the heart of this crisis. Dr. Eduardo's background in both Western and Eastern medicine makes him the person who can help bridge the gap in understanding where and why many of the current diet/exercise protocols fall short. Dr. Eduardo's authenticity, passion for ayurveda, and love for humanity are at the core of his work and set him apart from other *Vaidyas* (doctors). True inquiry and integrity with wisdom is a rare but powerful combination; this is who Dr. L. Eduardo Cardona-Sanclemente is, and this is the essence of his work."

MONA DOCTOR, COFOUNDER AND DIRECTOR
OF THE INTEGRAL SPACE, MUMBAI, INDIA

"I first became a patient of Dr. L. Eduardo Cardona-Sanclemente in 2006. I was suffering from obesity and anxiety. I received great support from his ayurvedic approach to diet and lifestyle. He encouraged me to join him for a three-week ayurvedic retreat in Coimbatore, India. It was a very special experience. In 2009 I had a serious fall. Eduardo was there immediately to treat me and help me recover quickly. His knowledge of ayurvedic supplements and Indian massage was very valuable in my recovery. His personal support and encouragement of self-discipline was exemplary. I still incorporate his ideas and approach into my life."

HEATHER ELGOOD, MBE, DIRECTOR EMERITUS OF THE
POSTGRADUATE DIPLOMA IN ASIAN ART, THE SCHOOL OF
ORIENTAL AND AFRICAN STUDIES, UNIVERSITY OF LONDON

"I have been a patient of Dr. L. Eduardo Cardona-Sanclemente due to my conditions of morbid obesity and diabetes. I had been taking pharmacological drugs for several years that did nothing but 'keep me stable.' Thanks to his support, I integrated his customized ayurvedic approach to diet, lifestyle, and other practices assigned due to my constitution. I can tell you that today I am a borderline overweight person and I am not taking any medication for diabetes. These changes, which initially were a great effort for me, are now enjoyable norms for my new healthy body and mind."

MARCO A. GARZON-ALFARO, ATTORNEY

Traditional medicine has played a central role in the success of human life on Earth, especially in China and India. We thank Dr. L. Eduardo Cardona-Sanclemente, who was a respected faculty member at our university, for publishing the wisdom of ayurvedic medicine to educate and inform readers how to achieve optimal weight and health in a natural and safe way.

RON ZAIDMAN, PRESIDENT OF FIVE BRANCHES UNIVERSITY
GRADUATE SCHOOL OF TRADITIONAL CHINESE MEDICINE

AYURVEDA
FOR OBESITY AND
GUT HEALTH

The Natural Way to Overcome Weight Imbalances for Your Body Type

A Sacred Planet Book

DR. L. EDUARDO CARDONA-SANCLEMENTE

Healing Arts Press
Rochester, Vermont

Healing Arts Press
One Park Street
Rochester, Vermont 05767
www.HealingArtsPress.com

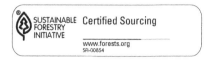

SUSTAINABLE FORESTRY INITIATIVE — Certified Sourcing
www.forests.org
SFI-00854

Text stock is SFI certified

Healing Arts Press is a division of Inner Traditions International

Sacred Planet Books are curated by Richard Grossinger, Inner Traditions editorial board member and cofounder and former publisher of North Atlantic Books. The Sacred Planet collection, published under the umbrella of the Inner Traditions family of imprints, includes works on the themes of consciousness, cosmology, alternative medicine, dreams, climate, permaculture, alchemy, shamanic studies, oracles, astrology, crystals, hyperobjects, locutions, and subtle bodies.

Note to the Reader: *The ayurvedic material provided in this book is not intended to serve as medical or therapeutic diagnosis or treatment. If you are interested in addressing body-mind health imbalances related to the obesity or gut issues described here, I advise you to discuss them with your physician or a certified ayurvedic doctor before starting any practice to avoid any kind of adverse events. Case studies presented here have been anonymized for patient confidentiality.*

Cataloging-in-Publication Data for this title is available from the Library of Congress

ISBN 978-1-64411-488-9 (print)
ISBN 978-1-64411-489-6 (ebook)

Printed and bound in the United States by Lake Book Manufacturing, LLC
The text stock is SFI certified. The Sustainable Forestry Initiative® program promotes sustainable forest management.

10 9 8 7 6 5 4 3 2 1

Text design by Virginia Scott Bowman and layout by Debbie Glogover
This book was typeset in Garamond Premier Pro with Gill Sans MT Pro, Hagin Caps, ITC Legacy Sans, and Kepler Std used as display fonts
Figures on pages 18, 19, 20, 21, 22, 28, 67, 69, 87, 113, 150, 155, 185, 201, 214, and 254 by Patrick Byrne
Line drawings in appendix 3 by Christina Wightman at Etching Trails

To send correspondence to the author of this book, mail a first-class letter to the author c/o Inner Traditions • Bear & Company, One Park Street, Rochester, VT 05767, and we will forward the communication, or contact the author directly at **EduardoCardona.com**.

CONTENTS

Part III. Ayurvedic Body-Mind Constitutions
Prakruti, Vikruti, and Manas Prakruti

Part IV. Participants That Are Fundamental to Life
The Unfolding Language of Our Gut

Part V. Main Structural and Functional Organs
Players in Your Bodily Imbalance

Part VI. Making Ayurveda Work for You
Rebalance via Proper Food and Diet

PREFACE

We will be companions here, traveling together among these pages, so let me first provide some personal background, starting with my early connection to this subject.

From a young age, it was endlessly fascinating for me to discover how diverse our human bodies are in shape and size; and yet, with all our many different physical manifestations, we seem to function much the same. Still, as a society, we make distinctions: how easy it is to put people into boxes or categories according to our preconceptions and prejudices surrounding "appearance." In addressing diet, gut health, and obesity through my scientific and professional work over decades, I found myself increasingly drawn to the relatively uncharted phenomenon of body-mind connection, as a way of explaining how dietary, mental, socioeconomic, and other imbalances affecting the emotional body-mind framework can shape our eating and weight issues. I write "uncharted" because in the Western medical scientific literature, it is only recently that we have witnessed an explosion in the quantity and quality of body-mind research being conducted through clinical and scientific exploration.

However, what I sought to learn and understand had, in fact, been transmitted orally and written down thousands of years earlier in the sacred Sanskrit texts that embody the Hindu philosophy of Vedanta and the ancient practice of ayurveda, in beautifully crafted expositions by scholars such as Charaka, Sushruta, and others. Vedanta is an ancient school of Hindu philosophy teaching the concepts of the soul (*atman*) and its relationship with the supreme God (Brahman), centered on the three canonical Vedic texts: the *Upanishads*, the *Brahma Sutras*, and the *Bhagavad Gita*. In addition, *Rig*, *Sama*, *Yajur*, and *Atharva* are the four Vedas (ancient Hindu scriptures), and ayurveda is a subsection of the *Atharvaveda*. In a testament to their timelessness, it is remarkable that the essence of these ancient texts remains highly relevant today. Whilst these texts are recognized as great philosophical and spiritual works, here we will only concern ourselves with their direct, practical commentary on diet, gut health, well-being, and weight-related issues. We will explore this, and its scientific application to our subject matter—but first what is needed for readers new to this ancient medical system is a modern scientific explanation of ayurveda, and a description of its efficacy. This I will furnish you with, in parallel to exploring how ayurveda uniquely addresses matters of gut health and related conditions such as obesity. My aim with this approach is to provide a recognizable framework within which to view ayurvedic practice, both for the newcomer and the seasoned health care professional.

My journey to ayurveda has been a long and gratifying one. I began my career in conventional Western medicine, conducting scientific research and teaching medical students in universities and hospitals throughout Europe. However, my quest to understand and address in a more holistic way the role of body types, genetics, habits, lifestyle, and psychological components in gut health and obesity drew me to the ayurvedic medical system, which for thousands of years has expounded, in crystal clear terms, how we manifest responses to physical and mental challenges and how our *prakruti*—our individual constitution type, determined at birth—dominates outcomes.

Fifteen years ago, I was invited to be an international speaker at the annual conference of the United States' National Ayurvedic Medical Association (NAMA) in Palo Alto, California, where I gave a talk about obesity.[1] Among the participants listening to my presentation were people directly concerned with the subject matter, for clear personal reasons, and this touched me deeply. Before that, I had mainly given seminars and talks in European countries, covering various topics within ayurveda—usually chronic conditions including obesity—to groups of forty to fifty academics or health care professionals motivated by their work interest in people who are overweight, obese, or suffer from other metabolic disorders. In the early days of these academic presentations, many of the participants approached the treatment of chronic conditions with a one-size-fits-all mindset, but my view is that today, mainstream Western medicine is awakening to the wider field of cofactors impacting our gut health generally, and our high incidence of obesity specifically. In particular, I've seen at my presentations, resonating with my Palo Alto presentation at NAMA, that there is a noticeable decrease in the social stigma associated with weight imbalance, with more focus being rightly placed on what causes it and how we address it individually, rather than condemning habits we often wrongly associate with its cause.

Research has shown that a culture of prejudicial behavior toward people with obesity and other metabolic disorders is linked with many negative outcomes like harassment, discrimination, and depression. As well, studies show that such prejudice makes it more difficult for some to seek a body rebalance strategy—not just for weight loss but also when it comes to other types of health care, such as mental health support. Contrast this with people suffering from, say, cancer, who rightly receive sympathetic support. Neither group is largely responsible for their condition. But one of these conditions is socially stigmatized, and it happens to be the one that is visible to the naked eye. This stigma is part of my motivation for writing this book. The more we explain health conditions in a rounded way, the more we can accept them with compassion, both as sufferers and as supporters of those who suffer. Let us treat ourselves with kindness as we address weight, gut, and related mental health issues.

WHY I WROTE THIS BOOK

I slept and dreamt that life was joy. I awoke and saw that life was service. I acted and behold, service was joy.

RABINDRANATH TAGORE

On several occasions I have been asked to write for the general public on the subject of the gut and metabolic imbalances, including obesity and being overweight, since I am considered by some to be an authority on the subject. This stems from over forty years of medical, scientific research at respected medical schools and universities, in my specialist areas of biochemistry, physiology, nutrition, diet, and the causes, nature, and effects of these in the formation and persistence of chronic disorders. So, what prevented me from writing such a book up to now? I had no problem writing scientific papers for journals, yet I felt a real difficulty in trying to formulate the beautiful but intricate science of gut health into material that was suitable for the general public. I also had very personal reasons for not confronting this challenge.

I am a private person, but I feel it is time to share my story before going further. For countless years, I had a secret lover. We lived quietly with each other and traveled together everywhere, from the Americas to India and many other places. We were inseparable. I learned a lot from our connection, and I grew up academically and as an adult through this close companionship.

In the late 1980s I visited India for the first time, for a period of six months, and had the experience of sharing daily in a culture where nutritional approaches, diet, and mental attitudes were completely different to those we know in the West—and my conceptualizations shifted as a result of engaging with ayurveda. As I researched and experienced ayurveda, my analytical, scientific mindset eventually assumed its proper role, helping me to gradually integrate and construct a more well-rounded understanding of how our health state begins in the gastrointestinal tract (GIT) and how our body imbalances are associated with it.

So, what of my secret lover? Let me be fair to you and end the mystery: my beloved was the one and only cholesterol. You see, my secret love was not exclusive to me; other scientists wanted to get to know her in detail. We lived under the umbrella of the metabolism of lipids and lipoproteins, and its connection with chronic diseases such as obesity, hypertension, and other risk factors of cardiovascular diseases. We were very attached.[2] Nowadays, metabolic syndrome and gut imbalances, which result in outcomes such as obesity or being overweight, are pandemic in both developed and developing countries, and are not only seen in the adult population but are also becoming more prevalent in adolescence. Given this explosion of gut metabolic imbalances, and my lifelong love for lipids (my beloved cholesterol), as well as the failure of current regimes aimed at tackling obesity to slow its increasing prevalence, I feel the need, through this book, to take a different approach that addresses these particular body imbalances and their treatment in a more holistic fashion. I hope my deep and lifelong affection and respect for this subject matter shines through as I take you on a journey that draws upon ancient systems to discover new ways of helping people who are overweight, obese, or suffer from declining gut health.

AIMS OF THIS BOOK

My aim is to show how ayurveda, the world's oldest continuously practiced medical system, can contribute powerfully, effectively, and economically to addressing the multifactorial characteristics of the present pandemic of obesity, poor gut health, and being overweight. I hope to provide a lively exploration of ayurvedic concepts, diagnostics, and treatments, and how these are becoming more accessible to you today as you address the problems of obesity or being overweight.

I also intend to share the practical knowledge, applications, actions, and ayurvedic strategies to rebalance body functions and achieve physical, emotional, and spiritual wellness by exploring the intersection between science, spirituality, and consciousness. I will establish approaches that integrate ayurvedic practice with corresponding aspects of modern medicine, based on accessible biomedical terminology, clinical research, and therapies, so we can translate and attest to the remarkable wisdom and efficacy of ayurveda. Previously, most ayurvedic instruction was presented from within the canons of the ancient Sanskrit texts. These have remained intact for thousands of years and are very difficult for the ordinary reader to use when seeking to understand not just whether this system works but also how it works.

I'll provide you with fresh perspectives for understanding your body-mind imbalances that are determined by your individual makeup. Good health is "simple, but not easy"; however, ayurvedic practices will support you in rebalancing your physical, mental, and spiritual health. In some cases, these practices will be restorative; in others they will prevent deterioration of body or mind conditions.

Moreover, I'll communicate to you the integrated concepts of nutrition, dietary behaviors, physical activities, hereditary factors, mindset, and other influences, to address body imbalances associated with food components such as carbohydrates, lipids or fats, proteins, and other related molecules—without further promoting any stigma.

This book also provides references to some of the latest scientific studies, as well as tables, figures, and images to support your understanding of ayurvedic principles. Relevant ayurvedic terms are defined in a glossary at the back of the book. I provide pertinent quotations and citations from classical ayurvedic Sanskrit verses (*slokas*), or other reference works that capture precisely—and better than I could state in my own words—specific tenets of ayurveda.

I dedicate this book to the following individuals, each of whom has had a profound influence on my life and work: My dear father, with deep affection, for his perpetual example of *satyagraha*. Indira and Mona Doctor, who in 1986 introduced me to their extraordinary country. And lastly, several dear Indian friends and colleagues like Eliam Thomas and Vinod Kumar, for their kind support in furthering my appreciation of their country and the science of ayurveda.

My thanks and gratitude go to Richard Grossinger for introducing me to the Inner Traditions team. I also wish to thank my dear friend and brother Patrick Owen Byrne for his professional support in polishing some of my fourth-language misdemeanors and for being a sounding board in regard to preparation and presentation.

PART I
What Is Ayurveda?

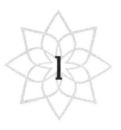

THE BASIC PRINCIPLES
OF AYURVEDA

Ayurveda is a holistic health care system that is approximately five thousand years old. Originally, it was passed on by oral tradition, and its earliest documentation is found in the ancient philosophical texts known as the Vedas, a profound component of Indian culture and history, and a cornerstone of Hinduism. Ayurveda has been practiced in hospitals throughout India for thousands of years, treating millions of patients. However, in the Western world, ayurveda is still considered to be a complementary or alternative medicine, despite its long-documented history and daily practice in India. The World Health Organization (WHO) has recognized ayurveda as a safe traditional medicine based on an extensive body of scientific evidence.[1]

Ayurveda's main objective is restoring balance within you. It is that simple, and the simplicity of this aim will be constantly reinforced throughout this book, because all components of ayurvedic medicine align to achieve this goal.

Ayurveda emphasizes the wholeness of each of us. It defines wellness as a state in which all bodily tissues, organs, systems, and functions are acting together interdependently to maintain the delicate balance between body, mind, and consciousness (spirit) so as to promote good health, in spite of many negative influences around us.

MAIN FACTORS OF IMBALANCE

When your gut is in a state of imbalance, its ability to manufacture and synthetize, as well as assimilate and absorb various nutrients, regulate blood sugar, and store fat becomes impaired. These imbalanced conditions occur most often due to overeating in parallel with low expenditure of energy. They become the cause for accumulation of lipids, in particular at the level of adipose tissue and liver. A deterioration in these basic functions can lead to putting on extra weight, or becoming overweight or obese. By maintaining balanced gut health, we can prevent or more easily manage such conditions.

In Western scientific terms, obesity is described as a multifactorial disease involving a complex network of physical, systemic, physiological, and mental factors. Your body accommodates excess calories—which normally come from carbohydrates, fats, or proteins—as forms of fat that may impair the maintenance of good heath, because this fat cannot be burned off through the usual channels. Many Western diets are high in calories, frequently from fast food and high-calorie beverages. People with body imbalances might need to eat more calories, or what we call "empty calories," before feeling full, or may eat more than is necessary due to stress or anxiety. The ayurvedic approach of personalized or tailored nutrition recognizes our individuality and is rooted in the concept that one size does not fit all. I am sure this perception resonates within you.

ENCOURAGEMENT

To encourage you to read further, let me set out some key challenges and explain how I approach the subject at hand.

If weight loss and rebalancing were easy, you wouldn't be reading this book. Given that you have started to read this book, you will be learning about your gut and how and when to communicate with it.

Weight loss, for most people, is not just a simple equation of eating less or exercising more. This book will support you by investigating the ayurvedic understanding of how your gut functions based on your individual body constitution (your prakruti) and its potential and limitations and will provide you with the most relevant tools and personalized activities to address weight and gut health issues naturally, economically, and effectively. In these pages you'll find recognition of yourself as you are right now, and if required, you'll be aided in your transition away from a "vicious circle" to a "virtuous circle."

The words *obese* or *obesity* have clear medical meanings, but they often appear with adjectives, such as "morbidly obese." However, the categories of "obese" and "overweight" in fact exist in various grades; one is not simply obese or morbidly obese—these distinctions are more nuanced than merely one or the other. As such, I will refer to grades of obesity where possible or helpful. One fundamental pillar of ayurveda is the respect for all creatures.

Awareness of your body imbalance and what it means for those who are trying to manage extra weight, or who are overweight or obese, is critical to making change. We will explore this in both ayurvedic and modern scientific terms, address specific gut health and weight issues, and present effective ways you can tackle weight and general gut health in your daily life, with minimal disruption to your regular activities.

Let me share that recently, I wrote a book called *Ayurveda for Depression*, and through the process of writing on this other pandemic condition, I was reminded of the many interconnections between these subjects. For that reason, here, I will sometimes refer you to the contents of my previous book to provide you some complementary information that may be helpful.[2]

A SOCIETAL APPROACH

Modern biomedical research seeks to provide answers as to how we can effectively address these physical, and mental, imbalances. However, these approaches tend to be more "macro" in their application—a one-size-fits-all prescription—irrespective of the reasons for a particular individual's being overweight or suffering from obesity. This can result in standard "guidelines" that cover virtually everyone but may not be ideal for many people.

Ayurveda differs fundamentally in its approach: you are a person requiring solutions tailored for you and your condition; you are not treated as a tiny replication within a larger pool of patients.

Also, let me note here that words matter: The modern language used in addressing pandemic or epidemic challenges is often the language of warfare—"the war on drugs," "the war on terror," "the war against cancer," "the battle against obesity," and more recently, "the war against Covid" It is the language of fighting, conflict, and confrontation. It is not the language of solutions. Perhaps it is time to stop "killing" and instead start noticing and learning to live based on the observation of our biological processes that lead us to these types of personal imbalances and participate actively from a nonviolent place within ourselves.

What we don't hear—and what I want to address more specifically in this book on obesity, under the light of ayurveda—is a more discerning language of change: "the answer to obesity" instead of "the war against obesity"; or "the connection to our gut" instead of "the war against calories." Connecting and sharing "the answer" is a step toward resolution of the challenge at hand. Nobody is at war with anybody here. This phrasing reshapes our expectations, showing us that we will not be fighting and killing but instead facing and solving the issues.[3]

We will also address and describe extra weight, being overweight, and obesity conditions as metabolic imbalances in order to differentiate them from the relatively new term *metabolic syndrome*, a cluster of biochemical and physiological abnormalities such as high blood sugar, high blood pressure, anomalous cholesterol levels, and surplus body fat around the waist—all of which are associated with the development of cardiovascular disease, including heart attack and stroke, as well as type 2 diabetes.[4] Most of the ailments related to metabolic syndrome have no symptoms, and they respond well to exercise, weight loss, proper diet, and other lifestyle changes like quitting smoking, which can eventually be supported by prescribed medication.

YOUR TREE

Like us, trees also come in all shapes and sizes, and they have the potential to grow healthier and thrive when planted on favorable and protective grounds. Looking at nature, we see that trees are nurtured through the elements of light, earth, air, heat, and space, and require a balance of these factors to grow. A mango tree will produce mangos, and their taste will be sweet, while a lemon tree will grow lemons with a sour or bitter taste. Even if they were planted in the same soil and received identical nourishment, their inner natures will result in fruits with specific characteristics. Of course, to create their fruits, these trees require special care such as the right soil and water, and the eradication of weeds. So, consider, if you were a tree, what type of tree would you be?

We have been and remain engaged in a process that is doing continuous damage to nature, which we lack the light or clarity to discern, and which as a result directly affects what is so beautifully described in ayurveda as prakruti—our individual constitution. Our human situation cannot be compared to trees well-nourished by exceptional soil conditions that allow them to grow, spread, and create worthy output. Independently of our prakruti, either by ignorance, misuse, or abuse, we allow the growth of many weeds around us in our daily lives, often in the form of habits. Additionally, we do not necessarily know the kinds of fruits that life has invited us to yield, and as a result, in the process of daily life, these weeds can proliferate, consume space, and use up our essential substrates, making us weaker and more imbalanced. Without taking care, we can end up being identified with the weeds we nurture within and around us.

The laws of nature—by means of the combination of our parents' DNA and external environmental conditions at the moment of conception—gives us each a unique prakruti. And ayurveda is a door to access awareness of ourselves and the possibility to understand and accept our own nature. At this early stage in our journey, it is appropriate to ask: What is the connection between all this and a condition of imbalance such as obesity? In the process of growing up and all through our adult lives, most of the time we do not have sufficient clarity to sense, discern, and breathe our real human condition. This is normal—we are not constant observers of our inner physical and mental health. For all of us, our likes and dislikes in terms of food, diet, behavior, and social pressures are conditioned either by our genes, families, or social and geographical environments. Unlike trees, we can move, and that sense of mobility gives us the impression of freedom. In fact, we do not realize—or we keep forgetting—that in reality we are not free, and our lives depend on food for our bodily and mental functions. The false impressions we derive from our physical mobility are a distraction impeding us from facing reality.

When we choose the food we eat, how much do we know, or even consider, about its real qualities? Here is where ayurveda provides an answer related to your personal constitution. Most people only occasionally become aware of their dietary choices' impact on their health, usually as they age, or under specific circumstances such as a traumatic experience. They then realize that the branches and trunk, once big and strong, are in fact troubled by lack of quality nutrients from the natural environment and perhaps too many junk, or wrong, foods resulting in the roots becoming weaker over time and affecting the entire bodily balance.

Many of us are concerned about the deforestation of our planet and the effects on the quality of our global environment. Rarely do we stop to consider our inner deforestation: the wilting of a once-thriving intestinal flora—nowadays more commonly called our microbiota—the vast array of microorganisms within the greenhouse of our gut, whose maintenance is essential to healthy living. Microbiota, and their arena of activity, the microbiome, are essential components of good gut health and weight management.

Ayurveda understood thousands of years ago this essential process of body maintenance and strengthening against the perils of everyday living.

Central to ayurveda is the notion that "the issues are within the tissues," a concept we will be discussing throughout this book. Life provides us the best surroundings to grow healthy, from the land to the other essential elements such as light, heat, air, and water.

> *But you must not forget it. You become forever responsible for that which you have tamed. You are responsible for your rose . . .*
> ANTOINE DE SAINT-EXUPÉRY,
> *THE LITTLE PRINCE*

My intention is to be the best possible gardener and work with you to take care of your tree and rose by explaining in clear and practical ways how to use ayurvedic knowledge in your active body-mind management process, in rebalancing and growing your tree or rose in a proper way.

However, remember that we, like trees, also come in all shapes and sizes, and ayurveda addresses your individual health needs, beginning in the GIT, by trying to keep your individual constitution and digestive fire in balance. Ayurveda understands how an imbalance leads to problems in various parts of the body, triggering symptoms, syndromes, and then finally disease.

We do not go directly from health to disease. The ayurvedic explanation offered in this book will help you understand the long chain and progression involved: just like overnutrition or undernutrition of the tree, obesity and being overweight fall under the same laws and processes of nature. This book will show you how to intervene and turn back toward better health.[5]

OUR BODY-MIND

Body imbalances leading to the development of extra weight, or leading one to become overweight or obese, are the result of lifestyle factors and the dynamics of diet, nutrition, food intake style, working conditions, physical activities and exercise, stress levels, socioeconomical factors, and social (media) pressure. Note that while there is a large menu of ingredients here, not all fit each of us the same. Ayurveda recognizes that—and, happily, I am going to present you with a personalized, practical, easy, and cost-effective way to tackle your individual needs and issues by combining profound ayurvedic knowledge and modern medical modalities.

In terms of food intake, we are all different: each of us has different ways to digest food based on our genetic predispositions and learned experiences, our intestinal flora, our patterns of food ingestion, and other aspects such as our external environment, climate, type of work, and family conditions.[6] By not taking care of these individual, distinctive factors, and not considering the totality of their impact when addressing imbalances of body and mind, we are approaching conditions such as carrying extra weight, or being overweight or obese, in a way that is neither holistic nor ultimately effective. There will be always something we have not addressed.

We all, to a greater or lesser degree, are looking for the components that represent living a healthy life: eating healthy, an active lifestyle, stress management, loving ourselves, powering our minds, and achieving a happy life balance. The ayurvedic scholars recognized that while we share many common facets, genetically we are all different and live under different circumstances and influences; for example, when considering just one aspect such as food intake, we see that each of us handles the food we eat, the time we eat, the disposition with which we eat, the amounts we eat, and the way we eat, in different ways. Subtle differences within each variable mean we each need tailored solutions based on our body-mind constitution and personal lifestyle. Environmentally, two people may work in an office, and one finds the temperature too hot while the other thinks it's just fine. While we share traits, at the micro and macro levels we all respond differently.

Ayurveda does not provide a cure for the masses; it treats the masses, one individual at a time. There is no "one size fits all." This is ayurveda's uniqueness, and contrasts with modern medical practices that develop a single pill or diet to treat millions of different patients.

It is my task to show you how internal and external factors play a role in your individuality, putting you at risk of moving from a state of balance to a state of imbalance with respect to declining gut health and its consequences.

As a summary, I will say that in nature we see large and robust trees. There is nothing wrong with being like them; what is wrong is to be an unhealthy large and robust one.

2

THE AYURVEDIC MEDICAL TREATISES OF THE *CHARAKA SAMHITA* AND *SUSHRUTA SAMHITA*

How Ayurvedic Founders Provide Timeless Wisdom

Ayurveda, one of the oldest complete systems of medicine, was developed in India around 2000–1500 BCE. The seers and scholars of India at that time used their observation, knowledge, and environmental facilities to formulate the outstanding system of ayurveda, which translates to the "science of life." The *Charaka Samhita* and *Sushruta Samhita* are the essential scriptures of ayurveda, and they have been supplemented over time by a large number of additions based on scholars' observation and experience.[1]

Historical records show that in our seven global regions commonly regarded as continents, every civilization has had its own medicinal tradition. Regrettably, all these systems suffered through invasions and colonization in one way or another, resulting in the destruction of most or all of the accumulated knowledge, in some cases entire libraries' worth. The Indus Valley, which today includes India, was no exception to this plunder. Despite this, ayurvedic traditional medical knowledge remains alive today, unchanged over the centuries due to its well-documented treatises. Ayurveda's authentic framework of knowledge describes the way we know things and the way things are. The Rig-Veda and Atharva-Veda provide centuries of documented knowledge collected by sages and scientists of each era, describing a tradition of healthy living rooted in a profound observation of the natural sciences.[2, 3]

In particular I will draw your attention to the existence of a number of texts addressing body weight rebalancing, as we embark on our journey into ayurveda. These classic texts of the ancient scholars are called the Samhitas in Sanskrit, a word that translates approximately to "treatise" or "compendium." I quote from the Samhitas partly because they contain, in the written word, the breadth and depth of ayurvedic scientific practices that have remained largely intact for thousands of years and are highly relevant to how we address obesity from an ayurvedic perspective. I also quote from the Samhitas because they contain the most profound, timeless wisdom. One sentence from a Samhita can capture the entire essence of a topic. The Samhitas are, of course, originally written in Vedic Sanskrit, and here I will use widely adopted English translations that hopefully are faithful enough to the original meaning. I should also mention that some of the language as translated is direct, archaic, and would be considered inaccurate and problematic if used in the context of describing a patient's symptoms or state of health. My role here is to convey how such descriptions were written, thus they have remained largely unchanged. Whilst some phrases appear judgmental, I will not take issue with that; I will simply pass on to you how ancient scholars described such things, without making judgments of my own.

As a final note, striking similarities have been observed, both in theory and clinical practice, between ayurveda and Traditional Chinese Medicine—as well as certain significant differences. Perhaps the influence of ayurveda was brought to China by travelers or missionary Indian Buddhist monks, and exchanges also flowed the other way. There are also historical reports describing interchanges between ayurveda and the Middle East.[4]

CHARAKA SAMHITA

In Sanskrit, the term *charaka* can be translated as meaning "a wandering scholar or physician," which is used to describe the ancient tradition of wandering physicians carrying medical knowledge throughout India. The treatise of the *Charaka Samhita* is a major ayurvedic compendium of medical theory and practice represented by eight *sthana* (sections) composed of 120 chapters covering principles of medicine, pathology, anatomy, study of the sensory organs, therapeutics, pharmaceutics, and toxicology.

Key for us is that the Samhitas also include chapters on the relevant topics of hygiene, diet, prevention, medical education, and physician-nurse-patient collaboration required for health recovery, as well as describing success in treatments using many medicinal recipes that originate from plants, animal products, minerals, and metals.[5]

Charaka, the physician whose updates to the *Agnivesha Samhita* resulted in the *Charaka Samhita*, is thought to have flourished sometime around the fourth century BCE and is considered in India to be the Father of Medicine: "Health and disease cannot be predetermined, and human life can be prolonged or increased by paying attention to lifestyle" is one of his famous quotes. Charaka described obesity (*sthoulya*) as "disgraceful persons" (*ashta nindita*), in *Sutrasthana*, chapter 21, explaining the diagnosis, origins, characteristics, diet, and treatment. Charaka also mentioned *athi sthoulya* as one of the diseases occurring only by kapha dosha alone and they are called *kaphaja nanatmaja vyadhi*. The scholars described twenty types of vitiated conditions and considered that they could in fact be innumerable.[6]

SUSHRUTA SAMHITA

The *Sushruta Samhita* has six volumes containing 186 chapters covering the study of health and pathology in India. This treatise examines more than one thousand ailments, among them those related to body imbalances such as obesity and other metabolic disorders. Sushruta describes the causes, symptoms, signs, and treatments of obesity.[7, 8] These detail-rich volumes, dated to around the sixth century BCE, include the study of seven hundred healing plants, as well as several formulations developed from animal and mineral origins. The writer, Sushruta, conceived original and novel procedures in reparative surgical interventions, indeed inventing the practice of cosmetic surgery with procedures such as skin transplants and reconstruction of amputated noses. Sushruta is also widely regarded as the Father of Indian Medicine and, beyond India, as the Father of Plastic Surgery.

MADHAVA NIDANA

More recently, Madhava, from the seventh century, wrote the *Rug-vinischaya*, later known as the *Madhava Nidana*, a volume of seventy-nine chapters containing verses and references explaining the causes of a disease, early symptoms, full-fledged signs and symptoms, aggravating and relieving factors, and origins of several body imbalances. He described obesity under a separate heading called *medo roga*, mentioning causative factors (*nidana*), symptoms (*lakshana*), and pathogenesis (*samprapthi*). The *Madhava Nidana* is considered mainly a compilation of much earlier works of ayurvedic scholars such as the *Charaka Samhita*, *Sushruta Samhita*, and other classics.[9]

YOGA SUTRAS OF PATANJALI

The written yoga sutras emerge out of the Vedic tradition of ancient India circa 400 BCE. They are a thread of concepts that are each generally conveyed as a single sentence, or sometimes strung together into two or three sentences. Before the existence of the written form, sutras were memorized, and teachers would expand upon them. Yoga is one of the six schools of Vedic philosophy, linked with Samkhya philosophy, but commonly followed in Vedanta. The scholar Patanjali outlined a path with eight (*ashta*) limbs (*anga*) to quiet the mind and reach reunification with the Divine. Patanjali Yoga is also named Ashtanga Yoga (The Eight Limbs) and Raja Yoga (The Royal Path).[10] A description of an essential precept of the yoga sutras is located in the second sutra at the beginning of the text: "*Yoga chitta vritti nirodha*." This renowned sutra means that yoga (union) is achieved when the disorders (*vritti*) of the mind (*chitta*) are removed (*nirodha*). Most of the other yoga sutras are guidance regarding how to calm the mind and attain this yoga state. Ayurveda and other pertinent Vedic disciplines are more interconnected than we normally recognize, especially in the West. Since, as Vedic sciences, they are part of an integrated stream of higher knowledge, we cannot fully grasp the knowledge of one of these systems without the others.

Ayurveda and yoga continuously reestablish themselves and adapt without ever abandoning their core structures. We can see the rise and vitality of yoga over recent years, practiced by millions all over the world. Few doubt the efficacy of yoga in helping to maintain good physical and mental health, a pursuit often embodied in fashionable meditative techniques called mindfulness that receive increasing acceptance and practice. These are all part of ayurveda's tool kit for rebalancing health without using toxic and unnatural substances. Both yoga and mindfulness share a common practical point with ayurveda: they are very cost-effective, requiring minimal expense to fully engage with.

AYURVEDIC TERMINOLOGY

To explain ayurveda in Western scientific terms and also integrate this ancient science with modern science, a full comparative collation and analysis is required of every source describing the core of the ayurvedic system and its conceptual framework. Unfortunately, the translation or transliteration of Sanskrit into modern languages is not so simple, since some of the ancient Vedic Sanskrit terminology does not have an equivalent word, and the potential interpretations will not necessarily carry the same meaning. For that reason, I will be describing the core of ayurveda in our modern language all the way through, limiting myself as much as possible to using only the essential, non-translatable words or terms that are required to allow such an integration. The good news is that even where we do not have an exact match to the Sanskrit word, we do have excellent approximations in meanings. This situation is the same either when addressing body-mind imbalances such as metabolic disorders (obesity, diabetes, etc.), or other physical or mental conditions that require certain specific terms to properly describe the ayurvedic conceptualizations. As with any language, a term or a phrase can convey several meanings, and Sanskrit is no exception, with exact meaning depending on the context in which the terms are being used.

Texts such as the *Ramayana* and the *Mahabharata* were written in slokas, the classical basis for epic Indian poetry used in traditional Sanskrit poems. Ayurveda, as one of the branches of the Vedas, follows the same format. The Sanskrit word *sloka* denotes a verse, poem, proverb, or hymn that uses a specific meter. The functional translations and explanations will be more than enough for your perception and use. As an illustration, the term *ayurveda* combines two Sanskrit words: *ayur* (life or vital power) and *veda* (knowledge or science). Thus, ayurveda means "the knowledge or science of life" (As. Hr. Su. 1/3; Su. Sū. 1/12).

Let me provide two more examples to show you how the meaning depends on the context: The Sanskrit word *meda* signifies the fatty tissues of the body, but also means adipose tissue, omentum, and sebum (skin oil). The Sanskrit word *sattva* is said to have one hundred meanings. It is helpful to work with the ancient Sanskrit texts because of their richness and precision in describing particular conditions, and how we can link these descriptions to the treatment of body imbalances and related conditions. Thankfully, that is not a task we will need to dwell on too much here. Where possible, we will match the translated terms to words you may be familiar with from modern medicine.

In the same way that books provide references for scientific reports or findings, this book presents the essence of ayurveda through original quotations translated from the ayurvedic scholars. Some examples from the scholars Charaka and Sushruta:

From Sushruta:

Su. Chi.: *Sushruta Chikitsasthana*

Su. Sa.: *Sushruta Sharirasthana*

Su. Sū.: *Sushruta Sutrasthana*

From Charaka:

Ca. Su.: *Charaka Samhita Sutrasthana*

Ca. Ni.: *Charaka Samhita Nidanasthana*

Ca. Vi.: *Charaka Samhita Vimanasthana*

Another example from the third major treatise on ayurveda:

As. Hr. Su.: *Ashtanga Hrdayam Sutrasthana*

The sixteen essential terms we will be using, as well as their meanings, are listed below.

BASIC AYURVEDIC TERMS

Sanskrit Term	Modern Use of the Term
prakruti	pra = primary; kruti = creation; DNA; your primary constitution
vikruti	state of imbalance in your primary constitution
doshas	three physio-psychological body energies: *vata, pitta, kapha*
vata	movement, bodily activities
pitta	energy for metabolism
kapha	body structure, cohesion
dathus	seven bodily tissues
meda	adipose, fatty tissues
sthoulya	obesity
agni	digestive fire; food transformer
ama	undigested food; incomplete mental thoughts or emotions
malas	bodily waste products that need to be removed
atma	spirit, the self, soul, consciousness
manas	mind (can be individual or universal)
gunas	three qualities of the mind: sattva, rajas, tamas
sattva	truth, equanimity, contentment, consciousness
rajas	action, energy, movement, dynamism, alertness
tamas	inertia, heaviness, unconsciousness, imbalance

We will integrate these terms progressively, starting with concepts such as prakruti, gunas, meda, and sthoulya together with vata, pitta, and kapha. All are essential to the perception and comprehension of ayurvedic knowledge when we are addressing body weight imbalances. Understanding these terms and their use will make it easier to build your knowledge of ayurveda when addressing the subjects of body weight, obesity, the gut, or any other topic.

THREE UNIVERSAL BODY ENERGIES

Vata, Pitta, and Kapha

At the core of ayurveda is the aim to be in stable good health, and we achieve this by striving for a balanced body, mind, and consciousness—a concept that parallels the actual definition of health by the WHO.[1, 2] There are three major causative factors of managing health (*hetu*) and disease (*roga*): they are features of an individual in health (*arogya*), under disease (*rogi*), and in regard to medicines, treatments, diet, and lifestyle (*aushadha*).

For ayurveda, this balance results from a dynamic adjusting of the following four participants. Each and every one of us is the result of a process of dynamic balancing of:

Dosha	Biofire (Agni)	Tissues—Seven Dhatus	Waste Products
vata	stomach/duodenum (*jataragni*)	plasma	feces
pitta	five basic elements (*bhutagni*)	blood	urine
kapha	seven tissues (*dhatwagni*)	muscle	sweat
		fat	
		bone	
		reproductive tissue	
		bone marrow	

PANCHAMAHABHUTAS
(THE FIVE ELEMENTS)
....
From Subtle to Gross Elements

The precept that the entire universe and all human beings are one, and governed by identical laws of nature, is the essence of ayurveda. Any alterations that could occur in the universe will also occur in the human body. Consequently, natural substances are concordant with the human body and support it in retaining the balance of its components. Ayurveda describes the universe and the human body as being made up of the same fundamental five elements (*panchamahabhutas*, see figure 3.1). Their balanced state in the body conveys health, while an imbalance causes illness. Let us look at these five elements within the perspective of ayurveda and its core teachings, which described thousands of years ago the correlation between the macrocosms of the universe and galaxies, and our microcosmos—the human body and cellular components.

Three Doshas

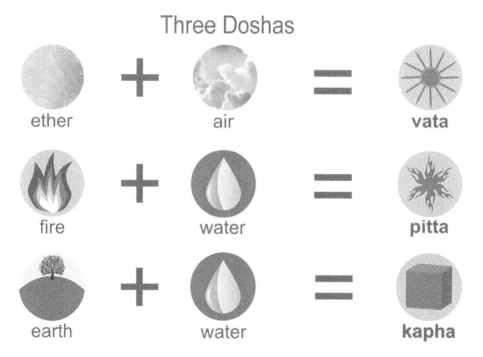

ether + air = **vata**

fire + water = **pitta**

earth + water = **kapha**

Fig. 3.1. Panchamahabhutas: Composition of the Three Doshas

AKASHA (SPACE)

Space is the dimensional extent to which objects and events have a relative position and direction. The human body requires space for free movement of nutrients such as oxygen to our lungs and general body as well as food constituents. The body could be considered as *akasha*: your visceral cavities provide space for your various organs and tissues to perform their normal physiological functions, in the same way that the space within a cell and between two cells allows intra- and intercellular communication, which permits all kinds of metabolic functions.

Examples of imbalances of akasha are increases, expansions, or dilatations such as cardiomegaly (heart enlargement), hepatomegaly (liver enlargement), aneurism (ballooning at a weak spot in an arterial wall), and varicose veins. A perpetual dance of millions of biochemical reactions is taking place, second by second in every cell, always with the goal of reaching and maintaining equilibrium despite the external pressures of entropy. In the same way that physics studies electromagnetic fields in space and the various energetic particles present, we can also visualize, according to specific circumstances, the intercellular space allowing the same kind of interactions via proteins called receptors. These receptors bind to signaling molecules present at the interstitial space between the cells of our digestive system, circulatory system, or even the skin cells, to allow passage and all kinds of metabolic processes such as utilization or production of fat in our systems.[3] For ayurvedic scholars, space is global and all-inclusive, a broadening of awareness.

VAYU (AIR)

Among the components of space, we have the invisible mixture of near-weightless, gaseous substances, mainly composed of nitrogen and oxygen, that surround the Earth. Ayurveda perceives air as the second manifestation of consciousness, a universal magnetic field responsible for the movement of the elements earth, wind, and water. Its qualities are cold, dry, rough, irregular, mobile, subtle, and light. *Vayu* or vata is considered the air-force, the control force and central government of our body mechanisms from which all activities begin and continue—everything from the blinking of the eyes, swallowing, and molecular transport to the evacuation of bodily wastes. For example, air—in the form of the oxygen we breathe—is essential for the normal functioning of all cells because it facilitates oxidation that supplies the body with the energy it requires. The resulting mixtures of gases also have oxygen and nitrogen, and their combination at a cellular level produces the essential molecule of nitric oxide (NO), which plays a pivotal role in vasodilation, allowing several essential cellular processes to keep our body-mind in a state of balance.[4] This aspect interests us particularly because the gastrointestinal system is one of the major producers of nitric oxide, and its vasodilating properties and smooth muscle-relaxing properties play a key role in the regulation of the general motility, mucosal blood flow, and gastric protection of the abdominal functions.[5] Nowadays one of its uses is as a popular recreational drug.[6]

TEJAS (FIRE)

Fire is the result of the chemical reaction of applying heat to a fuel in an oxygenated environment, which yields heat, light, and diverse reaction products. Our sun represents light or heat—forms of energy that are transferred from the sun to our planet, which keep life functioning on Earth. Fire provides warmth and enables life, and it can also burn and destroy. The element symbolizes great energy, power, activity, dynamism, creativity, passion, freedom, love, vision, anger, strength, will, assertiveness, and courage.

From the ayurvedic point of view, when your digestive fire, described as agni, is fully functional, you efficiently obtain the nutrients from what you eat as well as removing potentially harmful undigested compounds that could slow down your body and mind functions (*tejas*).

In the same way, at a cellular level, metabolic fire processes produce energy to keep our body alive and functional.[7] For instance, during metabolic processes, your body converts what you eat and drink, combined with oxygen, into calories to release the energy your body needs for normal functions. When your digestive fire (agni) is functioning properly, you obtain the nutrients of what you eat as well as removing potentially toxic undigested compounds that can slow down your body and mind.

AP (WATER)

While the oceans contain most of the planet's water, it is also found everywhere as ice, water vapor, and liquid. We can see the interconnection between air and water because air helps water move between these states. When water is heated by the sun, it evaporates into the air and becomes water vapor, a process known as the water cycle.

We need to drink water every day; and at the same time, our thermic cellular reactions that result from the digestion process also produce water molecules. This occurs because of the oxygen present in the air we breathe. Along with water, these reactions release energy through a process known as oxidation. These are essential flow processes required for proper functioning and for the satisfaction of all our physiological needs. The various glands in our bodies secrete gastric fluids and watery acidic digestive fluid—including hydrochloric acid, enzymes, and mucus—to support digestion and assimilation, and our bodies remove excess water in the form of urine and sweat, to eliminate the toxins that in ayurvedic terms are described as *ama*. It is well understood that scarcity of the water element can lead to drying out of the body and mind, causing conditions such as constipation, emaciation, and bitterness, and that body water retention is present in most cases of extreme obesity.[8] One brain region of our body has a clever way to detect how much water we should drink every day by combining signals from our gut, mouth, and blood.[9]

PRITHVI (EARTH)

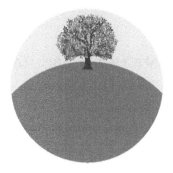

Earth can be thought of as the material composing part of the globe as well as the denser constituents that make up our bodies. Ayurvedic scholars describe earth, or matter, as the material manifestation of awareness as the result of the heating of fire and water. They characterize the qualities of the earth element as cool, stable, heavy, dry, rough, gross, dense, dull, and hard. The earth element accesses our bodies by way of the nutrients we eat. Earth provides underlying structure and foundation that allows for the growth and development of tissues. In conditions where fat or adipose tissue grows and spreads in the body, there is a broad increase in both liquid and structure, so they are interdependent in a way that increases the earth and water elements and results in a thickening of the structures of the body.

If we consider things that are not matter, or at least not matter in the terms we understand them today—such as our thoughts, feelings, emotions, or types of energies we can all recognize, like anger or fear—all these, in ayurvedic terms, represent even more subtle manifestations of the material panchamahabhutas or five elements.

Under ayurveda, the cosmos will manifest subtle effects and influences over our lives. Recall that the moon's gravitational pull impacts the tides of our oceans and other suggested physiological process such as menstruations, sleep patterns, or even our feelings and emotions.[10, 11, 12]

The attributes of these five elements or panchamahabhutas generate certain properties and modalities that ayurveda relates to organs of perception, as follows:

PANCHAMAHABHUTAS
The Five Elements

Mahabhuta	Attribute	Property	Organ	Modality
Space/Field	space	sound	ear	hearing
Air	motion	sound + touch	skin	touch
Fire	conversion	sound+ touch + form	eye	vision
Water	liquidity	sound + touch + form + taste	tongue	taste
Earth	condensation	sound + touch + form + taste + smell	nose	smell

THE TRIGUNA
Organization, Direction, Character

Another important ayurvedic concept is the view that regards all creatures as aspects of nature, and all beings as governed by the same laws of nature, described by three universal qualities known as the *triguna* that pervade everything. These may be considered highly refined ideals that convey direction, organization, and a character to that which they permeate. According to Samkhya philosophy,[13] your prakruti (body constitution) is composed of these three basic gunas.

These three qualities, known as the triguna, comprise everything in our physical nature and all energetic expressions within the universe. The following is a brief outline of the qualities of each member of the triguna. Samkhya philosophy describes your prakruti as being composed of these three essential gunas whose nature and behavior are a complex interplay, with each guna operating at various levels.[14] For instance, the conduct may be *rajasic* with a substantial impact by the *sattvic* guna; or, in some, it may be rajasic with a substantial impact by the *tamasic* guna, and so forth.

QUALITIES OF THE TRIGUNA

	Sattva	Rajas	Tamas
Qualities	truth equanimity contentment consciousness	action energy dynamism alertness	inertia heaviness unconsciousness imbalance
Examples	humility nonviolence compassion	passion challenge competition	repress emotions anxiety depression

PURUSHA (CONSCIOUSNESS) AND PRAKRUTI (BODY NATURES)

In our daily lives, we rarely stop to contemplate the physical and mental nature of our interactions with the environment. In the twenty-four hours of every day, we do not dwell much on the air we breathe, the water we drink, or the myriad of chemical reactions and processes in our bodies that ensure we are able to function; perhaps we take all this for granted. Furthermore, we are not conditioned by modern living to see how connected these things are either in a scientific or philosophical way. Ayurveda, on the other hand, treats these issues as central to its mode of operation, and at the core of its understanding is its view of the five elements in terms of look, feel, and function, describing the human being as a creation of the universe in accordance with prakruti and *purusha*.

According to the Samkhya school of philosophy—or the dualistic theory of creation and causation—two eternal principles called purusha and prakruti are recognized as the creators of the flow of the universe (*loka*):

▾ Prakruti is the dynamic, infinite, primal, creative natural force of the universe. It is considered the foremost cause of all the gross and subtle existing objects. It is your "perfect blueprint," and it is given to you at conception.
▾ Purusha (consciousness) is the spirit and consciousness. It is eternal, passive, pure, and permanent. It is energy without matter and has the ultimate healing power. It is your unmanifested potential and is behind everything in nature.

Purusha needs a vehicle to experience and express itself in the world, and when it joins with prakruti, your physical existence and senses come into being. Through your physical form and the senses, purusha experiences the world and plays a large part in the creation of health or disease. In that way, life starts passing through diverse transitional stages to reach a materially perceptive aspect: these are the five elements or panchamahabhutas, meaning five big first forms of existence.

GENETICS, EPIGENETICS, AND AYURVEDA

The science of genetics studies the role of the genes, the basic units of heredity that are parts of our chromosomes. They are made up of molecules of deoxyribonucleic acid, or DNA, situated in the nuclei of our cells. Each of us has two copies of every gene, one inherited from each parent. In living species, the difference between genes consists of some small molecules called bases (Adenine–Thymine, Guanine–Cytosine) in the DNA. Comprised within the letters (A, T, G, C) of the human genome are about 21,000 genes. Of the entire genome, only about 1–2 percent is made up of coding genes that are directly involved in producing proteins, which can affect the phenotype. The entirety of the DNA, including noncoding regions, constitutes the genotype of an individual.

The genotype denotes the part of the genetic makeup that defines a unique combination of characteristics in each of us. The genotype is constant and non-changing unless it suffers some damage. Biological or environmental factors can change gene expression, causing abnormality in genes and chromosomes, and they can be the cause of birth defects or different pathologies. The genotype is responsible for the development of the physical properties of an individual. These individual observable traits—including the organism's appearance, development, and behavior—are what we denominate under the term *phenotype*. Anything you do in your life, intentionally or unconsciously, disturbs the phenotype and alters the expression of the genotype. Among all the factors understood to affect the phenotype, the four major ones are lifestyle and behavior, diet and digestion, stress, and environmental factors.

Epigenetics is the recent science studying the external DNA modifications that switch genes on and off, altering gene expression without changes in the fundamental configuration of the DNA, by specific epigenetic processes—maternal effects, DNA methylation, gene silencing, position effect, reprogramming, and others. These alterations are reversible and do not change one's DNA sequence, but they can change how one's body reads the DNA sequence.

Many causal factors of diseases described by ayurveda are now explained by epigenetics. Ayurveda addresses these factors that affect the body (*deha*); the immunopsychophysiological constitution (prakruti), which corresponds to the phenotype; and indirectly, the prakruti at the moment of birth (*janma prakruti*), which corresponds to the genotype. Furthermore, by following an ayurvedic lifestyle, we can reduce or prevent these epigenetic changes.

When our bodies (*deha prakruti*) are in a state of balance, then health is maintained. If our activities or external events are not supporting our bodies in a positive way, then our bodies become imbalanced, creating *vikruti*, and illness can manifest. This entire progression occurs through mechanisms that epigenetics studies in detail. These epigenetic changes can be reversed in a positive manner by the integration of ayurvedic practices and protocols into your daily life—as will be described and analyzed in subsequent sections of this book.

YOUR BODY ORGAN SYSTEMS
Dhatus, The Seven Body Tissues

The moon wets the earth, the sun dries it;
joined to both, air sustains life.

Su. Sū. 4/7

The body is composed of no more than doshas,
dhatus, and malas.

Su. Sū. 15/3

Ayurveda defines the primary structures or organ systems formed by a conglomeration of panchamahabhutas that make up the human body (*sarira*) as: plasma, blood, muscle, fat, bone, nerve and bone marrow, and reproductive tissue. Each is seen as being interrelated with the others in a cascading effect, meaning that what happens to one impacts the following in the sequence. They nourish one another; so, at the same time, if one is weak it can cause a chain reaction, leading every layer of tissues to become unstable. The seven body organ systems are fundamental to understanding the relation between the organs and tissues in the body, and the sites where imbalances can occur. Furthermore, like most conceptions expressed in the ancient Vedic texts, these ideas are far more profound that we normally believe. The dhatus are composed of the five *mahabhutas* or elements. Consequently, the doshas, which are also made up of the five elements, support the equilibrium of the dhatus. A system of well-balanced doshas supports the balance of the dhatus, allowing for proper performance of the entire seven-organ system. According to ayurveda, sarira is divided into five sheaths (*koshas*) from gross to fine (physical, physiological, psychological, intellectual, and spiritual). Functional sarira is made up of three bodily humors (*tridosha*), seven tissues (dhatus), and three excretory products (malas). Let me give you a short description of how they function:

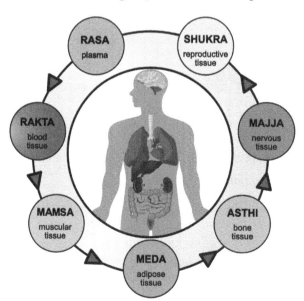

Fig. 3.2. Dhatus: The Seven Bodily Tissues

The Seven Dhatus

1. *Rasa dhatu* (plasma) provides nutrients and hormones to the parts of the body that need them and removes waste from the other dhatus. It is sustained by kapha dosha.
2. *Rakta dhatu* (blood) brings oxygen and nourishment to the whole body and strengthens all the cells and body tissues. It is sustained by pitta dosha.
3. *Mamsa dhatu* (muscle) responsible for movement by contractibility and is a physical support to fat. It is sustained by kapha dosha.
4. *Meda Dhatu* (fat) adipose tissue is the major storage form of energy in the body and for body lubrication and bone support. It is sustained by kapha dosha.
5. *Asthi dhatu* (bone) provides shape and mechanical support for the body, and development and storage of blood cells. It is sustained by vata dosha.
6. *Majja dhatu* (bone marrow) supports and strengthens our bodies and keeps rakta dhatu cellular functions. Majja dhatu nourishes the reproductive tissue sustained by kapha dosha.
7. *Shukra dhatu* (reproductive tissue) feeds the reproductive strengths of an individual (ovum and sperm) and is sustained by kapha dosha.

An understanding of the seven organ systems or dhatus is important when considering what can become out of balance in the body. We often hear "the bigger, the better," and lots of people hold this perception in relation to muscle mass. On the other end of the spectrum, we also hear, "less is more," which is often the conviction when it comes to body weight. Ayurveda stresses "all things in moderation." This also relates to our dhatus, which include muscles and body fat. Ayurveda accentuates the quality of the tissues much more than their quantity.

At present, Western medicine describes the human organism as comprising eleven organ systems interconnected and dependent upon one another to function: the skeletal, muscular, cardiovascular, lymphatic, respiratory, nervous, digestive, endocrine, integumentary, urinary, and reproductive systems. We will be discussing in more detail the way both sciences understand these systems' interconnections, as well as the implications of other potential body systems participating in the ongoing processes of our body-mind functionality and balance.

MALAS: THE THREE WASTE SYSTEMS

Ayurveda considers the specific roles of waste systems of the body to be as relevant as the organ systems for maintenance of good health, body balance, and longevity. Normal internal biological processes convert our food substances into micro-components that are compatible with our bodily requirements for each cell, tissue, and organ. As a result of our normal processes, we generate different kinds of waste materials, by-products, or metabolic end products (malas), which must be properly excreted for maintenance of good health. This is an ongoing process, and waste needs to be excreted out of the body at proper times and in the right quantities. If waste products remain in the body, they can be the cause of many disorders.

Ayurvedic medicine separates the waste system products into two main components: 1. body wastes (*dhatu malas*) and 2. metabolic wastes mostly originating from food (*ahara malas*). They are additionally subdivided into three groups: urine (*mutra*), stool (*purisha*), and sweat (*sveda*). Metabolic wastes are similarly subclassified according to the seven organ systems—that is, secretions from the eyes, nose, ears, and other components like hair and nails.[15]

Let me illustrate the importance of proper waste management by considering common "misbehaviors" I see with my patients. Instead of regular elimination of normal stools (purisha) in a semisolid state, a client presents themselves with one or more of the following: Several days experiencing constipation, continuous flatulence, diarrhea, and colic (often as a result of an imbalanced diet or lifestyle). Similar dysfunctional waste management can be seen in cases where urine waste product or mutra, under imbalanced conditions, manifests as urinary tract infections (UTIs), renal stones, or even renal failure.

In the case of perspiration or sweating (sveda), most clients underestimate the important thermoregulation and lubrication roles of the skin by shaving their armpits and using antiperspirant, thus causing irritation to the surface of the skin resulting in dermatitis, psoriasis, and reduced body temperature. Those antiperspirants containing aluminum are currently under study for their association with mammary cancer.

This ongoing process of waste excretion at a proper time and in the right quantity is fundamental. If waste products remain in the body, they can be the cause of many disorders. These situations described above can ultimately affect our tissular processes if our by-products are not formed in normal ways, processed, and eventually eliminated. I can tell you it is common for some patients to endure poor waste management function; in fact, it becomes part of their lifestyle because they believe they can tolerate some of the discomfort arising from a perpetuation of bad habits, and lifestyles choices built up over years, which may well be the cause of their health imbalances or diseases. This is one of the reasons why ayurveda among other things recommends cleaning your tongue when going to bed and once waking up in the morning using a tongue cleaner.

AGNI: YOUR DIGESTIVE FIRE

Agni, the ayurvedic concept of digestive fire or biofire, is critical to overall health. Fire is one of the five elements, and agni is one of its manifestations as an essential element for maintaining life. Agni is responsible for all metabolic functions—including digestion, absorption, and assimilation of ingested food—that require and produce energy in the form of the molecule adenosine triphosphate (ATP). As this digestive fire is increased or depleted, our body-mind biological functions respond accordingly. Agni is the force of intelligence within each cell, tissue, and bodily system, shaping which particles enter our cells and tissues, and which particles should be removed as waste.

Ayurvedic scholars describe up to forty types of agni, expressing that when the agni is extinguished, death soon follows. Despite these forty diverse agni, it is important to appreciate that in all forms, agni shares the same fundamental qualities existing in the whole body. It is hot, sharp, penetrating, light, spreading, subtle, luminous, and clear.

In general, agni is categorized into thirteen types based on their role and place of action, as described by Charaka (Ca. Chi. Su. 15/38):

bhutagni: five agni from five basic elements
jataragni: one agni manifesting in the stomach and duodenum
dhatwagni: seven agni, each one manifesting in the seven tissues

Among all of these, the mother of all agni is the digestive or gut fire (*jataragni*), acting as the central commander of all the other types of "micro-agni" in our bodies.[16]

Depleted or disturbed agni compromises the balance of your physical and mental health, manifesting in numerous ways. It is important to look beneath the symptoms and to address the root cause of your body imbalance, because the protocols required for body rebalancing are going to depend on which qualities of agni are most compromised, how they reached that condition, and where in your body the disorder is most active. Tailored protocols and programs to support and restore the quality of your agni, in parallel to addressing other imbalances, will be presented in the sections on nutrition and diet (see chapter 15).

Therefore, as a summary we can say that ayurveda targets maintenance of the equilibrium of dosha, dhatu and mala, *srotas* (channels), and a healthy agni. Let me give you four case studies of agni and body types. Remember that our agni is related to our body constitution, that is, the distribution of our vata, pitta, and kapha.

CASE STUDY
Tikshna Agni (Fast Metabolism)

Albert is a fifty-two-year-old man, who came to me describing his great appetite and ability to eat large amounts of food, becoming angry if he could not eat when hungry, and saying that under conditions of overactivity he can have heartburn and difficulty digesting fats. He is hypermetabolic (having an elevated resting energy expenditure, or more simply, faster than normal digestion) as per his intense fire, described in the ayurvedic texts as tikshna agni. This is an example of a pitta-predominant prakruti with sympathetic and parasympathetic nervous system participation, that can be supported by lifestyle adjustments such as respecting his digestive fire by eating cooling, grounding, nourishing, and satisfying non-spicy foods.

CASE STUDY
Manda Agni (Slow Metabolism)

Margaret is a sixty-year-old woman with a strong build and a heavy frame, who was complaining that she was still gaining weight despite eating less. This is a condition of slow metabolism that in ayurveda we call manda agni; it is as if you have your oven on but at a low temperature, resulting in a sluggish digestion. In simple terms, this is typical of kapha-predominant people: They have the slowest but most efficient digestion due to an increased parasympathetic nervous system, which stimulates the ability to eat food, but in parallel with a slow-moving digestive transit, allowing a more thorough absorption of food, resulting in gaining more body weight. In these cases, I suggest avoiding stressful eating, eating too fast, unhealthy foods, or eating close to bedtime.

CASE STUDY
Pitta Prakruti

Charlie has a pitta prakruti. During his consultation he described the need to lose weight and inability to understand why, if he was having only one meal per day, he remained obese and unable to achieve his goal. The issue was his only daily meal was at nighttime after a long working day. After explaining to him that even a pitta-type person with a strong digestive fire (agni) will have a reduced ability to metabolize big meals during the sleep period—when ingested food will have the tendency to accumulate as body fat deposits—he accepted the need to modify his food pattern intake by having breakfast, his main meal, at lunch-time and a small, light dinner. He managed to rebalance his body weight after some time. It is important to emphasize that issues arising from late eating applies to all of us if we do not listen to the natural physiological processes of our biological clock.

The practices that ayurvedic scholars developed to obtain a harmonic and vital balance of body weight are founded on these principles:

▾ a restorative system harmonizing body, mind, and consciousness
▾ a thorough systematic vision, down to the minute and even invisible levels
▾ importance of functionality of body systems, not only symptoms
▾ nourishment tailored to your constitution
▾ administration of remedies to rebalance your metabolism
▾ fresh, organic, and native prescriptions for rebalancing
▾ boosters for your natural defenses
▾ management of body-mind restoration and end-of-life care
▾ stress-related and subconscious conditions

The ayurvedic protocols for body-type balancing involve a number of factors: evaluation of your body constitution, lifestyle, diet, attitude, and beliefs; natural ayurvedic medicines; and tailored ayurvedic physical therapies. In assessing the degree of imbalance of your body's organ systems, ayurveda draws on a combination of factors, including the origin of the disorder, your strengths and weaknesses, and the seriousness of the symptoms you are experiencing.[17]

Ayurveda sees good health in the following way:

He is healthy whose doshas, agni, and the functions of dhatus and malas are in equilibrium; whose mind, intellect, and sense organs are bright and cheerful.

Su. Sū. 15/40

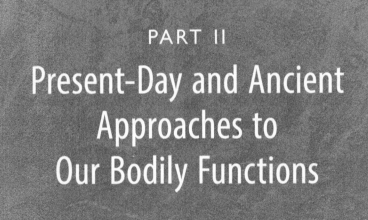

PART II

Present-Day and Ancient
Approaches to
Our Bodily Functions

4

BEING OVERWEIGHT AS IT RELATES TO THE GUT

How the Body Becomes Imbalanced

THE CELL

Every living organism is made up of cells, and we can consider them as the smallest self-contained unit representing the building blocks of life. The cells within the human organism are like rooms inside an enormous house, and our bodies contain around fifty trillion cells. Even just one of your toes has about ten billion cells of different shapes, sizes, and functions. In terms of size, some cells can be really long, such as the nerve cells that run the entire length of your back, but in general they are tiny and can only be perceived under a microscope. Our cells have three things in common, independent of their type: they have a cell membrane or selective barrier that separates the inside of the cell from its surrounding environment; a cytoplasm, a kind of jelly-like fluid; and DNA, the cell's genetic material (except mature red blood cells). Cells are composed of around 70 percent water, and their other components include carbon-containing (organic) molecules—such as proteins, nucleic acids, carbohydrates, and lipids or fats—as well as inorganic ions.

There are many types of cells carrying out different jobs; however, some of these jobs are common to all cells, such as making proteins and producing, delivering, and storing energy, and some jobs are specific to the type of organ where the cell belongs. Most cells have "little organs" called organelles, which are specialized parts of a cell that have distinctive jobs to perform. These organelles include: the nucleus, which contains the DNA; ribosomes, where proteins are made; lysosomes, the "garbage collectors" of the cell; and mitochondria, the powerhouses that make "energy molecules" or ATP to provide energy for all the cell's activities. As a more specific example, the heart's cells labor together to pump blood around our bodies.

In this section, you are going to learn a bit more about our different types of cells, addressing in particular the cells associated with the metabolism of fat—their constituents, their mechanisms of storage, and potential associated imbalances promoting body-mind pathologies such as obesity.

For our particular purpose of addressing the gut and metabolic imbalances like obesity, we could look at our human body and its components—cells, tissues, organs, and systems—in a way that relates to how today's society works:

cells: citizens

tissues: clusters or big groups of citizens

arteries and veins: rivers and canals transporting both nutrients and waste

immune system: patrol, inspection, quality control

organs: buildings

lungs, heart, and kidneys: filters and buildings

nerves: electric network for sending information

central nervous system (CNS): city hall or regulator center

gastrointestinal tract (GIT): plant or factory that processes the final products

The word *obesity* is derived from the Latin term *obesus*, whose meaning can be broken down thus: *ob* → by reason of; *edo* → I eat; *obesus* → have eaten or having eaten until fat. It is defined in medical terms as abnormal growth of the adipose tissue as a result of a growth of fat cell size (hypertrophy), or an increase in fat cell number (hyperplasia) or a combination of both.[1]

In ayurveda, obesity is described in the texts as *sthoulya*, which stands for "thick," "solid," "strong," "big," or "bulky"; and fat is described under the name *meda*. Charaka, Sushruta, and other scholars studied metabolic disorders such as obesity at a time when India was one of the most prosperous countries in the world, and described these disorders as the result of affluence and sedentary life factors. They defined obesity as a fat tissue disorder (*medoroga*) leading to "hugeness," caused mostly by an unhealthy lifestyle.

Before moving deeper into the ayurvedic understanding, let me describe in more detail the components of the gastrointestinal tract (GIT) or gut: the mouth, esophagus, stomach, small intestine, large intestine, and anus are the pipeline of the tract, and organs like the liver, pancreas, and gallbladder are equally part of the digestive system.

Our bodies require organs for filtering and cleaning, and their core purpose is to maintain a state of homeostasis so the body may function well. The kidneys, liver, lungs, bowels, and skin are the organs responsible for body cleansing. They clean and filter our blood while also transporting nutrients to the cells. In an idyllic state of good health, or balance, our tissues and cells must live in an uncontaminated environment, where the intra- or extracellular watery space—which makes up 70 percent of the human body's volume—is as clean and unadulterated as possible. In order to achieve that balance, our organs responsible for filtration engage in a constant process of purification of the volume transported, all day every day, from the instant we are born until the moment we die.

Alterations of the participation and functions of the different constituents, from the "citizens" to the "electric network" to the "factory," can occur due to an unhealthy lifestyle, including factors such as food intake. This will cause imbalances associated with metabolic dysfunctions such as obesity.[2]

Consider now, in general terms, the different cellular constituents and the way they function and organize themselves under their aqueous system.

LIPIDS/FAT
Definition, Classification, and Role

Lipids are a varied group of organic compounds, insoluble in water and soluble in nonpolar organic solvents. They occur naturally in a majority of animals, plants, and microorganisms, playing roles like cell membrane constituents, major energy storage molecules, insulators, blood clotting molecules, and hormones, among others.

They are components of adipose, skeletal muscle, bone, and visceral organs. The adipose tissue, whose role as a tissue or organ we will be discussing in more detail (see chapter 5), includes: adipocytes with collagen and elastic fiber, fibroblasts, capillaries, and extracellular fluid. Human adipose tissue is often assumed to have an average composition consisting of 80 percent lipid, 14 percent water, 5 percent protein, and less than 1 percent mineral; and of the 14 percent H_2O of adipose tissue, 11 percent is extracellular water. Adipose tissue has two main types, subcutaneous and internal. Abundant in subcutaneous sites is what's known to gross anatomists as superficial fascia, defined as the adipose tissue between the skin and the muscles. Adipocytes or fat cells serve as the primary storage site for triglycerides.

Their physical appearance can be solid or liquid: for example, there are fats or solid triglycerides with high amounts of saturated fatty acids, and oils or liquid triglycerides with high amounts of unsaturated fatty acids.

Examples of fats are oils, waxes, cholesterol, sterols, fat-soluble vitamins, glycerides, triglycerides (TGs), phospholipids, and others such as fatty acids (FAs). They are the building blocks of the fat in our bodies and in the food we eat. The most usual FAs contain twelve to twenty-two carbon atoms, though some are smaller, such as omega-3 and omega-6 fatty acids.[3]

Cholesterol is a fat-like molecule, a waxy substance essential for our lives. It is vital for our cell membranes, several hormones, vitamin D, bile acids (for the digestion and absorption of fats), and other substances. Many fats in our bodies—for reasons of their use, transport, and storage within the body—must go through a process of oxidation-reduction known as esterification.

ENZYMES

Our bodies produce proteins, called enzymes, to act as facilitators or catalysts of specific biochemical reactions—that is, the breakdown or digestion of fats (lipolysis) by the gastric and pancreatic lipases, acting under hormonal control.[4] Lipids are digested in the small intestine, and the bile salts (produced in the liver) play a key role in their digestion. Since lipid molecules are insoluble in water, bile salts make them water-soluble. We can visualize them as a kind of vinaigrette dressing after shaking—a mixed suspension that we call emulsification. During this process, bile salts facilitate a gathering of lipids in the form of droplets (micelles), which contain cholesterol, monoglycerides, and FAs, thus creating an easier way to transport lipid molecules in a body composed of approximately 60 percent water.

ABSORPTION

From the droplets (micelles), FAs, cholesterol, and monoglycerides disperse and are absorbed into the mucosa of the small intestine. The small FAs (less than twelve carbon atoms) disperse directly into the blood, which transports them to the liver as unesterified FAs. The FAs with more than twelve carbon atoms are reconverted into TGs. The residual lipids in the small intestine are grouped into molecules called chylomicrons by the activity of the external cells in the intestinal mucosa. Since chylomicrons are too large to pass through the blood capillaries, they enter the vessels of the lymphatic system and are transported into the blood system via the lymph.

TRANSPORT OF FATS

In our watery bodies, lipid molecules that dislike water (nonpolar lipids), such as cholesterol and TGs, need to be transported in combination with proteins, since these dissolve in water. The proteins used for this purpose are called lipoproteins and are spherical particles that contain thousands of molecules. For essential cellular interactions, the external shells of these lipoproteins act as networkers. The protein component of these lipoproteins, known as "apolipoproteins" (apo), is produced by the liver and intestines. They are designated by the letters A, B, C, D, and E, and each apolipoprotein has specific functions.[5, 6]

ORIGINS AND SIGNIFICANCE OF
CHOLESTEROL AND LIPOPROTEINS

The molecule of cholesterol has two origins: (1) exogenous, or via food intake, representing approximately one third of cholesterol, and (2) endogenous, or via biosynthesis, which represents two-thirds, mostly produced by the liver.[7] Fatty foods, even if they lack any cholesterol, will severely raise the blood cholesterol level in two possible ways. First, a large ingestion of fat from our food stimulates reabsorption of cholesterol-containing bile back into the blood, which means less cholesterol goes to feces.[8] Second, when saturated fats are broken down in the liver, our cells use some of these subproducts to make cholesterol.

In the mid-1980s, a blood cholesterol level of around 300 mg/dL was considered normal. The current belief is that you must keep cholesterol levels as close as possible to 200 mg/dL to avoid health complications.

FUNCTION OF LIPOPROTEINS

Perhaps you've had a checkup to evaluate your lipid profile, which shows the fats circulating in your blood. The lipid profile consists of an evaluation of various forms of lipoproteins playing various roles, but essentially acting like carriers of fats or lipids. Lipoproteins are also named based on their density, which varies with the ratio of lipids to proteins, from low density to high density. Functional categorization from largest and lightest to smallest and heaviest is as follows:

chylomicrons: carry TGs (fat from diet) coming from the bowels to the liver, skeletal muscle, and adipose tissue
very low-density lipoproteins (VLDL): pass newly synthesized TGs from liver to adipose tissue
intermediate-density lipoproteins (IDL): midway among VLDL and LDL
low-density lipoproteins (LDL) or "bad cholesterol": carry 75 percent of the total cholesterol from the liver to the cells of the body

high-density lipoproteins (HDL) or "good cholesterol": remove
cholesterol excess from our body's tissues, bringing it back to
the liver

Lp(a): similar structure and contents to LDL

LIVER FUNCTIONS

The roles of the liver in fat metabolism include breaking down fats to generate energy for other bodily functions; formation of lipoproteins; biosynthesis of large quantities of cholesterol and phospholipids; converting 80
percent of cholesterol into bile salts that will be secreted into bile, while
the remainder is carried by lipoproteins and transported via the blood to
every cell in the body; and lastly, conversion of large amounts of carbohydrates and proteins into fat.

THE FATE OF FATS

Lipids, like carbohydrates, change with the addition of oxygen—a process
called oxidation—to produce molecules of ATP, which is a molecule that
carries energy and is found in the cells of all living things. ATP represents
chemical energy obtained from the assimilation of food molecules, and
it gets released so as to fuel other cellular processes. When our bodies do
not require lipids, these lipids are stored in adipose tissue—the principal
metabolic organ in maintaining the whole-body equilibrium—as well as
in the liver.

The regulation of growth and regression of adipose tissue, which is
influenced by several factors, is still a subject of debate in the scientific
research.[9] Let me give you an example: On average a grown-up person has
thirty billion fat cells, representing a weight of 30 lb. or 13.5 kg. When the
person gains excess weight, their fat cells increase in size around four times
before dividing and increasing the total number of existent fat cells.[10, 11]
One of the main functions of adipose tissue is to remove TGs from the
macromolecules of chylomicrons and VLDL and store them until they
are required for energy production in other tissues and body organs. TGs

in adipose tissue are continually broken down and rebuilt. When excess quantities of carbohydrates are available in the body, carbohydrates are used as an alternative over TGs for energy. There are several motives for this "fat-sparing" effect of carbohydrates.

When the body breaks down lipids, which is called catabolism or lipolysis, TGs deposited in adipose (fat) tissue represent 98 percent of all body energy reserves and get split into glycerol and fatty acids by enzymes called lipases.

And when we rebuild lipids after eating, a process known as anabolism or lipogenesis, carbohydrates are converted into glucose, an instantaneous source of energy for the cells. Any excess of glucose gets stored in the liver as macromolecules called glycogen; or, with the help of the hormone insulin, this excess is converted into FAs, circulated to other parts of the body, and stored as fat in adipose tissue.

If we eat proteins in excess, they get stored as fat, while the surplus of amino acids is excreted, leading to extra weight over time, mainly if you consume too many calories while trying to raise your protein intake.

Our bodies are in a perpetual dance, a theme that will reoccur as we look at the gut and our weight through the lens of ayurveda. When required, carbohydrates and amino acids can convert to fat, and fat can also convert to carbohydrates and/or amino acids, according to the body's needs.

CAUSATIVE FACTORS

Intrinsic Factors
One of the difficulties when addressing the origins of body imbalances is discerning the different causative factors, due to their interrelation involving:

Age
Obesity can happen at any age, and generally its incidence increases with age. In overweight children, both the size and number of adipocytes increases from the time they become overweight, regardless of their age. Studies show that weight loss shrinks adipocyte size but does not affect their number.[12, 13] Ayurveda believes that obesity can happen at any stage

of life due to an imbalance between the metabolic power of the tissues (*dhatu agni*) and the main digestive fire (*jathara agni*).

Sex

Sex is an important variable in obesity analysis. Differences between sexes exist in obesity incidence and constitution, body fat distribution, drug efficacy, and different secondary effects of surgical procedures.

The prevalence of obesity is higher among males than females, but females have a higher percentage of body fat content compared to men, and sex appears to be an important factor in the manifestation of central (android) or peripheral (gynoid) obesity. Bearing in mind that adipose tissue is one of the factors affecting the distribution of many drugs, mainly lipophilics, sex differences might be expected in the physiological actions of anti-obesity drugs.[14]

Genetic Factors: Biochemical Levels

Hormones

Our appetite, metabolism, and body fat distribution are influenced by hormones like leptin, insulin, estrogens, androgens, growth hormones, and adrenaline, among others.[15, 16, 17] Obese people have hormone levels that incite the buildup of body fat.[18] For example, leptin produced from fat cells in adipose tissues and intestinal covering cells supports the regulation of energy balance by inhibiting hunger, which in turn reduces storage of fat in the adipocytes. Leptin also signals the brain, acting as a feedback mechanism to regulate food intake and body weight.

Control of Appetite

Two hormones, closely associated with the energy body's energy homeostasis, contribute to sensations of hunger and fullness. Leptin decreases your appetite, and ghrelin increases appetite while also playing a role in body weight. Studies have explored the consequences of missing out on lunch and confirmed that a lack of food makes otherwise manageable people "hangry." Hunger was linked with stronger feelings of anger and irritability and lower levels of pleasure.[19]

Energy Burning (Thermogenesis)

The process of body heat production occurs in particular tissues such as brown adipose tissue and skeletal muscle.

Genes

It is challenging to evaluate the role of genes in the manifestation of obesity, but it is commonly noted that obesity tends to run in families.[20, 21] Obesity can happen in families according to a clear inheritance pattern instigated by changes in a single gene. Until now, rare variants in about nine genes have been associated with single-gene obesity. The most-associated single genes are the ones codifying for leptin (LEP), leptin receptor (LEPR), and melanocortin 4 receptor (MC4R). Genetic alterations or mutations associated with obesity were linked to several clinical consequences including faulty immune system, cognitive deficiency, insulin resistance, and hypopigmentation.[22] Whatever the role of genes in obesity, environmental factors play an important part, as proven by the fact that famine prevents obesity even in the most obesity-prone individual.[23, 24]

Lifestyle Factors

Social Status, Ethnicity, and Occupation

A review of 333 published studies showed that lower socioeconomic status is correlated with larger body size for women.[25] In well-developed nations, the strongest association was with education and occupation, while positive associations for women in medium- and low-development countries were most linked to their income and material belongings. There is also a well-documented correlation between obesity, occupation, and ethnicity, associated with the quality and intake of nutrients.[26] Eating habits of overweight and obese people are variable and can cause disorders such as anorexia nervosa or bulimia nervosa that compromise nutritional status and health. Not all obese patients eat more than a regular individual, but overall they eat more than they need. It has been demonstrated that obese patients eat more than they admit to be eating, and in the long term, this daily excess can lead to a large buildup of fat.[27] Ayurveda considered obesity as an *adhyaroga* condition (*adhya* means rich), since affluent people have more opportunities to eat richer food, and larger quantities of food, and in general they are likely to have a more sedentary lifestyle.

Physical Activity and Drugs

Obesity is less common among persons who lead active lives. An obese person is inclined to expend more energy during physical activity, as they have a larger mass to carry. In general, however, obese people decrease their amount of physical activity. Corticosteroids and drugs used to treat psychological diseases may contribute to obesity with long-term use,[28] as they specifically play a key role in the genesis of obesity.[29, 30]

Environmental Factors

Interacting external factors include:

physical environment: food, air, and water
biological environment: living things such as microbes, insects, animals, and plants
psychosocial environment: customs, beliefs, morals, religion, education, lifestyles

Body Weight Type: Analysis and Markers

Weight Imbalance

Imbalances can be a cause of several chronic diseases, including being overweight or obese, which results from a combination of factors and can be classified as: primary obesity (exogenous), a typical result of excessive food intake, in which fat distribution is uniform although rather disproportionate under the chin and gut; and secondary, or glandular obesity (endogenous), when being overweight is the primary complaint, and an endocrine condition is occasionally the cause.

In both cases, obesity can be mild, moderate, or severe, depending on individual characteristics. The body distribution of fat can take different forms: generalized, central, superior, inferior, girdle, hard fat, or multiple lipomatosis.

There are two major types of fat distribution in adult obesity: fat accumulation around the hips and thighs, known as pear-shaped or gynoid; and fat accumulation in the abdominal area, known as apple-shaped or android distribution.

Abdominal Obesity

Your waist size (WS) is a good marker of the amount of fat you're carrying, mostly around the abdominal area, and is the best and easiest anthropometric measure of your total body fat. Some scientists consider it a more insightful measure of body fat than the body mass index (BMI), as BMI measures do not account for age, sex, bone structure, or fat distribution. WS is a locational measure; you are literally measuring a large amount of the fat that resides around your hips. It is also a simple, easy-to-conduct measurement, and studies show it is a strong predictor of disease and mortality when combined with BMI.[31]

Your WS could define the level of intra-abdominal fat mass that surrounds your internal organs, which is strongly associated with type 2 diabetes, heart disorders, and nonalcoholic fatty liver disease. Our subcutaneous belly fat is the excess skin and tissue that one can pinch with our fingers around our middle abdomen. High visceral fat or proper belly fat is that which accumulates at the abdominal area and between organs, and it is strongly linked with grave health issues.[32, 33]

Gut adipose tissue is associated with an increased risk of certain diseases, which could be a resultant effect of inflammation contributing to a higher risk of cardiovascular issues, even in those who are of normal weight but with abdominal obesity.[34]

Assessment of Body Weight Imbalances

You will find many formulations to assess obesity. The more current methods in terms of weight and fat content are body weight, BMI, ponderal index, Broca Index, Lorentz's formula, corpulence index (pinching the folded skin on the triceps by the use of vernier calipers), and waist-to-hip ratio (WHR). BMI is the more widely used and has established the obesity condition by categories. Class 1: BMI between 30–35, class 2: BMI between 35–40, and class 3: BMI of 40 or greater.[35]

To evaluate your waist size, just measure your waist around the smallest part below the rib cage and beyond your belly button. For men considered average height (this varies by country, but in the US, it is approximately 5 ft 9 in, or 175 cm), having a waist size of 37–40 inches is considered overweight, and more than 40 inches is obese.[36]

For women considered an average height (in the US this is approximately 5 ft 3 in, or 163 cm) a waist of 31.5–34.6 inches is overweight, and more than 34.6 inches is obese.[37] To calculate your own BMI, please look at a BMI calculator on the National Heart, Lung, and Blood Institute's Calculate Your Body Mass Index web page.

Treatments and Pathways

Today's modern medical approaches to treatment can be thought of in three measures:

1. **Non-Pharmacological**

   These include reduction in calorie intake, exercise, and behavioral modification therapy:

   Dietary control: This depends on changes in eating habits and reduction in calorie intake.

   Exercise: Weight cannot be lost by exercise alone, and we need to understand the principles of energy intake and expense. Exercise activities that boost energy expended should be actively considered, always based on absence of contraindications.[38]

   Habits: Changing or eliminating the wrong kind of habit formation. Mainstream medicine uses psychological techniques to support changes in patient behavior, to eliminate or reduce habit formation. Ayurveda does not separate body from mind; instead, it understands and addresses why psychological emotions such as stress, depression, anxiety, and fear kindle our appetite and why we seek security in consuming more food that could result in obesity (medoroga).[39]

2. Pharmacological

There are two main types of weight-loss drug treatments, both with side effects:[40]

Appetite suppressants (anorectics): Drugs that modify the biological chemicals which decrease appetite and food consumption, and promote weight loss. Diabetic drugs, such as Ozempic, act as appetite suppressants by mimicking the receptor of the natural hormone (GLP-1), producing significant weight loss.

Ozempic is FDA-approved only for the treatment of type 2 diabetes despite it being used worldwide for obesity. Clinical studies show that it can sustain glucose levels over 30–68 weeks, but no studies extend beyond that period.[41] Adverse effects include GIT intolerability (potential intestinal blockage, constipation, diarrhea, and nausea), hypoglycemia, kidney damage, gallbladder issues, and muscle loss.

Nevertheless, our gut microbiome has its own natural built-in Ozempic known as incretin hormones. Specific gut bacteria play an essential role in manufacturing and regulating these hormones by converting undigestible food (fiber, polyphenols), into molecules which stimulate hormone production to control appetite and metabolism. So, eating more fiber can have a semaglutide-like effect. What of long-term Ozempic (and similar drug) use on the natural production of 90 percent of serotonin by our intestinal microbiota, and resulting mental health issues?

Enzymatic disruptors: For example, inhibition of the enzyme pancreatic lipase blocks the normal breakdown of fats, causing weight loss.[42]

3. Surgical

Bariatric procedures such as laparoscopic sleeve gastrectomy, laparoscopic Roux-en-Y gastric bypass, laparoscopic adjustable gastric banding, and duodenal switch are the most frequently performed. These surgeries include stomach stapling, gastric bypass, and sleeve gastrectomy performed on the stomach and/or intestines to limit the amount of food that can be ingested. This procedure normally is used for people with a persistent BMI above 40, due to the long-term complications of such.[43, 44]

Many people struggle with body weight issues and other health imbalances that impair their ability to enjoy daily life to the fullest extent. Many take the route of pharmaceutical drugs and other conventional approaches to relieve their symptoms, but in reality, those options do not address the root cause of the imbalance. Instead they act like a Band-Aid, with zero or little active participation by the individual in addressing root causes and the risk of harmful or unpleasant side effects.

What most people do not realize is that they can significantly improve their body-mind health—without causing any harm—by changing their diet and eating habits and engaging in a more active physical life when possible. I know that's all easy to write, and if it were that simple, obesity would not be a pandemic, as we would all adjust our diets and lifestyle once we thought we were becoming obese. So, this book aims to provide a deeper understanding of the weight-related processes that actually take place within us and the external factors that play a role in our weight management. I will also provide simple, safe, and cost-effective suggestions for reestablishing weight balance. Being better informed may help us become more motivated to act to address root causes of becoming overweight or obese.

The following chapters offer you the possibility of achieving your goals, by introducing you to the concepts and simple practices of nutrition, diet, and other protocols illuminated by ayurveda.

5

MEDA DHATU

··

An Ayurvedic Perspective on Adipose/Fat Tissue

HISTORICAL BACKGROUND OF STHOULYA (OBESITY) IN INDIA

In this chapter we consider in more depth the ayurvedic visualization of our body in a broader way, as a means of understanding how ayurveda treats body weight issues and obesity of both the fat tissue or adipose organ and the gut. Ayurveda understands that our body-mind system functions as an ecosystem in which pressure on one part of the system affects other parts of the system. Further, we are not solid, unchangeable beings, and we have a pattern of energies orchestrated by our natural inner intelligence, an extension of ourselves and our environment.

Thousands of years ago, when India was one of the world's most affluent countries, the pioneers of written ayurveda cautioned against the harmful risks of being overweight or obese. They described obesity as the result of the combination of affluence and a sedentary life, a disorder of excess kapha dosha—one of the three body constituents, alongside pitta and vata. The excess causes a progressive decreased metabolism and decline of energy consumed by an individual at rest, generating weight gain due to the imbalance between high energy input via heavy foods and low energy expenditure due to lack of activities, including physical activities.[1]

In Ayurvedic medicine, the science of pathology, or *nidana*, studies the origin, causes, nature, effects, and courses of diseases, addressing the conditions and processes to understand the consequences of the structural and functional changes of a condition such as obesity. *Nidana* evaluates five clinical steps (*nidana panchaka*) or premonitory symptoms to understand the nature of the imbalance, as follows:

1. *nidāna*: cause/etiology
2. *purvarupa*: prodromal signs and symptoms or pre-stages of disease
3. *rupa*: cardinal signs and manifestations/symptoms
4. *upashaya*: therapeutic guidelines/response to treatment
5. *samprāpti*: pathogenesis, the origin and development of a disease

The practitioner's diagnosis is essentially achieved by specific examination and assessment of the patient's condition (*rogi pariksa*), which includes one or more three-, six-, eight-, or ten-point examinations. As an example, the eight-point examination of the disease covers:

▼ quality and nature
▼ quantity or magnitude
▼ causes
▼ premonitory symptoms
▼ signs and symptoms
▼ aggravating and pacifying factors
▼ prognosis
▼ complications or sequel of the condition.

Following these evaluations, the patient is invited to see the ability of the body to heal itself, the need or lack of need of outside influences (that is, drugs, natural medication, surgery) to restore or to prevent an illness (imbalance of the doshas), and to be an active participant to recommend lifestyle changes before the condition is allowed to deteriorate.

Ayurvedic health care is essentially aimed at maintaining the equilibrium of doshas and gunas (universal qualities) by means of a healthy agni. An equilibrium in the activity of these doshas is required for good health, so the imbalance of doshas can be considered a "disease state."[2] The psychological component relates to the qualities of the three parts of the triguna: sattva (essence, light, balance, and understanding), rajas (energy of movement and activity), and tamas (inertia, heaviness, and materialism). An intimate connection exists between the bodily and psychological constituents, so if one constituent is out of balance, the others are also out of balance.[3, 4]

Management of the condition includes diagnosing which tissues or systems are in imbalance and how they can be brought into equilibrium based on two principles: depletion (*karshana*) or repletion (*brumana*), determined by the individual's constitution and requirements. It involves cleansing methods that include five protocols called *panchakarma*, a type of therapeutic procedure useful for all medical conditions, which prepares the body for the stimulation of the process of elimination of toxic products, endogenous and exogenous, contributing to the overall management of a disease—as I'll describe in more detail later (see pages 252–54).[5]

AYURVEDIC DESCRIPTION OF THE FORMATION OF FAT/ADIPOSE TISSUE (MEDA DHATU)

Meda dhatu or body fat tissue is the fourth tissue among the seven dhatus, or body systems, and it is formed from muscle tissue (mamsa dhatu). Meda dhatu is then the precursor of bone tissue (asthi dhatu). While the term has a literal translation meaning "fat," conceptually it refers to the condensed waters of the body, revealing the nourishing nature of fatty tissue. Based on the five constituents of all living matter (panchamahabhuta), fat is essentially built from the water and earth elements, and the presence of earth reveals its role in sustaining the body-mind functions. According to modern medicine, adipose cells typically contain a large lipid droplet, occupying more than 90 percent of the cell volume, with variable fat and water contents, between 60–94 percent and 6–36 percent, respectively— which corresponds to the ayurvedic description.[6] Therefore, meda dhatu in one's physical body represents the body fat that contains water, and relates to the skin oil (sebum) and body omentum surrounding the intestines and other abdominal organs.

Let me share with you a description of fat/adipose tissue by Charaka:

When the small part of muscular tissue (*mamsa dhatu*) comes in contact with digested fat, then the digesting fire forms fat tissue. Due to the water quality present in fat tissue, the oily/unctuous quality is increased. Muscular tissue then can digest its own fat due to its own fire (*mamsa agni*) and the water present in it to form fat tissue (Ca. Chi. 15/35).

In other words, meda dhatu in our bodies represents the body fat formed as muscular tissue. It then flows into fat tissue if it is not required, and the oily skin secretions of sweat and sebum are just waste products.

QUALITIES OR FUNCTIONS OF FAT

Fat has heavy and oily attributes (gunas). It provides strength and body nourishment, makes oil/fat and sweat (sveda), and feeds the bones. It is remarkable that reports concerning the mathematical golden ratio or divine proportions attributed to Fibonacci, which were described many centuries earlier by ancient Indian scientists, are now validated and apply to the fatty acid structures, as verified recently by scientists of the Jena University.[7]

Ayurvedic descriptions of the types of lipids in the body:

meda: fat that is dense and thick like ghee
vasa: fat present in muscles
sthula asthi: yellow bone marrow present in long bones
anu asthi: red bone marrow present in small bones
medodhara kala: third layer of the skin that holds adipose tissue
(present in *udara* and *sukshma asthi*) (Su. Sha. 4/12).

QUANTIFICATION OF ADIPOSE TISSUE/FAT
(MEDA DHATU PRAMANA)

The method of quantification in those days was represented by the volume contained in the concavity when keeping both hands together (*anjali*), and in the case of adipose tissue was described as two *anjali*.[8]

Ayurveda describes the above conditions as medo roga (meda = fat, roga = disease), a disorder manifested by serious imbalance in the magnitude of accumulated fat tissue, because of alterations of body fat's metabolism that create complications, as described by the ayurvedic scholars Sushruta[9] and Charaka[10]

FAT/ADIPOSE TISSUE CHANNELS (MEDOVAHA SROTAS) AND ITS INJURED SYMPTOMS

Two types of fat channels are described in the ancient texts: sweat (*meda dhatu mala sveda*) (Ca. Chi. 15/18); and the ligaments (*meda dhatu upadhatu snayu*, or waste product) (Ca. Chi. 15/17).

Their symptoms of injury are sweating (sveda), oily body parts (*snigdhata anga*), dryness of palate (*talu shosha*), large swelling (*stoola shopha*), and thirst (*pipasa*) (Su. Sha. 9/12).

STHOULYA (OBESITY)

The condition called *ati sthula* or obesity occurs when an individual, because of excessive accumulation of muscles and fat in their body, manifests floppy buttocks, abdomen, and breasts; energy levels that are below normal; and muscles and fat tissue that are abnormally accumulated despite having been nourished and formed normally in childhood.[11]

Ayurveda also uses the term *ati sthula* for people who are "hyperobese" and includes them under the category of the eight groups of people who are, in the stark language of the scholars, "socially unfit" (*ashtau nindita*).

According to most scholars, the terms *ati sthula* or *ati sthoulya* both represent the imbalance of meda tissues, and as a consequence, these terms are used interchangeably.

Clinical Characteristics of Obesity

kshudra shwasa: gasping for air

trusha: excessive thirst

moha: delusion

svapna krathana: snoring

saada: exhaustion

kshut: excess hunger

sveda: excess perspiration

durgandha: foul body odor

alpa pran: short breaths

alpa maithuna: depleted sexual strength

PATHOLOGY OF OBESITY

According to ayurvedic scholars, as a result of blockages of the tissular passages or ducts, fat tissue starts accumulating, and therefore the successive dhatus (bone marrow and sexual organs) do not get suitable nourishment. This leads to further accumulation of fat (meda), so the different tissues and organs struggle to perform normal daily tasks.[12]

Fat deposition around the abdomen area occurs because of the blockages of the channels of organs (dhatus) such as the kidneys and part of the abdomen known as the greater omentum. As a consequence, the blockage of these channels is most probably the cause for the pendulant abdomen in sthoulya.

Ayurveda associates obesity with the individual's agni or metabolic fire. Let me integrate the ayurvedic concepts of meda, vasa, and sthoulya with the following case study.

CASE STUDY

Growth (Vrddhi) of the Fat/Adipose Tissue (Meda Dhatu)

Mark, a forty-year-old man, came to me seeking a consultation concerning his body weight. On visiting my consultation room, he appeared obese, and when walking, the fat movement of his pendulant buttocks, abdomen, and breasts were obvious. This condition in ayurvedic terms is defined as excessive vrddhi *(growth) of the meda dhatu (fat/adipose tissue). He presented* medodushti *(disorder of fat metabolism), a condition of* medovaha srotasa *(channels transporting fat), involving* meda dhatu *(fat tissues), as well as excess of fat in* vasa *(muscular tissue). In general, we can find two types of* meda vrddhi *(excessive growth of fat/adipose tissue) happening in our body:* baddha meda vrddhi *(obesity associated with adipose tissue) and* abaddha meda vriddhi *(resulting in dyslipidemia).*

In fact, Mark presented the condition of obesity associated with adipose tissue and dyslipidemia as per his long history of hypercholesterolemia, a borderline BMI of morbid obesity, and non-insulin-dependent diabetes, with no family history of the last two conditions. Studying his case, the whole pathology was associated with his lifestyle choices—a complete disregard for his body clock—no breakfast and one meal at dinner time, lack of physical activity, the wrong diet based on mostly fast food and fizzy drinks as well as the poor sleep patterns, which he described as resulting from his heavy workload as a lawyer.

Following my description of the risks of his serious ongoing condition for a forty-year-old man, combined with the habits formed in his lifestyle as a result of work patterns, he was willing to participate in an active way. I evaluated Mark as a vata prakruti, *and his* vikruti *as an altered predominant-dosha kapha-vata. My recommendations from the ayurvedic perspective focused on the importance of a tailored diet based on vata-appropriate foods to immediately address his* vikruti.

In addition, I recommended basic changes to the habits he had formed, to support Mark in addressing his vikruti *and body weight objectives together: regularized meal times and not a single, large daily meal; introducing physical activities into his currently sedentary routine; tailored herbal protocols; and strategies to calm his agitated state of mind via breathing exercises (pranayamas), relaxation and meditation activities—all to help Mark become more aware of his daily life and create more motivation for a healthier life going forward.*

AGNI: ENERGETIC CONSIDERATIONS OF THE DISTORTED METABOLISM

The ayurvedic view of agni (fire or biofire), previously discussed (see pages 31–34), covers the entirety of digestive and metabolic activities that generate ATP, the energy-carrying molecule.

Digestion and absorption activities carried out by our digestive fire (*pakvaagni*) and enzymes lead to the transformation of nutrients into various tissue materials, a transformation facilitated by tissue fire (*dhatuagni*).[13] The digested food must be absorbed by the intestine and circulated in the blood plasma, but equally must be absorbed by the local tissue cells to be assimilated by the body.

Ayurveda states that the seven primary organ systems or dhatus in the body are all made of cells that communicate between these systems via minute channels or ducts (*suksma srotas*) in charge of receiving and distributing nutrients as well as excreting metabolic waste products.[14] This ayurvedic account of cellular communication is consistent with the modern scientific understanding of intercellular uptake and release of substrates and metabolites.

Fat's role is offering the necessary lubrication and unctuousness to our cells, tissues, and organs, preventing wear and tear in the body. If the fat is retained in balanced proportions, its essence is good, and it can benefit our functioning. A short ayurvedic description of the energy dynamics between nutrients, digestive fire, tissues, channels of transport, and exchange in obesity is as follows:

An excess in fat-specific energy (kapha humor), and waste product of adipose tissues (*kleda*) blocks the channels. Due to the blocking by fat material in the tissues, vata dosha is increase within the alimentary canal (*koshta*). Vata influences the agni and leads to increase of agni (digestive fire). This leads to drying up of food leading to a quicker digestion, pushing the individual to crave food, thus indulging in binge eating, which in the long term will manifest in serious health imbalances.[15]

In modern idiom, when low metabolism is caused, with a progressive decrease of the basal metabolic rate, this generates body weight gain, leading to a dysfunction of the adipose tissue that we know as obesity.

CONTRIBUTING FACTORS OF OBESITY
(NIDANA)

Ayurveda describes obesity as the effect of an increase of fat tissue (meda dhatu), and explains that buildup of fat in the body, leading to obesity, is caused by:

avyayama: lack of exercise, sedentary lifestyle
divasvapna: sleeping during daytime, indulgence
shleshmala ahara sevana: intake of harmful foods and beverages that increase kapha dosha

Under these circumstances, the end-product of digestion (*annarasa*) becomes "sweet" by being digested but not properly assimilated. Broken carbohydrates are converted into high levels of sugar, resulting in accumulation of oiliness (*sneha*) and fat.[16]

The scholars of ayurveda describe in detail diseases resulting from obesity, such as heart disease (*hridroga*), diabetes (*prameha*), and other disorders that we cannot cover here in detail. However, let me give you one of the scholars' descriptions of obesity as a risk factor for heart disease: When the body pathways and channels get clogged by accumulation of morbid fat, the other body tissues are deprived of the nutrients required to continue building and maintaining themselves. Since this fat keeps accumulating over time, the fat tissue takes away all the nutrients in all the passages, causing depletion of other tissues—and this is why the individual becomes weak and impaired in doing any kind of work. As a result, they become afflicted by conditions such as excessive hunger, thirst, shortness of breath, intermittent dyspnea, unconsciousness, oversleeping, indulgence, body weakness, excessive sweating, body odor, lower sex drive, and decreased life expectancy (Ma. Ni. 34/2,3).

A fundamental pillar of ayurvedic philosophy is the concept of *loka-purusha*.[17] The universe (loka) and the human being (purusha) are subject to the same laws and exist on a continuum from the sphere of the universal to that of the smallest form of creation. They interact through the eternally shifting interplay of three factors that exist in both realms and form a bridge between loka and purusha. These three factors are: *buddhi* (intellect), *indriyartha* (sense objects), and *kala* (natural rhythms).[18] The continuously altering conditions both in nature and in the individual generate a dynamic harmony between the universe and the human being, a condition we recognize as good health. This interaction operates under the law of *samanya-vishesha* or like-increases-like. When there is greater deviation than can be tolerated between the individual and nature, that harmony is lost, and a state of imbalance, represented as something like obesity, can arise.[19, 20] The human being is a combination of sattva (mind), atma (soul), and *sharira* (body).

In ayurveda, the causative factors of any disease are classified as: exogenous or external factors (*bahya nidana*), which include food and daily regimen; and endogenous or internal factors (*abhyantara nidana*), these being the dosha and the tissues.

The ayurvedic protocols for rebalancing the doshas, dhatus, and malas, as well as igniting the biofire or agni of the different body constitutions resulting of multifactorial metabolic imbalances, involve the evaluation of your body constitution, lifestyle, diet, attitude, and beliefs; the use of natural ayurvedic medicines; and the application of tailored ayurvedic therapies. To give an example, ayurveda links obesity with a sluggish thyroid function, and guggul, known as *Commiphora wightii*, which is a yellow resin produced from a small thorny mukul myrrh tree, is a popular and widely recognized herb supporting weight loss, cholesterol and TG level reductions, and stress management, in India.[21, 22] The active ingredient in the guggul extract is guggulsterone, which appears to have powerful antioxidant and anti-inflammatory activities at the systematic and cellular levels, attributes that are under study but have been shown to alter thyroid function and improve metabolism.[23]

Also, in assessing your body's degree of imbalance, ayurveda draws on a combination of factors, including the origin of your ailment, present strengths and weaknesses, and the level of suffering caused by your symptoms.

To achieve a rebalancing, ayurveda address the root causes of the disease, bringing you back to your original constitution by building a comprehensive, personalized plan based on the actual condition of the patient (vikruti), allowing you to reach a balanced weight progressively and naturally.[21]

This approach requires taking into consideration the interconnection between the different body systems, and not only addressing the patient's concern about body weight issues and causes but equally helping the person to be mentally balanced. Ayurveda's philosophy will address the lifestyle of the individual by drawing awareness to daily issues such as diet and nutrition, physical activities, and all other factors that could be affecting the imbalance.

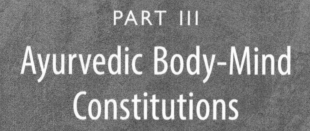

PART III

Ayurvedic Body-Mind Constitutions

Prakruti, Vikruti, and Manas Prakruti

6

PRAKRUTI

Your Body's Constitutional Characteristics

WE ARE ALL THE SAME, YET DIVERSE
Your Body at Birth

We each enter this world with appearances that are physically similar to one another, but over time, those apparent similarities give way to a range of evident differences in our shapes and sizes. Our genes develop muscles at different rates, burn fat from some parts and not others, and build varying bone structures. Our external appearances change, and we become taller or shorter than others, develop long limbs or a short torso, or perhaps short limbs and a long torso. And some of us grow up to become overweight or obese. Diverse body types also function differently, a subject we'll consider in this chapter. Hippocrates (ca. 460 BCE–ca. 370 BCE), is frequently credited with discovering the importance of the connection between our bodies and our emotions, with the theory of the four humors—blood, phlegm, yellow bile, and black bile. And in 1940, William Herbert Sheldon introduced another body typology: ectomorphic, mesomorphic, and endomorphic somatotypes that are linked with certain personality characteristics.[1]

We can also find classifications beyond the physical form, including variations in mental function (numerous classes of intellect), emotional reaction (degree of emotional responsiveness), social relationships (grade of necessity for connection or seclusion), and behavior predispositions (degrees of stress response).[2]

The notion of programmed fate, or karma, can be frustrating for those who seek to maintain and improve their body weight across their lives through attention to diet, nutrition, and level of physical activity. If your body is inclined to store a quantity of fat, you may find it more challenging to lose excess weight.[3] On the other hand, if your body is naturally inclined to be lean, you will find it harder to build muscle and bulk up.

In ayurveda, these bodily conditions equally apply to your mind, a concept we will explore to understand how metabolic, hormonal, and mental processes work with your distinctive prakruti and your condition of carrying extra weight, or being overweight or obese. We'll discuss how you can become an active participant if you are looking for improvement or rebalance.

To achieve this, we'll map out the fundamental framework of ayurveda, centered on the concept of the tridoshas, or qualitative energetic field types, that express your distinctive prakruti, or constitutional nature.

Ayurvedic medical science is supported by the basic notion of prakruti and doshas. Prakruti is explained in detail in three classic ayurvedic texts focused on different areas: the *Charaka Samhita* focused on internal medicine; the *Ashtanga Sangraha* focused on physiology and therapeutics; and the *Sushruta Samhita* focused on surgical procedures.

The assessment of an individual patient's prakruti involves a variety of methods used by the ayurvedic physician, such as a thorough physical sensory evaluation including visual, tactile, and olfactory aspects. It also includes an auditory estimation based on data collected by indirect means, including questions asked of the patient. Finally, conclusions are drawn from available information, knowledge, and experience.

To appreciate the customized system that ayurveda applies to the treatment and management of obesity, being overweight, and related conditions, we must first appreciate prakruti.

PRAKRUTI AND TRIDOSHA
Life in 3-D

In ayurveda, innate disposition, providence, time, chance,
cosmic order, and evolution are regarded as prakruti.

Su. Sa. 1/11

The Sanskrit word *prakruti* (*pra* = primary or first, *kruti* = creation or formation) explains the singularity of each person at different levels. Ayurveda characterizes the constitutions, or prakruti, in the following way:

CONSTITUTIONAL STATES

Prakruti Type	Constitution	Expression
Dosha	Physiological	biological energy at childbirth (vata, pitta, kapha)
Deha	Bodily	developed modifications amid fertilization and birth
Janma	Genetic	imprinted in the DNA (genes) at conception
Manas	Mental	personal state of awareness (sattva, rajas, tamas)

Our five elements (panchamahabhutas) comprise the body's structural features, but our functional aspects are governed by three anatomic-physiological expressions of the three elements (doshas) above, occasionally referred to as biological humors, which can be considered as distinctive functional electromagnetic energies or fields. The ayurvedic concept of jamma corresponds to the modern medical concept of genetic material, or DNA. In ancient India, cellular language and the naming of a molecule like DNA did not exist as we understand it today, but the role that such substances played in the life process was fully understood and described in the ayurvedic texts.[4]

Ayurvedic scientists thousands of years ago described internal and external cellular energies, functions, and concepts that align with the modern scientific understanding of DNA and functional genomics. These scholars considered our sophisticated human bodies to be controlled by varying combinations of three fundamental biological energies, or doshas, engaged in an intensive interplay that governs all the molecular, biochemical, and physiological body-mind mechanisms. Despite the effort to translate certain Sanskrit words accurately, it is useful to know that *dosha* originates from the word *dushya,* which means "disturbance" or "that which is vitiated."

The doshas, or three biological energies, can be represented as:

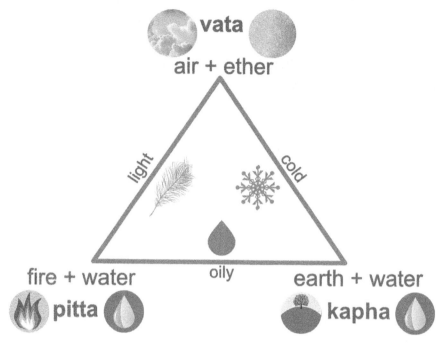

Fig. 6.1. Prakuti: The Doshas' Constitutions

DOSHAS, MAHABHUTAS, AND LIVING ROLES

Dosha	Component	Biological Type	Biodynamic Function
vata (breezy)	space + air	movement	bioprocesses stimulator
pitta (fiery)	fire + water	metabolism	biochemical transformation
kapha (earthy)	earth + water	configuration	structural provider/ preserver

Biological components of your body's constitution coexist in certain proportions and are in a kind of perpetual dance amongst themselves, collaborating to keep a harmonious body-mind balance. Vata (V), pitta (P), and kapha (K) preserve the general function of the human organism, working as a triumvirate with their different proportions, properties, and functions.

At the time of fertilization, the combination of your parents' prakruti (their DNA) determines your individual constitution, and both the ovum and sperm are equally influenced by your parents' lifestyles, diets, and emotions.

V-P-K is our 3-D triumvirate. It is present in every tissue in every human being, from the cellular level up to our bodily systems. These three biological functional energies govern all biological processes, comprising your physiological and psychological imbalances. Each one of us has a distinct combination and ratio of the three doshas, shaping our physiological, physical, and mental characteristics, with further classification into subgroups depending on specific dosha predominance. The 3-D triumvirate can vary according to lifestyle, diet, desires, and emotions. When any of these factors is not aligned with our internal makeup, body imbalances or illness may result.

Based on combinations of the three doshas, we find seven types of prakruti: There are three prevailing monotypes: V-, P-, or K-, in which one dosha is predominant and the other two are present to a minor degree. Secondly, three dual types—V-P, P-K, or K-V—are characterized by dual predominance. And finally, one type of prakruti, V-P-K, displays an even proportion of doshas (Su. Sa. 4/61).

When we have a primary and a close secondary dosha, the management protocols will generally focus on the primary dosha; however, it is not recommended to be too strict, as we must avoid aggravation of the secondary dosha, which could lead to more imbalance. As well, we are all made up of three doshas, so it is important to consider the metabolic approach of trying to raise the third dosha—in this case, to increase pitta dosha or the fire element that is so essential for all our digestive processes. Doing so is not complicated, and you will find your way by following the recommendations (see appendix 2) and enjoying finding the best food components that are required for your specific body type, condition, and goals.

The discovery of your prakruti is essential for a better realization of who you are, and to formulate a personalized program to rebalance your health. The three doshas are in an intensive interplay of motion (vata), chemical activity (pitta), and solid material structure (kapha) among

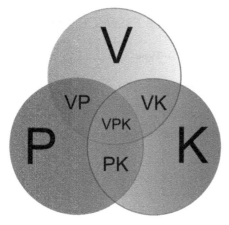

Fig. 6.2. Dosha Combinations: The Seven Types of Prakruti

themselves, and that interplay both governs our internal environment and responds to our external environment.[5, 6] Their shared interactions are essential for keeping an equilibrated state, even though disruptive influences may act upon them. The 3-D is the tripod upon which life rests. They craft your blueprint.

Keeping a balance in the activity of the doshas, as determined at conception—*the moment when your prakruti is established*—is required for good health. Although the 3-D coexist in determined proportions and functions, they can manifest properties that oppose one another, and this occurs because they are always in a perpetual dance. For instance, vata dosha cools the body's temperature, while by contrast, pitta keeps the body warm, based on fire as its major constituent. The refined movements of the doshas' constituents are responsible for the characteristics and functions that shape our bodily and psychosomatic temperament.

VITAL SUBTLE BODY-MIND ENERGIES

Ayurveda also defines three vital, subtle essences called prana (subtle life energy), tejas (subtle vitality, fire, or energy), and *ojas* (subtle immunity), which link to the vata, pitta, and kapha doshas, respectively.[7]

SUBTLE ESSENCE TYPES

Essence	Type	Manifestation
Prana	vital life force	pervasive expression of life stated by the breath
Tejas	biofire (agni), pitta dosha	expression of solar energy in the body
Ojas	preserve vitality of all body systems	the very seat of life

Ayurvedic scholars showed how the doshas, when aggravated by certain factors, affect the dhatus (tissues) and srotas (channels) of the body, eventually manifesting in disease. Translating the ayurvedic terms, this means that degeneration of the blood vessels is caused by increased vata in the blood vessels, which makes them hard, thin, dry, and rough. The irregular thickening of blood vessels as a result of deposits of lipids and calcium is a clear representation of the depositing of kapha (water and earth elements) in deteriorated blood vessels.

Increasing research has described patterns of association between each dosha type and physiological conditions, blood chemistry, genetic expression, and long-lasting illnesses.[8, 9]

One study shows that inflammatory markers positively correlate with the kapha constitution type, but does not suggest any significant association of pitta-kapha and vata-pitta prakruti with risk factors of heart disease.[10] Consequently, the detection of people carrying vata-kapha and kapha prakruti will help identify potential risk factors of cardiovascular diseases such as diabetes, dyslipidemia, hypertension, insulin resistance, inflammation, and others, and thus will allow people to take preventative action.

All prakruti types show a gene polymorphism correlation—in other words, a correlation relating to two or more possibilities of a trait on a gene—correlation with human leucocyte antigen (HLA) typing, and a matching laboratory evaluation test on HLA.[11] The pitta type correlates with a deficiency in the gene for the enzyme phosphoglucomutase 1 gene.[12] All prakruti types also have strong associations with blood parameters such as cell blood count (CBC) and blood groups, as well as being associated with distribution of lipids, hepatic function test lipid profile, and BMI.[13]

It is important to share that the concept of subdividing the population into individual categories is not exclusive to ayurveda. Kampo, the Traditional Chinese Medicine of Japan, as well as Sasang, the Constitutional Medicine of Korea, use the same concepts.[14]

If we interpret the process of epigenetics from an ayurvedic scholar's perspective, the concept of karma, the Sanskrit word for "action," could be represented at a cellular level by: "For every action there is an equal and opposite reaction," Newton's Third Law of Motion. Every cell has to go through this process, and conditions that could cause epigenetic modifications affecting gene expression can also be transmitted to the offspring. It is believed that about 90 percent of our existence is subject to epigenetic influence—the modifications in gene expression that manifest according to what we do all our lives.[15]

Ayurveda postulates that when a person acts in a way that is caring toward their body, deha prakruti, (our psychosomatic constitution), remains stable, and health is maintained. On the other hand, if the person's activities are not helpful for the body-mind system, deha prakruti becomes imbalanced, creating vikruti, and the imbalance manifests in the form of illness.[16] This process happens through epigenetic mechanisms. Yet such modifications can be overturned, and ayurveda plays a pivotal role in these rebalancing processes.

How? Well, ayurveda instructs us in how to tackle the mechanisms that trigger epigenetic modifications and that accordingly modify both the phenotype and expression of the genotype in an effective way. As adults, we are responsible for keeping ourselves healthy, and our actions can disturb our health in a direct and personal manner. Fortunately, we can counteract imbalances leading to ailments, through the practice of detailed ayurvedic guidance that addresses our prakruti and vikruti.

CHARACTERIZATION OF VATA, PITTA, AND KAPHA
Prakruti/Body Natures

BREEZY (VATA) PRAKRUTI

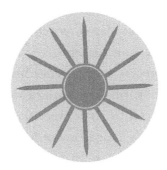

Vata physiological functions derive from the predominance of space and air elements. Vata can be considered as the biological "air" embodying the principle of movement within all beings. Movement in the body is indicative of the presence of life. The *Bhela Samhita*, an incomplete but reputed ayurvedic scholars' work earlier than the *Charaka Samhita*, states that life exists as long as vata lasts in the body to cause such movements.[17]

The word *vata* is defined by Sushruta as "the one having two functions": the first is movement; the second is knowledge, or how we handle information. These actions are no different from the essential body movements that keep all our body functions active—breathing, circulation, digestive motility, conception, fetal development, defecation, urination, and so forth—indicating that vata actions influence the other two doshas and the body constituents by regulating the body's movements through our nervous system.

Vata cannot be perceived by the sensory organs, due to its composition (space and air), indicating that vata does not possess color, taste, or odor. Modern scientists have been trying to link the existence of vata to our known bodily molecules, and the closest compound we can find is nitric oxide (NO), the tiny so-called "molecule of life." NO is synthetized by all kinds of human cells, and plays the role of vasodilator, widening the inner muscles of your blood vessels to allow relaxation.[18, 19]

As we've described, the two main functions of vata are motor (*gati*) and sensory (*gandhana*). To fulfil these functions, vata has to move throughout the body channels and vessels (srotas) that handle motor functions using muscles or other physical body parts (conative organs) as well as sensory functions of the body that are associated with the mind (cognitive organs).

Our mind is considered the regulator of all our sensory tissues and organs; as a result, both types of channels allow the transit of information through the mind. Our nervous structure consists of our brain and spinal cord, making up the central nervous system. The nerves in our bodies control everything we do by carrying information to and from the body and interpreting that information in order to determine a particular response.

The following table demonstrates the ayurvedic description of vata qualities (gunas), and their main characteristics as well as their functions in the body.

VATA (BREEZY) DOSHA FUNCTIONS

Elements	space, air
Qualities/Gunas	mobility, pervading, light, dry, clear, cold, rough*
Body/Mind Characteristics	slim body frame; light muscles/body fat; dryness (hair, skin, colon); nervous
Biological Functions	sparks all organ movement: voluntary and involuntary (i.e., inspiration/expiration); tissular circulation
Metabolic Transformations	vata motion controls pitta and kapha, body tissues and functions

*As. Hr. Su. 1/11; Ca. Su. 1/59

The ayurvedic scholars divided the *vatavaha srotas* (nervous system) in two types according to structure: *samvrta*, consisting of concealed or myelinated nerves fibers, and *asamvrta*, made up of open or unmyelinated nerve fibers.

Vata's characteristics of being minute (sukshma), intangible (*amurta*), self-derived (*swayambhu*), and volatile (*anavasthita*) allow it to move through channels and passages that can be just one micron thick. These features let vata control our body's voluntary and involuntary movements (*gandhana*), which include the secretory roles (gati), allowing us to assume that vata is the process of nerve impulse and its epicenter is the nervous system.

The ayurvedic scholars described vata even further, demonstrating a profoundly detailed understanding of its functions. These are described in the table below as subdivisions of vata dosha, and their locations in the body are defined, along with their distinctive roles (Ca. Su. 18/49). Also, *Ashtanga Hrdayam Sutrasthana* 11:15 described the symptoms that manifest from the abnormal function of vata.

VATA (BREEZY) SUB-DOSHAS: LOCATION AND FUNCTION

Vata Sub-Dosha	Location	Distinct Dosha Function
Prana	heart/brain/head/chest, CNS	perception/insight/thought/ATP
Udana	neck/throat/lungs	upward drive, inspiration/expiration, memory
Samana	navel/stomach/intestines	digestive rhythm of peristalsis, biofire
Vyana	nervous/vascular systems	epidermal/skin, circulation fluids, motion
Apana	colon/lower abdomen	wastes removal (urine, menses, feces, etc.)

CASE STUDY
Prakruti/Vikruti: Breezy (Vata) Dosha

François was a sixty-two-year-old, quite tall, with a slim body frame, light muscles, dry skin and hair, poor circulation (cold hands and feet), nervous movements, and unsure speech when expressing himself. He came for a consultation in an anxious state, sharing his main complaint of constipation and hard feces, with phases of bleeding and hemorrhoids. This is quite a typical case of a breezy or

*vata dosha–predominant person, and in his particular case, his main affected
sub-doshas were apana and udana.*

The vagus nerve is considered by some scientists to be a potential bio-
marker of relevant activities of vata dosha, such as preserving the balance
of the respiratory, neural, and digestive systems; regulation of mental well-
being and behavior; and sustaining the gut-brain link via the lower gut
(*pakwashaya*), the major regulatory location for vata dosha.[20]

For the purpose of understanding the process of body-mind imbalances
and the role of the gut, we will focus on the vagus nerve and vata dosha
to appreciate the various process that involve the gut-brain axis. Even better, we'll explore the alignment that we can call the gut-heart-brain axis.
Researchers have confirmed the existence of 40,000 "brain cells" in the
human heart, and there are more nerve cell connections in the gut than in
the brain. Even more interestingly, these connections communicate with
each other.[21] In our Western culture, we are educated to listen only to our
heads, and consequently we are missing the crucial connective information
coming from our other two "brains."

FIERY (PITTA) PRAKRUTI

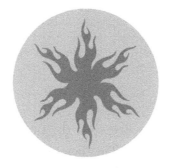

The word *pitta* originates from the Sanskrit verb-root *tapa santape*, denot-
ing the fire, the energy that produces heat in our bodies. Its major role is
cooking or combustion, so we can call it the biofire or the energy responsible for the biological transformations that occur in our bodies.

The ayurvedic scholars' principles reflected that everything under the sun manifests through fire, and they understood that pitta breaks down food and processes it to integrate it into our bodies. They described the body as the product of food, which can be eaten, drunk, licked, and masticated, and can leave impressions on the body (Ca. Su. 28/45).

The concept of agni in ayurveda means "the fire within us." There is ongoing agni activity in every cell, and according to ayurveda, the success of these activities is dependent on the quality and quantity of the fire in each of these cells.

The following table gives an idea of the ayurvedic description of pitta qualities (gunas), their main characteristics, as well as their functions in the body.

PITTA (FIERY) DOSHA FUNCTIONS

Elements	fire, water
Qualities/Gunas	hot, sharp, light, liquid, sour, oily, and spreading*
Body/Mind Characteristics	soft, warm, oily hair/skin; strong appetite/digestion; outspoken, sharp mind, memory; vitality, courage
Biological Functions	biofire; rules all metabolic processes: digestion, absorption, assimilation, hunger, thirst; body heat; intelligence, insight
Metabolic Transformations	produces energy from breaking down food

*As. Hr. Su. 1/11; Ca. Su. 1/60

The ayurvedic scholars described the functions of pitta at an even deeper and more detailed level. They described subdivisions of pitta dosha, defining their body locations where pitta plays a distinctive role. *Ashtanga Hrdayam Sutrasthana* 11:7 also described the physical manifestations of the abnormal function of pitta.

PITTA (FIERY) SUB-DOSHAS: LOCATION AND FUNCTION

Pitta Sub-Dosha	Location	Distinct Dosha Function
Sadhaka	brain (gray matter), heart	thinking, memory, understanding, emotions
Alochaka	eyes	good optical perception/ thinkers
Pachaka	GIT (stomach/small bowel)	initiate digestion, assimilation of food
Ranjaka	red blood cells/liver/spleen	balance nutrients, blood and detox, produces bile
Bhrajaka	skin	skin aspect, luster, radiance, temperature

For the purpose of better understanding the processes of body-mind imbalances and the role of the gut, we will be focusing in more detail on the digestive processes (biofire or agni) as well as the participation of the intestinal flora (microbiome). But first, let me illustrate a typical pitta person.

CASE STUDY
Prakruti/Vikruti: Fiery (Pitta) Dosha

Peter was thirty-five years old with penetrating eyes, oily skin and hair, early hair loss, a sharp mind, and a hearty appetite. He was outspoken when describing his complaints and was clearly focused on finding a solution to them. He requested a consultation for GIT issues, which included a burning sensation, a general feeling of thirst, and episodes of skin irritation. He also dealt with adrenaline rushes and insomnia, especially when under pressure at work. Peter is a classic case of a fiery or pitta dosha—predominant person, where in his particular case the most affected sub-doshas were pachaka and bhrajaka.

EARTHY (KAPHA) PRAKRUTI

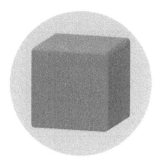

All the liquid and solid constituents of our bodies are kapha in origin, since water and earth are their constituents (mahabhutas). Kapha represents all functions associated with the fluid balance of the body, not only in intra- and extracellular spaces but also in making and nourishing our body structure and mechanisms.

KAPHA (EARTHY) DOSHA FUNCTIONS

Elements	earth, water
Qualities/Gunas	heavy, slow, oily, liquid, dense, thick, static, cloudy, cool, sweet, salty*
Body/Mind Characteristics	strength, stamina; heavy and strong bones, muscles; tends toward fat sensitive, patient requires incentive
Biological Functions	nourishment and lubrication of body structures: tendons, cartilage, muscles, ligaments; mental balance
Metabolic Transformations	nurture/regulate pitta and vata functions

*As. Hr. Su 1/12; Ca. Su. 1/61

Ayurveda describes the essential role of kapha at the level of five of the seven main tissue elements: plasma (rasa), muscles (mamsa), fat (meda), bone marrow (majja), and reproductive tissue (*shukra*). At a physiological level, kapha provides body unctuousness; supports our tissues' building and healing; connects the diverse constituents of our joints, providing stability to our body's general structure; enables strength and stamina for both physical and mental tasks as well as sexual function; and provides resistance to ailments and bodily decay. At a psychological level, kapha provides patience, endurance, intelligence, and warmth.

The following table represents a summary of the insightful observations of the ayurvedic scholars and their ability to discern the subdivisions of kapha dosha, their locations in the body, and their various functions. *Ashtanga Hrdayam Sutrasthana* 11:8 describes the physical manifestations of the abnormal function of kapha by symptoms.

KAPHA (EARTHY) SUB-DOSHAS: LOCATION AND FUNCTION

Kapha Sub-Dosha	Location	Distinct Dosha Function
Tarpaka	brain, spinal fluid, myeline sheath	CNS: nourish brain/spinal cord, memory
Bodhaka	tongue/mouth	saliva, swallowing, taste perception, speech
Kledaka	stomach, GIT	gastric secretion, digestion, absorption
Avalambaka	heart/chest/spine	nourish heart, support lungs/spine/emotions
Shleshaka	joints, synovial fluids	joint nourishing and lubrication

CASE STUDY
Prakruti/Vikruti Kapha (Earthy) Dosha

Betty was forty years old with thick hair, a strong body frame, well-formed bones and muscles, strong digestive fire and appetite, soft and slow speech, and a low level of motivation. Still, she came searching for a solution to her state of lethargy, feeling of heaviness, excess salivation, cold limbs, indigestion, and tendency to overeat, sometimes without feeling hungry. This a succinct example describing a fairly typical earthy, kapha person where the primary affected sub-doshas are bodhaka and kledaka, leading to being overweight and the associated implications.

For the purpose of understanding body-mind imbalances and the role of the gut, we will be focusing in more detail on the digestive processes (biofire or agni) as well as the participation of the intestinal flora (microbiome).

DUAL-DOSHA CONSTITUTIONS

We all manifest three types of energies or doshas, previously described as seven types. These include the predominant types (vata, pitta, or kapha), the dual doshas (vata-pitta, vata-kapha, and pitta-kapha), and the tridoshic vata-pitta-kapha.

Many people are dual-doshic, so perhaps you are dual-doshic as well. This can create confusion when you attempt to reconcile these often-conflicting diet recommendations and management practices intended for a single dosha. Please take this into consideration when reviewing the recommended food tables included in appendix 2.

Given the existence of the dual-dosha types vata-kapha and pitta-kapha prakruti, a certain degree of complexity faces us when we are addressing conditions of increased ponderal body weight and their potential reduction via diet. In fact, the first thing to consider is your prakruti and your present body imbalance (vikruti), and to what degree this imbalance is associated with your natural constitution (prakruti), or whether your present vikruti has been created by a wrong lifestyle. Let's discuss in more detail two of the three dual-doshic types.

Earthy/Breezy Kapha-Vata and Breezy/Earthy Vata-Kapha Types

If an ayurvedic professional describes you as vata-kapha type or kapha-vata type, that designation means you have an equal or nearly equal predominance of vata and kapha doshas. Since we are all different, and management protocols are individualized and not mass-produced, it is important to take notice of which is the preponderant: vata-kapha or kapha-vata.

Vata and Kapha Dosha Qualities and Main Characteristics

Tatra rukso laghu: sita:khra:susksmascalo'nila.

Vata is dry, light, cold, rough, minuteness,
and movement.

....

As. Hr. Su. 1/10

*Snigdhah shita gururmandah shlakshno mritsnah
sthirah kaphah.*

Kapha is unctuous, cool, heavy, slow, smooth,
soft, and static.

....

As. Hr. Su. 1/12

The main qualities (gunas) of both doshas show their similarities and differences: Vata is airy, light, dry, mobile, and cold. Kapha is earthy, heavy, oily, immobile, and cold.

As you can see, vata and kapha are fairly opposite (light vs. grounded), making a pretty changeable combination. However, both doshas share the quality of cold, so warming and heating practices will be balancing for the vata-kapha dosha. In this case, the cold quality is not as sensitive as for the vata dosha type, because of kapha dosha's lining.

The generally slender and bony body type of a vata person mingles with the solid body type of a kapha to either create a mixture of the two or to look like either one of them, not unlike the medium, athletic build of a pitta type.

Vata has the quality of mobility, so vata people are quick and efficient when working. Kapha has the quality of stability, so kapha people are determined and steady when working. This blend makes a vata-kapha dosha individual an excellent person for completing complex projects.

Regarding body-mind character for this dual-doshic type, frequently a vata-kapha person will shift between vata and kapha mental characteristics. For example, a vata individual is often changeable, fervent, and inclined to overdo things, while a kapha person is calm, relaxed, and averse to change. This leads a vata-kapha person to disregard the pitta qualities of will and discernment. If a kapha person is stressed, it could lead to withdrawn behavior and feelings of frustration and depression from time to time, while a vata person habitually expresses fear, anxiety, and nervousness under stress. These shared qualities in a vata-kapha person often manifest as deep feelings of hurt, and a tendency to struggle with overcoming upsetting situations.

Kapha-Pitta (Earthy/Fiery) and Pitta-Kapha (Fiery/Earthy) Types

If an ayurvedic professional describes you as pitta-kapha type or kapha-pitta type, that description means you have an equal or nearly equal predominance of pitta and kapha doshas. Again, it is important to take notice which is the preponderant: pitta-kapha or kapha-pitta. Nevertheless, the following applies equally to both. Since we are all composed of three doshas, it is important as well to try to raise the *third* dosha, in this case to increase vata dosha or the movement element, which is vital for all our digestive processes. You will learn to rebalance your body by following the recommendations and enjoying finding the best food components for your specific body type, condition, and goals.

Earthy or Kapha and Fiery or Pitta Dosha Qualities and Main Characteristics

Pittam sasneha tikshnoshnam laghu visram,
saram dravam.

Pitta is oily, sharp, hot, light, flesh-smelling,
spreading, and liquid.

As. Hr. Su. 1/11

Snigdhah shita gururmandah shlakshno mritsnah
sthirah kaphah.

Kapha is unctuous, cool, heavy, slow, smooth,
soft, and static.

As. Hr. Su. 1/12

The main qualities (gunas) of both doshas show us their similarities and differences: Earthy or kapha is earthy, heavy, immobile, oily, and cold. Fiery or pitta is liquid, light, spreading, oily, and hot.

Before discussing diet for this kapha-pitta type, let me give you an example of the important role of these qualities. Since the individual doshas kapha and pitta share the common trait of being oily by nature, consequently foods, drinks, and spices that are considered dehydrating will be beneficial for both dosha types. While pitta is hot and kapha cold, hot spicy foods—which are kapha's delight—most probably will aggravate your pitta, and cooling foods, which are pitta's delight, will be sure to increase your kapha. Thus in order to be cautious, the best approach will be to seek out foods and spices that are neutral or warm by nature.

The pitta-kapha type's character is the strongest, healthiest, and most resilient among the seven constitutional types. These qualities permit the person to adopt management roles with confidence. Their pitta quality of perseverance will offer enough energy to promote and carry out long-term plans, and the grounded kapha quality will offer a state of balance.

Breezy (vata), fiery (pitta), and earthy (kapha) describe the ayurvedic classifications of the three fundamental body types. Here, we observe a correspondence with modern perceptions of the nervous system. The autonomic nervous system (ANS) works with the endocrine system to control all the body's automatic or involuntary functions. The ANS comprises the sympathetic and parasympathetic nervous systems (SNS and PSNS). The SNS is responsible for regulating actions when the body enters what's commonly known as a fight or flight state—that is, when we perceive danger and in response we increase our heart rate, or our blood vessels constrict. And the PSNS is responsible for regulation functions while the body is in a "rest and digest" state, performing food digestion and the expulsion of waste, actions best undertaken when the body is resting.[22]

Based on the above descriptions, the primordial embryonic layers can be understood thus: the breezy (vata) type is ectomorph, or sympathetic dominant; the fiery (pitta) type shows mesomorph or sympathetic-parasympathetic coregulation; and the earthy (kapha) type is endomorph or parasympathetic dominant.

It is quite extraordinary to appreciate how ayurveda matches the doshas with the primordial embryonic layers and the modern scientific description of the autonomic nervous system.

WHAT IS YOUR PRAKRUTI
(BODY CONSTITUTION)?
....
Vata, Pitta, or Kapha

Your constitution is determined at conception by a specific combination of the three doshas—vata, pitta, and kapha—that comes from your parents. Each person has their own individual prakruti, just as we each have our own DNA. Your constitution and psychosomatic temperament are primarily genetic in origin. The combination of your parents' constitutions at the moment of conception will be your individual body prakruti, and throughout your life this combination will be under the influence of factors such as diet, lifestyle, environment, and emotional experiences.

Besides the fact that we all have our combinations of the doshas vata, pitta, and kapha, each dosha also has diversity in the twenty qualities (gunas) that are predominant in a person's constitution. Therefore, our uniqueness is not only the result of our particular combination of the doshas but also the unique combination of the qualities of those doshas. To better understand how this works, appendix 1 provides a prakruti evaluation (see pages 271–77) for you to complete. After completing the prakruti evaluation, you may find that, for example, you are kapha-pitta predominant. The interesting question then becomes, which qualities of kapha or pitta are more influential in your constitution—earthy, heavy, immobile, oily, and cold from kapha or hot, sharp, light, liquid, sour, spreading, and oily from pitta?

Recognizing your body constitution is crucial to making ayurveda work in your daily life and to addressing the condition of body-mind imbalances, because ayurveda's helpfulness depends on managing an individual's concerns based on their prakruti. Knowing your prakruti makes it possible to work out a tailored diet based on the qualities (gunas) that relate better to your predominant prakruti, and in this way, crafting a lifestyle that is more suitable for you. Most of the time, people have one predominant dosha, but some individuals have two predominant doshas. Less frequently there are individuals with equal levels of the three doshas.

Now, if you are a vata-pitta, vata-kapha, or pitta-kapha, how do you know which dosha you have to balance, which nutrients to eat, and which qualities to nurture? To address this question, adopt the suggestions in the sections on both the doshas that are codominant in you (see chapter 3).

Prakruti Evaluation: Understanding Your Body Constitution by Self-Assessment

The prakruti evaluation (see pages 271–77) indicates your inherited doshic predominance, with a view to assisting you in learning about yourself so as to understand your body-mind tendencies better and thus accept them without judging, which will enable you to take action. Additionally, the evaluation helps you to understand why you and others around you act and react the way you do, and how you can identify and work on different aspects of your relationships through recognition and acceptance of other people's prakruti.

The prakruti evaluation will never be 100 percent accurate. One of the reasons is that, in the case of illness, pathological processes affect the body in ways that mask some of the factors evaluated in prakruti diagnosis. Furthermore, we all change from good health to reasonable health to bad health and back again at different times in our lives, which will also affect the evaluation.

This prakruti evaluation will indicate your personal distribution of the three doshas. If one of the doshas is too high, ayurvedic procedures will guide you to rebalance or fortify the other two constituents through recommendations regarding diet, lifestyle, and other practices such as physical activity, yoga, meditation, and relaxation, to balance the three constituents and attain better bodily and mental stability.

VIKRUTI

···

Your Current Abnormal State

Why are so many people carrying "extra baggage"? It is a question that researchers have been working on diligently since obesity prevalence started to spike in the 1980s. In ayurveda, vikruti refers to those cases in which a person reaches an unnatural or modified state, and they are not aligned with their prakruti. The ayurvedic perspective on how the body functions classifies the vikruti state as a condition of imbalance that can manifest as different metabolic alterations generating numerous pathologies.

Recent studies show that our DNA may be affected by everything in our surroundings from the moment of our conception, and it is disturbed by our experiences, attitudes, and beliefs, causing modifications in our gene expression.[1]

The Sanskrit meaning of *vikruti* can be broken down thus: the root *vi* means "after," and the root *kruti* means "creation." Vikruti is the state of disturbed and distressed physiology of the physical body and mind, which causes body-mind imbalances such that the individual becomes more susceptible to either physical or mental ill health.

BEING CONSCIOUS OF YOUR WEIGHT IMBALANCE CAN CHANGE YOUR GENETIC EXPRESSION

It is not uncommon to feel disappointed or even depressed when our efforts to reduce weight do not yield the results we hope for, despite much work and commitment.

Conversely, sometimes we have these feelings because we can't find the motivation to make an effort. I believe that through working to see ourselves in a new light, it is possible to acquire knowledge of how a thriving, centuries-old health system can address our weight issues. Through ayurveda we can bring about the necessary change, either mentally or motivationally, to create the conditions for sustainable weight management through a daily practice.

Understanding our vikruti, or present body imbalance, is a giant leap forward on that path.

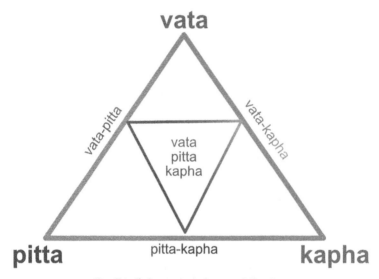

Fig. 7.1. Balance-Imbalance of Doshas

Let us explore in more detail certain generalities regarding what vikruti imbalance means in terms of abnormal function for vata, pitta, and kapha doshas, in light of Charaka's definition of health and disease:

Any disturbance in the equilibrium of dhatus (tridosha,
body tissues, and waste products) is known as disease.
The state of their equilibrium is health. Happiness
indicates health, and pain indicates disease.

CA. SU. 9/4

UNDERSTANDING AND BECOMING RESPONSIBLE FOR YOUR VIKRUTI (BODY NATURE IMBALANCE)

Let us start by explaining more aspects of the concept of prakruti and vikruti defined by the ayurvedic scholars based on doshic characteristics, before moving on to describing vikruti in fuller detail. As previously discussed, ayurveda sees every person as indivisible from the entirety of creation and manifestation of life; and at the same time, we all are microcosms of the macrocosm of the entire universe. According to ayurveda, all the existing elements within the world we know, and in the universe, are composed of the panchamahabhutas: space (ether), air, fire, water, and earth.

The presence of these five elements and their interactions, from the most subtle to the densest, supports functional processes and movements in the body that allow our organs to accomplish actions such as digestion, absorption, and assimilation of nutrients to create or rebuild the body continuously. Each of us has a distinctive ratio of these five elements. How they combine and work together in your body makes up your combination of doshas, and if the environment is not favorable, this will affect the properties and qualities of all your systems including the gut.

EPIGENETICS FROM AN AYURVEDA POINT OF VIEW

Understanding Factors that May Cause Epigenetic Modifications

Let me describe the concepts of human genetics and epigenetics from both modern and ayurvedic perspectives. Current biomedical sciences show us that the difference between living and nonliving things is the presence of deoxyribonucleic acid (DNA) in living species. The DNA in the nucleus of living organisms is composed of four different nucleotide bases: adenine (A), thymine (T), guanine (G), and cytosine (C). These bases pair up in specific ways—adenine with thymine and guanine with cytosine— to form the rungs of the DNA ladder. The sequence of these base pairs encodes the genetic information and determines the structure of genes.

The human genome involves approximately 21,000 genes, spread out along 3 billion base pairs of DNA, spread among 23 chromosomes. People carry two sets, one from each parent, from which on average we carry between 100–400 abnormal genes. These are known as the genotype or genetic features. The genotype is stable and non-changing—unless there is toxic harm—and corresponds to that part of our genetic makeup that defines specific features of an individual. Meanwhile, we each also have a phenotype or physical properties such as individual appearance, development, and behavior.

The genotype is responsible for the development of the phenotype of the individual. Our daily actions can disturb the phenotype and may change the expression of the genotype accordingly. The major factors disturbing our phenotype are lifestyle and behavior, digestion and diet, environmental factors, and stress. Obesity is a chronic multifactorial, multi-organ, multi-hormone, and multi-mechanism condition where genetic and environmental influences control adiposity and weight gain. These factors are highly relevant in their own right and the analysis of the tissues and organs, hormones, and mechanisms involved in becoming overweight or obese will be described in more detail in other sections, due to their importance when we discuss metabolic issues and their connection with body weight and excess body fat.[2]

Epigenetics outlines the dynamic association between gene expression and our environment, dealing with almost everything that happens to the expressed genes in the phenotype along our life cycle of experiences or in different phases of life. It addresses our lifestyle, diet, nutrition, stress, and environmental conditions including exposure to toxins, and how these impact the expression of genes.[3] Epigenetics refers to the external DNA changes that turn genes on and off, influencing their expression—crucially, without modifications to the basic structure or sequence of the DNA. This process creates a change in the phenotype without an alteration in the genotype and implicates components such as protein histone changes, methylation, mRNA molecules, and other processes that we mention here but will not dwell on.[4]

Ayurvedic scholars understood epigenetics and proposed that

this important mechanism needed to be addressed within the study of prakruti.[5] The scholars describe the deha (body) prakruti (immunopsychophysiological constitution), which relates to phenotype, and indirectly the janma prakruti (birth constitution), which corresponds to the genotype. Specifically, the janma prakruti or birth prakruti does not change and is the basis of the immunopsychophysiological constitution or deha prakruti (body prakruti), characterized by their changeable and dynamic properties. In that case, in ayurveda, the genotype corresponds to the birth prakruti, and the phenotype corresponds to the deha prakruti.

The imbalances or disorders in the deha prakruti are described as vikruti, which correlates with disorders and diseases in our modern medical system.

DEHA PRAKRUTI

Altered Current State Vata (Breezy) Functions

When space (ether) and air come together as a functional process in the body, they are described as vata dosha, vata being translated as physiological movement. Every existing object is contained in space. When we consider our food intake, the gastrointestinal tract motion starts from the moment we are chewing our food (in a space, with movement), progresses to the creation of a kind of bolus, and follows its transit down into the stomach where it encounters peristaltic contractions, which keep going all the way until the end of the GIT. Vata dosha is equally responsible for the transportation undertaken by the microscopic villi in your small intestine, which take these very small, entirely dissociated particles of food—now fully digested into the basic units of life—and allow them to be absorbed and brought into your bloodstream for use by the different tissues and organs of the body. Following the absorption of food as basic units, the large intestine absorbs water and electrolytes, serves as a site for the fermentation of some of the food matter indigestible by the intestinal flora, forms feces, and propels it toward the rectum for elimination.

All these dynamic motions are under the control of vata dosha. If any of the described functions are altered, then we have an abnormal function of vata, which can manifest, for example, as vitiation of the joints—that is, rheumatoid arthritis (RA) (*amavata*).[6]

Altered Current State Fiery (Pitta) Functions

When fire and water come together, they create pitta dosha, which physiologically can be translated as digestion and metabolism. This digestive fire or agni is present inside each and every one of our previously created cells. The intelligence of our existing cells performs the conversion of molecules of food into energy (ATP) in our digestive system. The digestive fire in your gut is described as the combination of fire and water because of the release of two main compounds—hydrochloric acid (liquid fire), and our digestive enzymes—responsible for breaking down food particles and thus producing energy, a process that creates fire through molecular alterations. These metabolic activities are cyclical processes that produce energy for the creation of new molecules, and support further metabolic activities or cellular synthesis for our various organs involved in digestion of food. All these processes are going on in that ocean of water containing small molecules that, with the participation of metabolic fire, get converted into small new structures through biosynthesis, and transported by that ocean of water for eventual cellular absorption.

These dynamic motions are under the control of pitta dosha, and if any of the described functions is altered then we have an abnormal function of pitta.

Altered Current State Earthy (Kapha) Functions

When the elements water and earth come together after food absorption, inside the cell membrane or barrier, they create kapha dosha. This originates new small physical structures that gradually become functional and start reorganizing themselves to construct carbohydrates from single molecules of sugar, proteins from the fundamental units of amino acids, and lipids from the basic units of fat—such as triglycerides and cholesterol—creating big lipid particles. By that time, your body has reached the level at which all these brand-new carbohydrates, proteins, and lipids are synthetized, and are available for incorporation by the entire body, starting with single cells transported by the vessels, and moving on to dense existing structures such as muscles and bones. In this exquisite dance of the five elements that make up your three doshas, it is also necessary to cool the system to provide lubrication for a suitable maintenance of the tissues.

For that reason, the watery aspect of kapha now plays the role of cooling and lubricating the system to prepare the ground—the lining of your stomach and other tissues—for the subsequent process of digestion of food due to occur over the coming hours. This process of cooling is also very important in preventing these hot strong secretions of gastric juice (composed by hydrochloric acid, enzymes, electrolytes, mucus, intrinsic factor and water) from eating right through the wall of your stomach, perhaps creating ulcers; equally important is the role of enzymes in reabsorption by the cells so that lubrication for protection along the whole GIT can take place. Conditions such as asthma, or *swasa*, are the most widespread in kapha people since these illnesses are precipitated by an excess of cold, heavy, moist foods, and overeating.[7]

As we've seen, here we have to break down all the above mechanisms and their interactions in order to describe and comprehend all these processes, but in real life all these processes are going on simultaneously and continuously, thanks to the perpetual interaction of the five elements or panchamahabhutas. Now, we can see the interconnection of the three bodily constituents or doshas—vata, pitta, and kapha—and how they participate in the process of digestion. They can act quite independently, but at the same time they engage each other in a harmonic interdependency since they need each other to keep cellular and body functions in a state of balance in order to perpetuate our existence.

The most important point to know at this level is the ratio of the three constitutional doshas in your body and the potential implications of any imbalances that may result in biological harm. When imbalances of the ratio exist, for example due to genetic reasons, this can result in body imbalances as well as mind imbalances—for example, a lack of proper connection with our senses. As an example, an excess of pitta can generate inflammatory conditions at various cellular and tissular levels. It can create burning up of the lubrication and protection of structures such as the cover of the lining of nerve cells, where this excessive pitta heat will cause demyelinating disorders, affecting the nervous system or other systems such as the immune system. Any imbalance of this trio of doshas can cause body-mind dysfunction that ayurveda recognizes as vikruti.

VIKRUTI: ALTERED FUNCTIONS

Vata Vikruti

An overabundance of vata may result in excess skin and hair dryness, cracking joints, and a dry colon. People with too much vata may become mentally and physically too mobile, thus creating a state of worry, anxiety, and overwhelming tiredness, leading to a kind of depression triggered by depletion.

Added aggravation of vata can lead to mood swings, indecisiveness, and impulsive actions. The main symptoms include tics, tremors, insomnia, and/or incessant talking. Aggravation of vata also causes stuttering or harsh speech, dryness of both hair and skin, body aches, debility, and desire for warm objects and substances.

A decrease in vata manifests principally in symptoms of body debility, including loss of physical ability, speech, awareness, and consciousness.

Imbalances in vata-predominant people tend to manifest as constipation as well as neurological, muscular, and rheumatic problems.[8]

Altered Fiery (Pitta Vikruti) Functions

The most applicable manifestations are poor digestion, cold and clammy feet, and changes in the complexion and radiance of the skin. Decreased pitta also manifests in bitter and sour tastes; fainting attacks; debility; inflammation/exudation, or pus formation; increased yellow coloration of the skin, eyes, urine, and feces; and excessive hunger and thirst. It may cause acid indigestion, loose stools, ulcers, hot rashes, fevers, insomnia, and a tendency toward hypertension.

Pitta-predominant people love knowledge and are excellent at organization and leadership. In general, they are instinctive, gifted people and perfectionistic, so they can also be controlling and domineering with a tendency toward comparison, competition, and ambition. The aggravation of pitta can make them aggressive and hypercritical.

In term of ailments, pitta people tend to show imbalance in the form of inflammatory diseases.

Altered Earthy (Kapha Vikruti) Functions

Kapha dosha is the slowest and steadiest of the three doshas. Its oily quality allows for smooth joint function, but if prominent, it can lead to excess fluidity or indisposition. Coolness, moisture, inactivity, and/or consumption of heavy food can push the kapha constitution into a state of imbalance.

Aggravation of kapha causes imbalances that can result in obesity, bad habits, persistent consumption of a wrong diet, lethargy, complacency, and depression rooted in past emotional issues.

YOUR VIKRUTI
Body Imbalance

The vikruti evaluation (see pages 277–81) will assess any imbalance of your three doshas based on your prakruti evaluation taken previously. It will help you better understand the concept of vikruti. When addressing the body imbalance revealed by the results of the vikruti evaluation, it is important to start by readjusting the dosha that is most out of balance at the moment. The way to establish which dosha is most out of balance is to define which dosha-relevant qualities are provoking in you the most varied effects.

An imbalance in your primary dosha is usually the easiest doshic imbalance to rectify. You can be imbalanced in any one of the three doshas, but it is most likely that the imbalance starts in your primary dosha. Let me present you some very short hypothetical examples of how people with a codominant dosha constitution can address dosha imbalances:

▼ A vata-kapha person may emphasize balancing vata during periods of travel or when feeling anxious but should shift to balancing kapha when feeling unenthusiastic, sleepy, or sluggish, or if putting on some weight.

▼ A pitta-vata person should pay attention to pitta when feeling angry, hot, irritated, or harsh toward other people. On days when this person feels jumpy, anxious, nervous, or less grounded, it will be important to focus on balancing vata dosha.

▼ A kapha-pitta person could focus on kapha foods to reduce body weight and boost vitality, but if the person is manifesting mostly aggressive or irritable feelings, then the focus must be on balancing pitta.

For everyday life, remember that we all have three doshas within us, so even our least dominant dosha can manifest in an abruptly excessive way depending on various internal or external conditions such as overeating, oversleeping, or excessive worrying. When you are approaching a treatment, it is important to take into consideration the dominant dosha in parallel with the reestablishment of agni and a proper kapha-pacifying diet.[9]

Vikruti, or your current state of imbalance, can mask your prakruti. Recall the case of Mark. This is a typical example of how vikruti can mask our prakruti. He had a vata-pitta prakruti, but due to his lifestyle he was exhibiting a kapha-vata vikruti (as his current state of imbalance), at the time of his first consultation with me. The role of ayurveda was to bring him back to a state of balance where his pitta dosha was back and active.

As a scientist, and on a personal experiential level, I observe our bodies under a sort of overarching plan that is "predetermined," a plan of dynamic systems that are highly sensitive to initial conditions that always invite us to a state of balance, despite the external forces and outside pressures in the world that can push us toward chaos. Yes, there is chaos in today's world and in ourselves, but consider for a moment that chaos need not be random, that, in fact, chaos sits somewhere on the spectrum of randomness and predictability. If for whatever reason we break or disconnect from nature's plan, we stop living in harmony with our systems, thus triggering body-mind imbalances and creating "new altered systems" within ourselves. It will be a new chaos, and the energy of the new chaos will have its specifics. Chaos in order is cellular intelligence, and illness is disarray or disorder of it. For that reason, in ayurveda, health is considered as the arrangement or order of energies, elements, rhythm of life, despite that chaos is inherent in all compounded things, and the theory of the three basic doshas provides the relation between the microcosm (the cell) and macrocosm (the body), which can be applied to physiological and pathological states. Modern science observes that even chaos has to respond to laws; some modern chaos theories state that within the seeming randomness of chaotic complex systems, there are basal patterns, interconnection, endless feedback loops, replication, duplication, and self-organization.

The following condensed case studies of patients with a dual main constitution, or dual doshas, are intended to give you an idea of how ayurveda addresses their conditions in cases of body-mind imbalances. If you would like to go deeper with respect to this analysis, take into consideration the qualities (gunas) of both doshas in terms of how much they could complement each other or, on the other hand, their potential antagonism.

The short ayurvedic diagnosis (*trividha pariksha*) is described here. In all cases it involves:

1. *Darshana:* visual observation of the patient including eyes, skin, hair, behavior, and so forth
2. *Sparshana*: a physical checkup using touch in which the ayurvedic professional checks the pulse, palpation, percussion, and auscultation
3. *Prashna:* Q&A concerning medical history, symptoms, lifestyle, and other relevant aspects, whether preexisting or related to the particular health issue being addressed.

CASE STUDY

Kapha-Vata (Earthy/Breezy) Dual Constitution

Sarah was forty-eight years old, ate a normal diet, didn't smoke or drink, and had body weight issues.

Main complaints: *Sarah's issues included fatigue, muscular and knee pain, and a BMI of 29.8, indicating borderline obesity. Her past history showed an absence of hypothyroidism, hypertension, and diabetes mellitus but a family history of overweight and obesity on both the paternal and maternal sides—her family were termed as "good gourmands." After working hard to maintain a normal weight* all her life, she adopted a sedentary lifestyle: she got little exercise, took daily naps, and ate an excess of sweet and oily foods at the wrong times of day for food intake. This had been going on for six years, as a result of her depression due to her divorce and other family issues.

Ayurvedic diagnosis: *K-V obesity affecting circulatory, muscular, and adipose tissues.*

Recommendations: *I encouraged Sarah to improve her irregular and improper dietary habits, abstain from daily naps, and integrate daily yoga, breathing exercises (pranayama), meditation, and other relaxation techniques. I advised her to take specific oral medication tailored for her K-V body-mind constitution, with bimonthly follow-ups.*

Outcomes: *Sarah rapidly learnt to enjoy the daily integration of a K-V diet and previously absent dietary tastes (in her case, bitter and pungent flavors), and to respect food intake times and forego snacks. She lost twenty-two pounds in a period of less than eight months and saw a significant decrease in her pain. Equally important, she experienced improved motivation to live a dynamic life, participated in more activities, and saw continued steady weight loss.*

CASE STUDY
Vata-Kapha (Breezy/Earthy) Dual Constitution

Hope was a sixty-one-year-old nonsmoker, drank socially, and ate a normal diet.

Main complaints: *She had a BMI of 31, along with walking difficulties, severe joint pain, swelling and tenderness in the joints due to rheumatoid arthritis (RA), breathing exertion, weak digestion, stress-related sleep troubles, and phases of constipation. She described her complaints as the result of lack of her small body frame's inability to manage her heaviness. There was no significant relevant family history.*

Ayurvedic diagnosis: *V-K obesity affecting her mobility, fat tissue, and mental state.*

Recommendations: *Two main lines of action were implemented in order to restore her body-mind balance: First, lifestyle changes including a proper tailored*

V-K diet, alcohol reduction, use of spices and ayurvedic herbs for her constitution and rheumatoid arthritis, and bimonthly follow-ups. And second, craniosacral therapy, lymphatic drainage, yoga asanas, vata body oleation (application of oils), breathing exercises (pranayama), and relaxation and meditation protocols.

Outcomes: *After a period of around one year, the results of the integrative therapy were very encouraging. Following an initial challenging period of adaptation, she started feeling the ignition of her metabolic fire, and enjoyed a better-quality sleep as a result of changing her food intake quantity, quality, and times. She now always ate her main meal at midday and later had a small, quality dinner, to reduce ama.*

Her lifestyle changes had a positive impact. She saw a drop in her stress levels and musculoskeletal pain, and she had better lung and evacuation functions, flexibility, and general movement.

Final recommendations: *I advised her to remain on a V-K diet and to incorporate a regimen of yoga, craniosacral therapy, pranayama, and gentle exercise. She was encouraged to pursue an ayurvedic detox program or panchakarma (see pages 252–54) involving oleation, sudation (inducing sweat), and purgation (inducing vomiting), to support her RA (amavata) and obesity-related disorders, to keep them at bay.*

CASE STUDY
Kapha-Pitta (Earthy/Fiery) Dual Constitution

At the time he requested a consultation, Paul was a fifty-five-year-old man who was single, a social drinker, and an ex-smoker of five years. He had a strong appetite, slow digestion, and a tendency toward overeating.

Main complaints: *Paul had been recently diagnosed as borderline diabetic. He had asthma (swasa) and had seen a continuous body weight increase for the past two years due to long hours spent driving to work. His daily diet consisted mainly of heavy takeout foods.*

Ayurvedic evaluation and diagnosis: *K-P obesity with enlarged abdominal fat tissue affecting mobility, and creating fatigue, shortness of breath when exercising, and loss of self-confidence. Assessment showed a BMI of 32.5, also indicating obesity.*

Recommendations: *Kapha people have an increased insulin response to carbohydrates, which sets up their metabolic reactions for fat storage, rather than fat burning for bodily functions. As a result, a complete change of lifestyle based on a wholesome kapha diet, specific to his primary dosha, and a diet of mainly home cooking was recommended to reduce kapha imbalance, a major causal factor of his weight gain. An evaluation was conducted of his food intake quantities, which led to recommended dietary modifications. I also advised him to change his work location so he could use the time previously spent commuting for badly needed activities such as physical exercise, yoga, breathing, relaxation, and meditation drills. I also encouraged him to take ayurvedic herbs to support and stabilize kapha. Treatment for his borderline diabetes needed to be coordinated with his main physician. Once his kapha was relatively stable, his pitta digestive fire could then be supported by a healthy pitta-kapha diet and pitta ayurvedic medication. A detox program was also badly needed.*

Outcomes: *I worked in a team with his main physician and with Paul himself, who was fueled by his motivation for radical change. His glucose levels normalized after a period of five months, and he gradually reduced his BMI to 27 over the course of one year. He moved to a location closer to his work, became physically active to help control his asthma through regular swimming, and took better care of his state of mind.*

Being conscious and proactive about our weight imbalance can transform our genetic expression—as the science of epigenetics shows us—and can even redress our inherited metabolic programming. We must keep our eyes wide open and trust in our inner selves.

VIKRUTI EVALUATION

The vikruti evaluation (see pages 277–81) will support you in better understanding your present body weight imbalances, their potential connection to incorrect food intake habits, and the possible role of your mind's relation to these habits. In the same way, by understanding the reasons for your own body's changes, you will better appreciate the reasons for changes in people close to you and understand why others react the way they do as a result of their own imbalances.[10] This knowledge is an important instrument that can help you identify and work on diverse aspects of your personal relationships as well as addressing your body weight. As being overweight or obese are not "balanced" conditions, we expect the vikruti evaluation to yield results that align with the factors needing to be addressed through ayurvedic treatments for weight management.

As with the prakruti evaluation, the vikruti evaluation will not be 100 percent accurate, but it will provide you with a basis for understanding which doshas are most misaligned with your nature.

After your vikruti evaluation, I will introduce you to the set of tools ayurveda offers to regain your body-mind balance. I hope the evaluation of your constitution and imbalances will be the starting point in your journey toward understanding your situation through a more holistic framework so you may work toward good health and rebalance your body weight.

Since this vikruti evaluation is not intended to provide a static profile, I suggest you repeat it at least once. The first time should be based on a long period of your recent life, such as two or three years, and the second time should be based on how you've been feeling over the last two or three months. Then, calculate both scores. This will help you understand whether recent life changes or challenges are reflected in the levels of your doshas—and you can also be a witness to your own gradual shift toward rebalancing. I encourage you to come back to the vikruti evaluation from time to time, as life conditions change for you.

8

MANAS PRAKRUTI

···

Foundations of a Healthy Brain-Body

MENTAL CONSTITUTION (MANAS PRAKRUTI) AND BODY-MIND IMBALANCE (MANAS VIKRUTI)

According to ayurveda, good health is a balance between body, mind, spirit, and social well-being. The best possible manner to understand mental constitution (*manas prakruti*) within ayurveda's definition of balanced health requires an analysis of the following:

▾ 3-D: the three body constitutions/doshas (vata, pitta, kapha)
▾ digestive fire (agni)
▾ body tissues (seven dhatus)
▾ secretions (feces, urine, sweat)
▾ physical and mental activities

and

▾ clarity of perception (senses and ability to focus)
▾ mental purity and integrity
▾ a happy, gratified soul

All factors are directly linked to the exchanges between the 3-D and the triguna—that is, between the tridosha (vata-pitta-kapha) and sattva-rajas-tamas—since our mental constitution follows from our DNA.

When there is an imbalance between energy in (food intake) and energy out (consuming of calories), weight goes up or down. By eating more than you burn, you increase weight—at times straightaway. It is a consistent observation from my professional practice: a large percentage of my clients who are overweight or obese have in common bad dietary habits and a high intake of unwholesome foods.

If you are dealing with obesity or other body weight issues, the material in this chapter and some material from my previous book will explain which foods may be contributing to your weight issues and stopping you from making progress.[1]

Ayurveda offers this very simple and straightforward advice: Eat the right foods, in the right quantities, at the right times and places, and with the right attitude. Nature will take care of everything else. If you follow this simple advice, you may take a giant leap forward in addressing your body weight imbalance. It sounds easy to say this, but perhaps you feel it is hard to put it into practice and change habits. Well, habits are most probably what got us here, and we need to change direction to restore balance. Addressing obesity through diet and lifestyle changes in a planned, methodical way is just like many things in life: it's more achievable when done step by step and not rushed. Change takes time.

It is appropriate here to describe the ayurvedic understanding of nourishment and digestion:

> The world around us is digested by our five senses; ideas are digested by the mind and intellect; the body digests feelings and wholesome foods. Nourishment—the process of extracting information and energy from our environment to make it available to our body-mind physiology—is received and perceived via our five senses, as well as through our minds and emotions (Ca. Su. 8/13, 8/15; Ca. Su. 11/11, 11/25, 7/60).

You can appreciate that the ayurvedic perception goes further than just biochemical description of digestive metabolic processes, to address other subtle energies via the science of energetics. The ayurvedic view involves our feelings as well as our environment—conditions that all of us experience when ingesting food, even though we are often unaware of them.

BRAIN-BODY CONNECTIONS

Manas prakruti is the triguna manifesting in the form of mental or psychic constitutions. Ayurveda uses the triguna to help us understand the various types of psyches and the potential imbalances of the mind that could manifest as disorders of our physical body, from states of anorexia to obesity, all associated with various types of mental imbalances.

Vedic philosophy categorizes human personalities one step further by examining the psychological and moral temperaments in relation to the triguna:

▾ sattvic: truth/purity mental constitution
▾ rajasic: action/movement mental constitution
▾ tamasic: inertia/heaviness mental constitution

Manas prakruti is part of your DNA; at fecundation, the fertilized zygote carries the combination of both parents' prakruti. According to ayurveda, the zygote also carries sattva from the universal or cosmic mind, as well as variations of the other two qualities, rajas and tamas, from the parents' minds. These qualities thus create the individual mind, which becomes manas prakruti or mental constitution.[2]

In ayurveda, the infinite mind maintains qualitative and quantitative equilibrium of sattva, rajas, and tamas as part of the laws of order of the universe. The classic texts describe how cosmic tamas creates darkness, cosmic rajas creates the movement of the Earth, and cosmic sattva creates the rising of the sun. In conformity with the laws of destiny (karma), at the time of conception, a particular blend of the three gunas arises in the consciousness of the fertilized ovum. The description of those processes varies across different philosophical schools—for the Samkhya philosophy, the mind is derived from the pure essence of sattva, but without rajas and tamas, the mind cannot function.[3]

These individual variances in psychological natures, and their responses to physical and sociocultural environments, are very well explained in the classical texts of ayurveda as principles in nature that govern the mind and emotions. The three gunas are essential drivers of the mind that differentiate individuals on the basis of their psychological constitutions. Ayurveda sees imbalances related to body-mind biological interactions and transformational energies as being the result of innumerable biochemical reactions. The totality of the triguna is defined as consciousness, rather than spirit or soul, because we are exploring our awareness of our surroundings. Modern science has demonstrated the existence of higher cosmic energies, putting this matter to rest—and even early scientific experiments concluded that the field previously called ether does exist, as per the studies conducted by the European Organization for Nuclear Research (CERN) using the Large Hadron Collider.[4, 5]

Ayurvedic scholars say that everyone is connected through an enigmatic net, or field, that bridges time and space through consciousness. Ayurveda integrated these concepts of consciousness thousands of years ago, visualizing our whole body as a tool that works only with the application of force or energy, and conceiving consciousness as a higher cosmic energy. Similarly, higher consciousness is vital for the body to work, and even though we don't see it, it is there.

Body balance is maintained by a cellular consciousness that keeps the human organism healthy. In other words, your body, composed of forty trillion cells and approximately two hundred different cell types, has a plan that requires functional harmony. If that harmony is somehow disturbed by lack of care or awareness of your real basic needs, proper body-mind functioning is not possible, and conditions such as obesity can manifest. Higher consciousness is that potential part of humankind that is capable of transcending animal instincts. To some extent, we can say that in a natural way, all of us have a regular material—or lower—consciousness, but a higher consciousness also exists.

Ayurvedic scholars subclassified manas prakruti into sixteen subtypes: seven for sattva, six for rajas, and three for tamas. For our purposes we are only covering the three main classifications. "The soul is essentially devoid of all deformities The soul is the cause of consciousness through the mind and the specific qualities of the basic elements (touch, shape, smell, taste, and sound). He is eternal. He is an observer. He observes all activities" (Ca. Su. 1/56).

AYURVEDIC TYPES OF MENTAL CONSTITUTIONS

The three kinds of psyches are explained as born from virtue, anger, and delusion, and are thought to be superior, medium, and inferior, respectively. The principal qualities of the three mental constitutions are explained as follows:

Sattva

components: truth, purity, understanding, balance, harmony, positive attitude

constitutions: constructive, righteous, peaceful, compassionate, loving, good

Rajas

components: alertness, dynamism, drive, overactive mind, overconfidence, irritability

constitutions: competitive, passionate, controlling, individualist, self-centered

Tamas

components: inertia, ignorance, imbalance, distorted mind, skepticism

constitutions: lazy, inactive, ignorant, disordered, reckless, selfish

Ayurveda's understanding of the perpetual interplay among these three qualities in the individual consciousness explains that the relative prevalence of either sattva, rajas, or tamas is accountable for distinct psychological constitutions being part of our genetic code.[6] Let me give you an illustration of each of the variances in psychological dispositions for the three main kinds of expressions.

According to ayurveda, we cannot be only sattvic, only rajasic, or only tamasic. Our nature and behavior are the result of a complex interplay among all three, fluctuating to varying degrees. In some, the disposition is rajasic with a significant influence of sattvic guna; in others it is rajasic with a significant influence of tamasic guna. For example, the rajasic manifestation of feelings of safety is dependent on external influences, particularly the attention of others. The reaction of the rajasic mind will be self-protection by assuming rajasic activities, like ambition and self-serving endeavors. In our younger years, we realize that through accomplishment and acknowledgment from others, it is possible to feel safe. Thus, the initial sattvic experience of a full heart and a free mind is substituted by the drive toward sensory stimulation of different kinds. The reality is that we are stuck in the material world of rajas and tamas. Yet we can find relief from tamas and rajas by self-monitoring our problematic states, such as lethargy, agitation, desire, and temptation.

As a result of becoming satisfied through rajasic activities and drive, our minds can burn out, and by gathering transient gratifications through the senses, we retreat into safe, protective cocoons. If people with a rajasic constitution stay on that path, they can become lonely, bitter, and angry, and eventually may seek indulgence in food, drugs, alcohol, or other dependencies, trying to keep the illusion of the safe cocoon, manifesting a tamasic constitution. Once we exist in that state of inertia and dependency, it becomes difficult to leave, and doing so demands the cultivation of sattva qualities to offer a hint of the lost experience of truth, joy, and happiness. It also requires the renewal of rajas to provide the necessary energy so we can make adjustments and take the proper actions.

Let me illustrate some examples of the three mental or psychic constitutions described in ayurveda as sattva, rajas, and tamas based on patients I have gotten to know quite well.

CASE STUDY
Sattvic Mental Constitution

Serena is a seventy-five-year-old woman, mother of four children, ayurvedic learner, with a vata prakruti. Each prakruti has its virtues and limitations. In

Serena's case, by understanding and accepting the "downsides" of her vata-predominant constitution (such as erratic or fluctuating mind, constipation, and eventual abdominal ballooning), her life became a continual search for awareness and connection to her name: serene. By taking good care of the challenging characteristics of her vata prakruti and accepting her age and limits in a dignified way, she was the example of a caring, humble, joyful, and compassionate person.

This is what ayurveda calls a knowledgeable, spiritual, sattvic mental constitution.

CASE STUDY
Rajasic Mental Constitution

Anna, a fifty-year-old woman, single, educator, with a pitta-kapha prakruti came to me with concerns about her obesity. She described how much she enjoyed her very active professional life and social position. Her body weight was a physical concern for her, but not a big mental issue. Anna was always a perfectionist in her work life, a busy person working very hard and in a competitive way, but remaining friendly, patient and loving to her staff and the people who helped her. She was a very kind person not necessarily open or connected to her potential inner awareness.

This is an example of the rajasic ayurvedic mental constitution, full of movement and activity.

CASE STUDY
Tamasic Mental Constitution

Javier, a fifty-seven-year-old man, father of two children, professionally active and with a strong pitta-vata prakruti is an example of what ayurveda calls a tamasic mental constitution based on heaviness and inertia. He was somebody very focused on himself, with a strong avidity to garner and accumulate possessions and he would describe his professional governmental job as an excellent opportunity to make the minimum of effort, and with as little as possible responsibility. He spoke openly about being unkind to others and becoming aggressive at the level of being able to harm people if they were affecting his interests. You can appreciate in this case the heaviness and level of inertia of a tamasic mental or psychic nature.

APPLYING THE AYURVEDIC MASTERY OF FOOD AND DIET TO YOUR OBESITY

The triguna can be perceived in everyday life. They are in constant interplay within us, affecting our lives, and their expressions are responsible for individual psychological constitutions. Let me describe them here:

Sattvic Prakruti (Purity/Knowledge)

physical/mental: active, very strong body-mind relation in all aspects of life

intellect: creative, intelligent, humble, respectful

emotional: happy, joyful, aware, alert, and fresh, doesn't get angry or upset easily

spiritual: intuitive, humanitarian, caring for all kinds of life

Rajasic Prakruti (Activity/Movement)

physical/mental: perfectionistic; enjoys power, control, and prestige; egoistic; proud; tends toward having a life of sensual enjoyment and pleasure, while avoiding pain

intellect: hardworking, active, restless, competitive, doesn't plan or have a clear direction

emotional: jealous and ambitious, leading to stress and fear of failure

spiritual: loving, friendly, faithful, unsure of inner awareness, calm when supported

Tamasic Prakruti (Inertia/Heaviness)

physical/mental: thoughts tend to focus on themselves and their possessions

intellect: short attention span, enjoys work with low obligations, feels tired quickly

emotional: greedy, selfish, attached, irritable; a gourmand who drinks, sleeps, and has sex

spiritual: careless, able to harm others in self-interest; tends toward laziness, lethargy, and oversleeping, even during the day

This newly acquired information allows ayurveda to invite you to live differently: you are now in search of awareness. Try not to give any color to that awareness; just be a witness of your observations by neutrally accepting the process. Years of accumulated scientific data suggest that what you eat is not only critical for your body composition, metabolic health, and performance but is equally significant for its effects on mood and mental well-being. Let me tell you, though, it is not easy to change your ways, and it takes practice to avoid letting your feelings interfere with your reflective processing.

After completing the first two evaluations in appendix 1, you should now have a clear idea of the way your body-mind functions—firstly in terms of prakruti, which reveals your predominant dosha; secondly, as relating to vikruti or dosha imbalances, which have various potential causes that you can see. Finally, you will be completing the manas prakruti evaluation, which will help you to perceive transitory mental conditions potentially associated with obesity.

MANAS PRAKRUTI EVALUATION

Just as you were able to assess and recognize your prakruti type and evaluate potential imbalances by using the vikruti constitution evaluation, we can similarly assess and comprehend the state of balance of the mental constitution by evaluating our manas prakruti (see pages 282–87). Try to express your true feelings as you answer the questions. What matters is to capture your real nature, instead of what you would like it to be.

An imbalanced mental constitution can change very rapidly, even over a short period of time. Some days, a person may have a more sattva mindset after hearing or viewing an uplifting talk; a few days later, the same person could be more rajasic due to a frantic working day. An individual born with a primarily rajasic or tamasic quality can make their mental prakruti more sattvic by practicing meditation, yoga, and noncompetitive exercise activities, as well as receiving proper guidance. So, in repeating the manas prakruti evaluation over time, do not be alarmed if your profile changes from previous attempts. In fact, this is to be expected as we never stay in the same, constant mental state.

Keep in mind the triguna is continuously changing; thus, the evaluation is not intended to provide a static assessment. The reason for being aware of the three gunas' qualities is to attain greater understanding of your tendencies or state of mind in the moment. This will help open your eyes to your protective patterns of behavior originating from external influences at various stages of your life, which created strong and lasting impressions.

MANAS PRAKRUTI CALCULATION

The goal of studying these three mental types is to offer a greater sense of self-awareness regarding your mental state, by observing potential recurrent protective lifestyle patterns such as a passive life, food cravings, sleeping patterns, and other areas that could be affecting your body balance. Through this understanding, you can develop strategies to address your body weight imbalance.

- ▾ A sattvic nature is deep in contentment and truth, free of continuous desire.
- ▾ A rajasic mind is active and needs stimulation, usually through the senses, to be satisfied.
- ▾ A tamasic type is more vulnerable due to their lethargic tendency and the likelihood of being under the influence of inertia.

Most people fit in the middle or the rajasic area, which is the main state in our active and outgoing modern culture. But if your tendency is more toward a tamasic state of mind, please do not judge yourself; it could be just a phase, and the important part of this exercise is having awareness of your path and learning how to readjust your lifestyle.

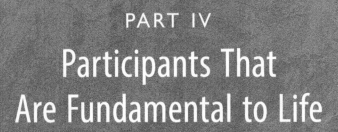

PART IV

Participants That Are Fundamental to Life

The Unfolding Language of Our Gut

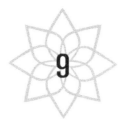

YOUR GUT AND BODY REGULATIONS

An Ayurvedic View

I feel the need to put things into a wider context before addressing this new section about our gut. In other words, I wish to put our house in order, as this is about our inner world: the gut. Today we believe that we are the sovereign leaders of our planet Earth, but in fact our planet is home to more than three trillion trees that belong to over 60,000 species. While they may seem extremely vulnerable to environmental changes, since trees cannot get up and leave when the climate no longer suits them, trees have been around for about 400 million years and have survived many battles with extinction threats. Trees can break down rocks, create soil, siphon carbon dioxide from the air, and exchange it for oxygen, making our planet habitable for us. Despite their apparent immobility, they also have a vascular network of communicating, interconnecting tissues and organs for transporting water, minerals, nutrients, and diverse signaling molecules throughout the plant body. Trees only need sunlight and water to produce their own supply of food and can live for thousands of years growing slowly taller and wider. And while to some of us they look like solitary individuals competing for access to sunlight with their neighbors, in fact if we look deeper, to the roots, instead of staring at the top and getting distracted by squirrels, birds, and other inhabitants of the forest, we can see that right under our feet, trees are sharing resources, passing on warnings, and handing down information over generations. They are a network of talking trees, thanks to the underground forest of fungi; both forest trees and fungi are engaged in a continuous and active exchange.

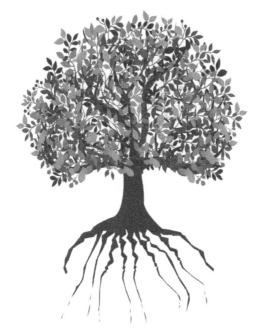

Fig. 9.1. Root and Branch: The Unseen and Seen

For that reason, let me tell you a bit more about the external forest before we address our own body forest. Ayurvedic scholars understood the interconnection of all organisms in nature, in the same way that, in 1885, the botanist Albert B. Frank proposed that plant roots and the fungi around them were functioning together. Due to the lack of scientific evidence in those days, he was held up to ridicule, only to finally be recognized as correct in this past century.[1]

We now know more about the specialized mutualism or symbiotic associations between the roots of plants and fungi, called mycorrhizal associations. Fungi collect water and nutrients from the soil, including phosphorus and nitrogen—both of which are vital for plant growth—and transfer them to their plant hosts. In exchange, the plants transfer to the fungi part of their photosynthetic labor: their sugars produced by photosynthesis. This association is the pillar of all our plants on Earth, and without it, life on Earth as we know it may have never occurred. Imagine how contaminated water plays a role in damaging this association.

In the early 1980s, scientists realized that not only do individual trees and fungi have a symbiotic relationship when it comes to reciprocating their resources, but the trees themselves also associate via this intricate, vast network, "talking" and cooperating by sharing resources. The studies showed that two different species are able to share nitrogen and other resources in both directions, depending on the season and conditions. The two species exist in an alternate feedback system, helping when the other needs it, which allows them both to remain healthy. There is also evidence that trees of the same species experience some form of recognition of their "relatives" through their fungal networks. They can identify which trees are most closely related to them and direct more supplies toward those trees.[2, 3]

So, trees are not solitary individuals but live in a cooperative harmony with one another, challenging the prevailing theory that cooperation is less important than competition in evolution. It might seem like the law of natural selection would cause trees to only compete for resources, but their cooperation is not purely selfless. If adjacent trees die, spaces open up in the protective forest canopy, allowing penetration of more sunlight, and the remaining trees can carry out more photosynthesis. Yet they are also more vulnerable: Hotter sunlight spreads along the forest floor, warming up and dehydrating the cool, damp, uniformly controlled microclimate that forest trees need. The forest becomes more accessible to breezes, and, deprived of nearby tree crowns to help stabilize conditions, the possibility of being uprooted rises. Therefore they have evolved to help neighboring trees live longer and reproduce more often in a health-giving, steady forest. If we can understand this network and embrace its philosophy of surviving and thriving under optimal conditions, we can minimize some of the worst impacts we humans have on the planet.

We see how, on our planet, mutualism is an essential part of many organisms' biology: the partnership between soil fungi and land-living plants, bees gathering nectar from flowers, the spider crab and its tenant algae, the corals and photosynthetic algae, and the sea anemones and clownfish. As it is with trees, so it is within us.

Now, let us move on to our reality as humans. As a result of our Western cultural beliefs we think that our lives do not depend on anybody, perhaps based on our past as nomads and hunters in the forests and on the plains. However, we moving beings also have that very common dependence that trees experience daily. We depend on and benefit from the sources and powers of our environment, such as good quality food from the earth, water, sunlight, and air, the four elements contained in the space (panchamahabhutas). And when we live in harmony with the Earth, both the Earth and its species prosper.

Furthermore, there is another world living within ourselves that we cannot see, which is also composed of the same five elements, a world of microorganisms that we host in our bodies. These microorganisms, mostly located in our gut, are the real essence of our lives: our intestinal flora. We live in continuous interdependency, mutualism, or symbiosis with them.

We need to learn to love and honor who we are and who they are, by actively searching for harmony within ourselves, such that we can be aware of this inner/outer universal nature and properly appreciate and respect it.

Nature reminds us that we are more than the physical body we see in the mirror, that we are whole and connected.

YOUR GUT
Body Regulations and the Role of Ayurveda

Ayurveda possesses practical wisdom in its approach to body weight imbalance, and it offers corrective protocols to restore us to a healthy state. The question is: was ayurveda able to understand these processes thousands of years ago and recommend tailored lifestyles to keep people balanced despite the lack of today's sophisticated technologies? I would like to ask you another question. Please keep it in the back of your mind as you read the following sections: Are we just habits? What—or who—within us controls them? I will be focusing on these deep questions because I believe ayurveda can provide the answers, and these answers are linked to our intestinal flora.

This section connects various themes from previous parts of this book. It is intended to give you a well-rounded ayurvedic vision, together with scientific information, to understand what is really going on in our body-mind-consciousness processes, so we can address body weight imbalances effectively through ayurveda. For ayurveda, the main issue of our biological body or mind imbalances is the direct connection with agni, our digestive fire that allows us to digest and integrate food components and their energetic powers, as well as to eliminate waste products. Do we understand how these processes occur in our constitutional bodies and how they can affect the structural balance of our body shape? Is it a one-person job? Are these processes connected to our intestinal flora? Do we know what inputs are required for our bodily processes to function properly, based on our individual constitutions? Do you feel resonance with these questions, or are they present only when there is an imbalance expressed as a problem like stomach pain, cramps, or organ failure? We are unaware of what happens beneath the surface; our tendency is to assume everything is fine until an imbalance manifests as illness. Even then, we are prone to blame external conditions: "That food was off," "it's due to the cold climate," "I'm under stress," and so on. Perhaps we even try to "sort out" the issue with a quick fix using pharmaceutical drugs.

Science tells us that more than one billion years ago, the first multicellular microbes were formed from unicellular ones. The bacteria, viruses, and phages present in our bodies and highly concentrated in our intestines are invisible to the naked eye; we cannot see them unaided, and it was only between 1665 and 1683 that we became aware of their likely existence.[4] The first scientific proof that our microbes are part of our natural human system appeared around the end of nineteenth century via the observation of a bacteria present in the intestinal flora (subsequently named *Escherichia coli*) and the Tobacco mosaic virus discovered in 1892.[5]

Medics in countries like India and China have understood gut function for thousands of years. It is only recently, through the combination of integrative and functional fields with conventional medicine, that we've been given a modern scientific interpretation of this ancient knowledge, creating a major shift in the comprehension of our body framework and metabolic imbalances. This knowledge is contributing to a recognition and deeper interpretation of the role of our intestinal flora, now fashionably called the microbiome. You probably did not hear of the microbiome being widely discussed fifteen years ago. Although the microbiome has been known to Western medicine for more than 300 years, it only reached prominence as a "health phenomenon" in recent years when gradually we discovered its vital importance to our well-being, mobilizing scientists to engage in the state-of-the-art research of novel gene sequencing, which has given us greater awareness of the role of the microbiome in our gut.[6]

MICROBES (KRIMI) AND OBESITY

Ayurveda is a manifestation of our own nature, balanced or imbalanced, and of the nature around us. This manifestation's aim is to restore balance, and a large part of achieving that is how ayurveda perceives and utilizes *krimi*—our microbiome. We humans, like plants, also depend on beneficial bacteria to survive, and our gut flora have a selfish interest in overcoming innumerable obstacles to keep us alive. This discrete ecological relationship established between the host and the microbiome is now termed as the *holobiont*.[7]

The microbiomes of the human gut and of plants control significantly more than just species survival. Microorganisms support and regulate plant and human beings' physiology, including digestion, biochemistry, immunity, growth, and even our psychological conduct—and, up to a certain level, plant behavior too. Today a growing arena of research known as psychobiotics is taking shape. It refers to the ingestion of live bacteria in suitable quantities to potentially provide a mental advantage by affecting the gut microbiome of the host system. The role that bacteria play in the gut-brain axis is now being actively researched to understand the key pathway associations, with psychobiotics being used to produce a gut-brain-body response at the levels of the digestive nervous system, immune system, and vagus nerve.[8, 9, 10]

Ancient Jain scriptures dating from 600 BCE questioned the existence of unseen microbial life.[11] During the Vedic period (ca. 1500–ca. 500 BCE), ayurvedic experts (*acharyas*) passed down what they understood through memorization from a regular oral practice, and then by writing down their knowledge, even mentioning the term *krimi* in the *Atharva Veda*.

(A. V. 5/23/3; A. V. 2/31/4; A. V. 4/20/9). Further reports by scholars such as Charaka and Sushruta described the classification, causes, symptoms, and treatment of krimi. The *Charaka Samhita* gives recommendations about how to keep quarantine at home in case of epidemics and indicates that they arise as a consequence of anomalous settings in nature, such as the planets and stars disturbing the nature of the seasons and elements.

Conceptually, these scholars theorized that everything existing in the world and universe is composed of our five elements (panchamahabhutas). They believed that the disruption of four factors including air, water, region, and time, alongside a troubled mind ("loss of integrity"), would aggravate vata dosha and potentially cause an epidemic. The ancient Ayurvedic scholars understood that a pure heart and mind (sattva mind) would resonate with the forming power of the cosmos. An imbalanced mind and heart absent of virtue would intrude and disturb the very delicate rhythms of nature that are crucial for our survival. Due to the developing research on epigenetics, the microbiome gut-brain connection, and our emission of photons of light, there is support for the view that our beliefs and feelings are powerful enough to resonate through nature's interconnections, provoking either a consistent or a dissonant result.[12]

What is the meaning of all this? Well, the ancient term *krimi* in the ayurvedic literature refers to all microorganisms such as bacteria, viruses, protozoa, and helminths; and the term *krimirogas* means diseases caused by pathogenic microorganisms.[13] Yet today, there is still some difficulty in correlating the term *krimi* with mainstream understanding, because of a scarcity of detailed description of individual krimi. In plain words, we could say that the term *krimi* broadly represents all microorganisms, which from the viewpoint of modern science include our concept of the microbiome. What is remarkable is how ayurveda also incorporates the idea and function of dietary fiber. Somehow, through visual observation of the presence of fiber in their feces, and by trial and error—since they lacked the ability to characterize it using technology—they understood that fiber is the part of plant-based foods (vegetables, fruits, grains/nuts, and beans) that the body is unable to break down and digest, since we don't have the proper enzymes to do it. They observed that fiber passes through the body undigested, keeping the digestive tract clean and healthy, facilitating bowel motion, and cleansing undigested food and harmful components from the body. On that basis, we can understand the great importance they gave to types of foods and their functions in preventive and curative protocols. They inferred that of all the different major nutrient groups that we eat, fiber is the component of our diet that directly feeds our microbiota. Let me present to you in more detail their profound microbiological knowledge, even more impressive considering the lack of modern biomedical technology available at the time.

Classifications of Krimi

Ayurvedic scholars described more than twenty types of krimi, including our congenital microbiome called *sahaja*. Ayurveda holds that sahaja is part of our biological nature at the time of birth, and that most of its components are friendly—they do not cause any diseases, and they have an important functional role for keeping the body in a state of balance.[14] Krimi were classified in two groups: *bahya* (external) and *abhyantara* (internal), with further subclassifications.

Within the abhyantara or internal group, ayurvedic texts described the various subtypes of internal microorganisms (abhyantara krimi) as most probably present in or coming from impure blood or *raktaja*, mucous or *kaphaja*, and excrements or *purishaja*. In the case of raktaja krimi, the scholars mentioned the word *adrashantor*, which refers to invisible worms (*adrishya krimi*). Although nowadays we know that microbes reside in every body part and cannot be seen with the naked eye, in ayurveda microbes were believed to come from feces (*purishaja krimi*) and from kapha disorders (*kaphaja krimi*).

In the bahya or external group, scholars described atypical bodily secretions (malas) as an invitation for the production and proliferation of microorganisms. Examples of these outward waste substances (*malaja krimi*) include:

anna mala (**urine**) in the case of urinary tract infections
rasa mala (**mucus**) resulting from respiratory and digestive infections
majja mala (**lacrimal secretion**) from conjunctivitis
mamsa mala (**other secretions such as ear wax, nasal discharge,**

and tongue coating) are caused by ear infections, sinusitis, and oral infections

Ayurvedic scholars believed that excess production of these secretions (malas), along with excessive body fluids (kleda), was either the cause of diseases, or their manifestation, since they invite krimi by providing a substrate in which to proliferate. We can understand them as an accumulation at the level of tissular vessels, blocking the passage of the normal channels of secretion (srotas).[15]

Treatment of Microorganisms (Krimi) in General

There are several signs of krimi infection mentioned in the ancient ayurvedic texts, such as ear or eye suppuration.[16] Charaka explained a threefold treatment when microbial infections (krimiroga) were manifesting as visible body secretions.[17]

This treatment included:

apakarshana: removal or elimination from the body
prakritivighata: destruction of the producing causative environment
nidanparivarjana: exclusion of the causative factors that are allowing the microbes to grow

It is fascinating to see how ayurvedic scholars inferred the existence of microorganisms in general and their effects either in creating good health or causing illnesses. They even explained diseases such as smallpox, which they called *masurika*, and other conditions like leprosy (*kustha*).[18]

Ayurvedic protocols and treatments for body cleansing or detoxification (*samshodhana*) are the initial treatment of krimiroga before any kind of rejuvenation protocol is started.

CASE STUDY

Krimi

John, a fit and active eighteen-year-old rugby player, came for a consultation, complaining of anal itching, discolored and itchy hands, bloating of the abdomen,

*and reduced appetite. After a thorough ayurvedic examination (including assessing
John as pitta-vata prakruti), all aspects were pointing toward a worm infection.
Sputum microscopy confirmed a pinworm infection (*Enterobius vermicularis*),
quite possibly because of his rugby activities (frequent contact with the soil in
damp areas), and also perhaps associated with poor hygiene and sanitization. The
ayurvedic management approach to this condition of krimi included anthelmintic
medications and a more hygienic routine, with satisfactory results observed in a
follow-up consultation.*

AYURVEDA'S ROLE IN ADDRESSING OBESITY AND OTHER BODY WEIGHT IMBALANCES

One of the many questions that scientists are currently trying to answer is
how intestinal bacteria are involved in body weight imbalances such as obesity. From the modern scientific point of view, we are still in the process of
trying to understand which particular species of microbiota are essential for
our well-being. Since there are so many different species, we need to recognize the ones that support our digestion, produce essential components
for food assimilation, and get disturbed by unwholesome foods, leading to
an abnormal increase in the overall bacterial population and causing small
intestinal bacterial overgrowth (SIBO). At the same time, we must understand how to avoid the flourishing of opportunistic, harmful species that
can proliferate in our large intestine. And we have to be careful when considering studies focused on the role of particular species in conditions of iso-
lation. It is quite possible that some species perform better and serve various
functions if they work in cooperation with other species, and in that case,
their cooperation would be not easy to identify when they are isolated as
stand-alone species of bacteria for the purpose of analysis.

Again, as always in ayurveda, what's important is to see the whole
picture—and in this case, we have far too many pieces in the puzzle. But
that is the beauty of science: to discover. We have the impression that we
are on the brink of a beneficial microbiome therapeutic revolution as a
result of recent discoveries.[19] Biomedicine has a duty to focus on the wel-
fare of individuals suffering from body-imbalanced conditions such as

obesity, being overweight, and many other body-mind imbalances. My personal view is that a new bridge is being built, leading the way to a more productive exchange between the science of ayurveda and modern biomedical sciences. This bridge is made possible by the arrival of newer disciplines such as epigenetics, chronobiology, pharmacogenetics, nutrigenetics (personalized nutrition), psychobiotics, and metabolomics (the scientific study of chemical processes involving metabolites)—all of which are changing the generalized minimization view of modern medicine into a more appropriate, novel biomedicine. It is encouraging to realize that some Western scientists are engaged in ayurveda-based clinical trials developed through integrative protocols. An example of how we are deriving benefits from novel therapeutic methodologies is the creation of personalized nutrition treatments (nutrigenetics) according to the patient's phenotypic information, such as age, gender, physical activity, and social conditions. Such treatments are considered state-of-the-art science.[20, 21]

For today's ayurvedic scholars and scientists, the above example of innovative modern scientific approaches is simply a very clear expression of one thing: pure ayurveda. The current conception of personalized medicine essentially embodies the prakruti-based maintenance of personalized health that is well known in ayurveda.

Normal eating behavior is coordinated by the strictly regulated balance between intestinal and extra-intestinal equilibrium, and potentially risky desires to consume solid and liquid foods for the purposes of pleasure and in the absence of physical hunger—the hedonic mechanism (HM). By contrast, food substance addiction is a complex, defective eating behavior that reflects alterations in brain-gut-microbiome (BGM) interactions and a shift of this balance toward the HM. Each component of the BGM axis has been implicated in the development of food addiction, with both brain-to-gut and gut-to-brain signaling playing a role. Early-life influences can lead a child's gut microbiome and brain to food addiction, which might be further boosted by increased antibiotic usage and dietary patterns during adulthood.[22] The copious availability and promotion of inexpensive, highly palatable, calorie-dense food substances can further shift this balance toward hedonic eating.

This occurs through physiologically altering both central (disruptions in dopaminergic signaling) and intestinal (e.g., vagal afferent function, metabolic endotoxemia, systemic immune activation) changes to the gut microbiome and the total number of intermediate products of metabolic reactions, called metabolome mechanisms.

OUR DOSHA AND MICROBIOME

So far, we have been discussing only your balanced or unbalanced body type (prakruti and vikruti) and your mental type (manas). Let's now turn our attention to asking whether you also have a unique ayurvedic gut type—and what about if that gut type function specifically corresponds to a core gut microbiome according to your prakruti constitution? We can explore those aspects with the help of scientific integration, starting with the existence of a group of gut types.

There are so many dietary plans that you might hear about from friends, relatives, or as the latest diet trend. Most diets are variations on a theme, some new book or article telling you how this or that regimen worked miraculously for the author within weeks, and it is not uncommon to find yourself following a diet or trying all kinds of different food protocols. As ayurveda sees it, the basic fallacy in this method is that it applies a one-size-fits-all solution to a collection of individuals. Ayurveda takes a different approach, understanding the individual at a physical, mental, and gut level, then tailoring specific treatments or regimens to suit that profile. More specifically, the wisdom of ayurveda focuses first on your gut type so that you can personalize your body-mind type, your own nutritional protocols, and other ayurvedic practices including recognition of seasonal factors. Keep in mind that the desire to ingest food simply for the purpose of pleasure, without physical hunger, is different from the complex maladaptive eating behavior of food addiction—the latter reflects alterations in BGM interactions, and modifications of their balance with mechanisms of pleasure, as well as changes in bacterial groups (genera).

For example, recent studies in India have recognized what is called a main gut microbiome involving *Bacteroides, Faecalibacterium, Prevotella,* and *Ruminococcus* as a major core of the gut; nevertheless, some types of prakruti display a particular increase of a few bacterial genera.[23]

FOUR GUT TYPES ACCORDING TO THE TYPE OF AGNI (FIRE) AND YOUR MICROBIOME

Ayurveda describes a linkage between your prakruti composition, in terms of your dosha distribution, and your gut quality by defining four biological manifestations of gut types as follows: *vishama agni* or variable type, *tikshna agni* or sharp type, *manda agni* or slower type, and *sama agni* or balanced type.

The vishama agni or variable gut type tends to manifest as a variable appetite, where one feels irregularly hungry at different times of the day, and this hunger is not necessarily associated with the normal periods of time related to our body's regular cycles of food intake. As a result, people with a variable gut, or vishama agni, can have drier stools, may have a hard time trying to eliminate them, and possibly do not eliminate feces every single day. They may even suffer from frequent constipation, or they might eliminate multiple times in an irregular way, instead of a normal daily evacuation of the bowels—which ayurveda describes as one or two bowel movements daily with a soft, ripe texture and a floating banana or sausage shape. Frequently, if the air element of vata is disturbed, the mobility can cause gas and bloating.

The second gut type is tikshna agni, or the sharp gut type. Tikshna agni is connected to pitta and to the fire element, and basically manifests as very fast biochemical breakdown of food and its transformation into energy—in order words, a hypermetabolic tendency. If tikshna agni is very strong, it can also lead to a hyper-acidic stomach due to excessive heat affecting the stomach lining; with a lack of proper lubricants, this may manifest as ulcerations. This is often the situation with conditions such as irritable bowel syndrome (IBS). A person with IBS may have either variable gut type or sharp gut type, or a combination of both, depending on the imbalance of these two agni types.

A general observation for those cases when IBS does not fit one specific category is that the condition includes elements of both gut types and will not fit into just one of these four gut categories. People with the sharp gut type (tikshna agni) also may tend to have low blood glucose (hypoglycemia), which manifests as often being hungry, or in some cases, feeling like they cannot eat enough, since they metabolize food very quickly. They also tend to have cravings, need to eat a lot of food, and cannot go for many hours without eating, especially if under stress or pressure. They can get irritable if they skip meals. Finally, someone with a sharp gut type can have the tendency toward looser, runny stools or various bowel movements throughout the day, since a sharp gut type is also related to disturbances of the fire/water elements of pitta.

The third type is manda agni or the dull/slow metabolism type (hypometabolic tendency). Essentially, *manda* means the slowest of the gut types. This dull type of agni is typically present in people who, despite hardly eating anything, increase their body weight, and their bodies have the tendency to keep increasing weight regardless of their level of exercise. The manda agni or dull, slow gut type is associated with the kapha type, being overweight, high levels of triglycerides and cholesterol, and high blood sugar. Someone with the dull and slow gut type could also have mucus in their stools, which may be more of a banana shape. They also might have sluggishness in their bowel motion.

Lastly, the fourth gut type is sama agni or the balanced type. In ayurvedic terms this means harmonious or well-adjusted and stable, with positive emotions and creative energy. When eating and after eating they feel light and invigorated. They also feel satiated and gratified with everything they eat, since they can eat pretty much anything without having a harmful digestive effect, and in general they don't have strong cravings.

If we try to establish a general comparison between the sama agni or balanced gut versus the other three gut types, we see that those gut types can vary between feeling either exhausted or overstimulated after eating.

Let me give you a brief overview of the emotional state of the other gut types, since ayurveda sees us as a body/mind/spirit unit that is difficult to separate, except with the intention of understanding its processes. Remember, according to ayurveda, everything physical or physiological always has a mental and emotional connection.

▼ Vishama agni or variable gut–type people are more prone to feelings of fear, tend to constantly experience self-doubt, and often feel isolated and alone.

▼ Tikshna agni or sharp gut–type people can feel greedy for protein and fat, but their system does not necessary digest fat very well.

▼ Manda agni or dull/slow gut–type people, after food ingestion, may feel like they need to take a nap, and their minds can get blurry and dull. They have a tendency to feel down and unhappy for no clear reason, and over time they may gradually find it more difficult to get motivated. They have to use a lot of willpower to gather the energy to participate in physical activities or just to complete their daily duties, and they may commonly feel a sense of unhappiness.

All gut types can feel a craving for carbohydrates, protein, or even fatty fried foods when there is a body-mind imbalance. It is important to take into consideration that if you are having strong cravings and if you are not the balanced gut type, you could be experiencing a nutritional deficiency that the body is trying to sort out.

I hope that after this short biological description, you will be able to recognize yourself in one of these four gut types and begin to harness the wisdom of ayurveda in recognizing the perpetual dance of the five elements of nature, and how they connect to your body and gut type. These natural metabolic processes, known as circadian rhythms, are periodic, and when you respect the right time for food intake—breakfast, lunch, dinner, and snacks if required—as well as eating the right portions and compositions, you can truly optimize your digestion. You will then be able to avoid causing a lack of nutrients that leads to undernutrition, or anorexia, or creating excesses that, sooner or later, manifest as extra weight and in the long term will express as obesity, resulting from kapha accumulation in your tissues.

If we relate recent scientific findings to the ayurvedic knowledge of following a natural diet based on wholesome foods largely from the vegetable kingdom, we can see that for thousands of years, these ancient discoveries have been protecting the balance, or homeostasis, between healthy microbiota and the body-mind, for people in India and other Eastern civilizations. In other words, our gut type correlates with our dosha type, and it is supported or regulated by our microbiome. We will be discussing this issue in more detail, but for now we could postulate that there is a cellular agni and a microbiome agni and that the result of a well-balanced interaction between them, when following an appropriate lifestyle, will guarantee proper body-mind functions. Both are our GIT agni!

Ayurveda has been saying forever that the foundation of all diseases begins in the gut. Today we can see that in cases such as inflammatory bowel disease, irritable bowel syndrome, neurological disorders, asthma, allergies, autoimmune issues, obesity, diabetes, heart disease, and other difficulties, there is a connection with the gut. When examining celiac disease conditions, we know very clearly what happens for certain people who have a genetic susceptibility to gluten, associated with a compound called gliadin.[24]

For ayurveda, it is not only about you having to practice a certain lifestyle, but also about learning its logic, being willing to participate, then enjoying living your natural balance. We cannot be our own enemies; this is the invitation from ayurveda.

The ayurvedic concepts offered here are simple, basic, functional, cost-effective, and can be readily applied to support and stabilize body rebalancing. In this process of learning, in the same way we stand up to protect our planet from deforestation, we need to understand and protect our gut from deforestation, which occurs due to our wrong habits and the many external pressures of modern life affecting our five elements. We also require good quality air, fire, water, and earth. We have to try consciously and courageously to use all possible tools to understand nature's network and unlock its secrets, if we want to reconnect with nature as a whole, and our own nature, to bring balance to our body-mind systems. Hopefully the wisdom of ayurveda presented here will guide you toward achieving balance and harmony with nature, so that you may grow well and reach your fullest natural potential.

AYURVEDIC RECOMMENDATIONS

Since microbiome diversity is critical for protecting us from body imbalances and from the weakening of mind alertness, remember that we can obtain a diverse, high-quality microbiome by following daily lifestyle advice and practices that ayurveda recommends.

Your body is constantly trying to communicate with you, and perhaps you are not listening properly, or you do not know how to listen. So, here's a short account of some tailored practices that will help you learn to communicate with your gut.

1. Seek out food variety. Embrace a diversified diet to give to your microbiome a better chance to flourish, rebuild, and thrive. Scientists advise that you eat diverse fruits and vegetables. Ayurveda has been telling us this for thousands of years.
2. Eat the right foods for your particular microbiome. This book proposes specific natural, unharmful foods based on the type of fiber that aligns with your constitutional needs. Put it into practice and experience it— but also remember that you could have a dual constitution.
3. Pay attention to your bowel movements. Monitor your schedule to identify when you could be constipated—a major cause of body imbalance. If you are not regular, you could be retaining food for days. Ayurveda describes in detail how undigested food becomes toxic material when moving around in your body longer than it should, causing body-mind disorders.[25]
4. Regarding junk food, you should avoid heavily processed foods and instead eat organic and natural foods that are rich in fiber. Studies have shown that adopting a plant-based diet for even short periods of five days can significantly alter human gut microbiota composition and gene expression, followed by return to baseline composition microbiota diversity two days after the end of the five-day diet.[26]

5. Avoid additives. Studies have shown they deplete the microbiota by harming the intestinal barrier, triggering intestinal inflammation, metabolic deregulation, and weight gain.
6. Incorporate physical activity. Engage in active pursuits. It might be difficult to start exercising, but it will pay off immensely in terms of body balance. Options like yoga, swimming, or stretching may be beneficial, and in some cases can be done from home or outdoors.
7. Cultivate awareness. Ayurveda offers so many options to anchor us, such as breathing exercises, vocalizations, yoga, and walking in nature.
8. Reduce stress. Your body and mind are interrelated via your gut. Stress alters your microbiome, so respect your body. Eat slowly and steadily, and relax your mind to reset your gut.
9. Be careful of drugs. Polydrug therapy, biological rhythms' disruption, smoking, heavy drugs, alcohol, and other stressors can lead to intractable problems and complications.
10. And finally, avoid antibiotics except in the case of serious health conditions. They destroy harmful bacteria, yes, but at the same time they destroy the good bacteria in an indiscriminatory way.

Do not disregard the microbiota that live with you, their host. The microbiota require care from you, in the form of proper physical and mental food. They are living with you—and you are living with them. In exchange for good quality "food," they will provide you plenty of health benefits on your path to restoring a healthy body weight and balance.

THE MICROBIOME

A Modern Understanding of the Gut

ARE WE JUST INTELLIGENT BACTERIA?

If So, Who Are They?

The moment we breathe outside the womb for the first time, we are covered by trillions of bacteria, and the predominant nature of our microbial colonization depends on the type of birth delivery we undergo.[1] When we are born via the birth canal, we are colonized by fecal and vaginal bacteria first; if we are born via cesarean delivery then we are exposed to a bacterial environment closely related to human skin and the hospital room environment, which may have a long-term impact on our microbes.[2] Whatever the circumstances of our delivery, we come into a world where microorganisms instantly colonize the interior and all surfaces of our body's tissues and organs, including the gut, skin, lungs, urinary tract, and reproductive organs.

Collectively, bacteria and other microorganisms in a host are known as flora. Although microflora or intestinal flora are historically used terms, the word *microbiota* is now common, and it is important to differentiate between two similar terms in current use. The term *microbiome* pertains to all microorganisms, and their genetic components, living in our bodies. The term *microbiota* applies to communities of microorganisms present in the body's various environments such as the gut, lungs, kidneys, and skin. At the gut level, microbiota establish themselves deep in our bowels, in our intestinal epithelium, as an inner forest of 10^{14} or one hundred trillion microorganisms, including at least one thousand species of known bacteria that enter an arrangement with the human body, receiving lodging and protection in exchange for mutual health.[3, 4] In other words, the microbiome basically declares to its host (you) in a friendly way, "We are smaller than you, but we are far more numerous, let's coexist in harmony." So that's what we are, combined beings, composed of trillions of microbial cells and trillions of our own cells functioning intimately with us, their host, to do metabolic functions useful to our health.

A couple of examples of the roles that our microbiota agni play to accomplish metabolic roles that have direct impact on our health are, firstly, carbohydrate-active enzymes (CAZymes) present in gut microorganisms, which provide us energy from dietary fibers (polysaccharides). These enzymes are not present in our human genome. They will support the processes of breakdown, digestion, and absorption of food.

A second example is found in comparative gut metagenome (beyond the genome) studies, which show that some enzymes—porphyranases and agarases—which break down dietary fibers, are common in the Japanese population as they come from seaweeds, a basic component of Japan's daily diet.[5] This is an example of the benefits resulting from symbiotic adaptation by the microorganisms of the Japanese gut to seaweed enzymes which are not in abundance in other population's diet due to the absence of these seaweeds as food substrates.

The gut, also known as the intestines, the enteric system, the bowels, the viscera, and the belly region—and often called the "second brain"—is now receiving significant research resources, which have led to very important scientific findings. These findings align with the ayurvedic ideas expressed as digestive fire (agni), individual constitution (prakruti), individual imbalance (vikruti), and the mind (manas).

Our gut is not just part of the viscera; it's a hub of intelligence, a lodging for neurons. Scientists are rediscovering what common sense knew for a long time: people of a nervous disposition get butterflies in their stomach, cowards lack guts, and we sometimes act on gut instinct with the gut feeling of fear in the pit of our stomach. Sometimes we're well aware that our brain is not the only captain on board and that some decisions result from an interplay between the gut and the brain. Why? Well, because the hundreds of billions of bacteria in our gut furtively influence the millions of neurons controlling our activities and personality.

The bacteria existing in the human body represent two to six pounds of weight, and the way they are studied is by the analysis of our feces. As an example, one single gram of feces contains more bacteria than the number of people on the entire planet. There is very clear evidence of a strong individual component to the composition of the gut microbiota. Approximately 30 percent of our microbiota is shared between all of us. But around 70 percent is distinct to each of us, so our intestinal microbiota could be considered a clear identity card. Recently, scientists coined the term *enterotypes* based on the bacteriological classification of living organisms that form an ecosystem in the gut microbiome—known as human-associated microorganisms. By categorizing the microbiota, we can understand their diversity and the ways they provide innumerable functions to protect and improve our health.[6]

There are several phyla in the kingdom of bacteria. Among the one hundred trillion bacteria in our gut, the predominant gut phyla are Firmicutes, Bacteroidetes, Actinobacteria, Proteobacteria, Fusobacteria, Cyanobacteria, and Verrucomicrobia. It has been calculated that human microbiota consist of more than 1,000 different species of microorganisms, and that the human gut microbiome contains more than 160 species of bacteria.[7] In a healthy gut, Firmicutes and Bacteroidetes constitute 90 percent of our gut microbiota, and the way they take care of you depends on the balance between them. They are working together for our good health but in constant competition with each other—a kind of wrestling between them based on the types of foods we supply them—and a takeover by one of them depends largely on us. If under any circumstance we are feeding harmful bacteria, then toxins and inflammation will occur and can even destroy a healthy gut lining.[8]

Not only are the microbes within us essential to our well-being, but their detailed study also opens up new avenues for the understanding of many diseases. Today we know that the gut houses more than 70 percent of our immune system, which makes sense given that the lining of your gut is the barrier between your inside and outside worlds. What if the future of medicine is centered in our belly, as ayurveda postulated thousands of years ago? Are there significative connections between the gut, the adipose/fat system, the immune system, and the brain? Can we improve our physical and mental imbalances by varying our eating patterns and the types of foods we eat? Is there a link between the presence of bacteria (especially in our gut), the foods we eat, and the ways in which a wrong combination puts our physical and mental health at risk? Well, these questions will be answered in this section—and then later we will focus on the potential link between our food intake, its breakdown and absorption, our body imbalances, and our gut inhabitants. We'll address all this through the lens of ayurvedic knowledge.

MICROBIOME: THE BIG PLAYER

From comparing bacteria present in the intestinal flora of hundreds of individuals, we know that microbiota vary from one individual to another. Despite the fact that microbiota are present everywhere in our bodies, the vast majority of them are found in the digestive tract, with an exponential population increase in the lower gut or colon—also called the large intestine, which is much wider than the small intestine. The length of the intestines can vary significantly among individuals. Various studies indicate that the combined length of the small and large intestines is a minimum 15 ft in length, with a small intestine measuring around 9–16 ft, whereas the large intestine is about 5 ft long.[9]

Our friendly microbiota have a number of relevant characteristics and roles. Most bacteria, in fact, are friendly—they guard us against germs. Our microbiota also serve many digestive and metabolic functions in the assimilation and absorption of food, such as supporting the digestion of tough carbohydrates including cereals, potatoes, and legumes, and facilitating the fragmentation of proteins and the degradation of bile acids and short-chain fatty acids (SCFAs).[10] These SCFAs are crucial energy sources for the colonic cellular layer and influencing bacterial gene expression.[11] Our microbiota also produces almost 95 percent of the human body's total serotonin in the intestinal lumen, help the body absorb mineral nutrients such as calcium and iron, and synthesize vitamins such as B and K_2 and other important bioactive metabolites. Further, the microbiota help to keep the gut well developed and to maintain its wall integrity—the wall being around twenty to thirty feet long and housing 80 percent of the immune system—and train the immune system by coaxing T cells to see them as friends. Finally, our microbiota make up a second nervous system containing one hundred million nerve cells, allowing all kinds of interactions.

Very interestingly, the distribution of the microbiome varies according to the individual and their community. A healthy gut often has a pattern of bowel movements, but of course this varies from person to person and according to their microbiome composition. It all depends on factors such as the level of fiber intake, dehydration, immune factors, stress, thyroid factors, and others. For example, with conditions like celiac disease, there is evidence that certain bacteria will destroy a particular part of the gut wall (*Pseudomonas aeruginosa* could increase inflammation of the mucous membranes in combination with gluten) or create alterations due to constipation.

Research conducted in two areas completely isolated from the modern world—the Amazon region and part of Tanzania—has shown that the diet and fecal microbiota of populations in these areas presented a richer and more diverse intestinal flora than those of city dwellers in Japan, China, the United States, and France.[12, 13] And, in fact, other comparative studies of the microbiome between the United States and other Western countries make us aware of the fragility of our intestinal flora, and how greater diversity turns out to be highly important for longevity. Some of the current research is directed toward understanding whether the abrupt rise of disorders such as inflammatory bowel disease, obesity, type 2 diabetes, depression, and autism may be associated with this impoverishment.[14, 15] What we understand so far is that the microbiome of one in four people is impoverished by a decrease in total bacterial load of important groups such as the *Lactobacillus*, *Bifidobacterium*, and *Eubacterium* genera.

Considering the scientific and medical data on the gut microbiome, we can ask ourselves: Could the recommended ayurvedic practices of consumption of good fiber handle potential microbiome imbalances? Could the understanding of our belly provide the answers for addressing modern chronic diseases? It all comes back to the questions: Are we just intelligent bacteria? Who are they? Who am I? Am I first- or second-level intelligence or wisdom?

INTERDEPENDENCE AMONG THE GUT MICROBIOME, FIBER, AND MODERN LIFE

Fiber is the most crucial ingredient for gut health needed to feed our intestinal microbes, and we've started to understand that having low fiber intake is a greater cause for concern than low protein intake. The well-being of our bodily systems, and in particular our digestive tract's proper functioning, leans on our interaction with the environment. When ayurveda was presented to the world, populations were living in real, direct contact with nature, free of the contaminants we encounter today. More significantly, they were eating natural foodstuffs that carried their full fiber content. We can deduce that they had a very rich microbiota, as is shown by the studies of the isolated populations of Tanzania or the Amazon, where diets have remained unchanged for centuries. Nowadays, from the moment we are born, the origins and quality of the foods "unprotected by nature" that we consume until our death have an effect on our GIT, playing an essential role in how our metabolic fire (agni) processes our food and affecting our body-mind system.

Studies in humans investigating the effects of whole grains show that when given whole-grain brown rice, barley, or a blend of both for a period of one month, people experienced an increase in bacterial group diversity. Additionally, the changes of gut bacteria groups were accompanied by a decline in systemic inflammation in participants' bodies.[16, 17, 18, 19] When we eat fiber, especially the kind present in vegetables, some bacteria pay us back by producing small fatty acid molecules to protect us against inflammation and other obesity-linked metabolic impairments.[20] A scarce food-fiber intake means reducing richness and diversity of our intestinal microbiome, leaving us in a more fragile situation overall. As you see, our crowd of bacteria who live with us require fiber, so it's better not to take away their preferred feast substrate, or we may deprive ourselves of all the beneficial healthy substances they produce for us. Our symbiotic bacteria are furnished with the proper enzymes to degrade fiber. By depriving our microbiome of its main substratum—dietary fiber—we are altering their colony size, composition of various species, and their enzymatic fermentation processes. Fiber contained in our food passes through the intestines largely undigested, aiding the shape and structure of stools, promoting regular bowel movements, and feeding the bacteria and making them flourish, both in number and kind, so they become a vital dietary component for good body-mind health.

Prebiotics and Probiotics

Prebiotics are specialized high-fiber foods or nondigestible nutriment constituents that act like discriminating "fertilizers" stimulating the growth of healthy, beneficial bacteria in the colon, which can improve the host's good health. In other words, prebiotics are no different from the dietary fiber that supports the growth of microorganisms in our intestines. Since we cannot break down prebiotics in the stomach or small intestine, they are the microorganisms' nutriment. Upon their arrival in the large intestine (colon), they are fermented by the gut microbiome, stimulating production of diverse SCFAs. Three SCFA types actively participate in keeping the gut cells heathy—in terms of structure, digestion, and absorption—and once they are absorbed by the large intestine, they will support around 70 percent of our immune system activity. In other words, you don't need to take a prebiotic if you are pursuing ayurvedic dietary principles in your daily life.

Probiotics are food products or supplements that contain live microorganisms intended to maintain or improve the "good" bacteria in the body by carrying enough viable microorganisms to adjust your microbiome and create potential health benefits. Probiotics are a mixture of live bacteria and yeasts that can be beneficial for your digestive system if used properly. They can also be used to treat conditions such as constipation, acid reflux, diarrhea, gas, and eczema.

Nowadays, prebiotics and probiotics are substances intended to support a healthy microbiome or reestablish balance in cases where bacterial imbalance has been triggered by ailments, an improper diet, or side effects of medications. That is the central theme of ayurveda: safeguarding equilibrium through bacterial homeostasis, by the intake of wholesome foods integrated into your diet containing all those natural, nondigestible fibers present in vegetables, legumes, cereal grains, nuts, seeds, and fruits. It is my vision, supported by modern research and the trial and error of thousands of years of practice in India, that probiotics can aid in keeping your gut healthy—but if you already have healthy gut bacteria and you are following the ayurvedic dietary values, then your body does not require these supplementary probiotics. Don't add what the body doesn't need.

Brewed foods and certain varieties of cheeses and breads support gut health by providing healthy living microorganisms that enhance absorption of minerals and increase the nutrients we get from food. Some popular examples of providing probiotics in a natural way, as fermented foods, include yogurt, kefir, sourdough bread, sauerkraut, kombucha, pickles, kimchi, tempeh, miso, and certain traditionally made cheeses.

Emerging data suggests that altering the composition of the gut microbiota through probiotic, prebiotic, and synbiotic (a mixture of probiotics and prebiotics) supplementation may be a viable auxiliary treatment option for obese individuals.[21] However, more studies are required to fully explain the cellular mechanisms of action of probiotics and prebiotics on human health, and to clarify the link between microbiota and obesity causality, using well-designed, long-term, and large-scale clinical trials.[22] We should really ask ourselves, do we need to take these man-made products right now?

The same applies to the many other products advertised by the food and supplements industry: does it benefit us to create one more kind of dependency? Perhaps instead we should just appreciate the thousands of years of Indian trial and error, by which that country's people found the way to promote good health through a natural wholesome diet, until very recently when the food industry invaded with Western sugary foods and many more synthetic products.

REPERCUSSIONS OF OUR MODERN LIFESTYLE ON THE MICROBIOME

In the early 1900s, scientists discovered that each person belonged to one of four blood types (O, A, B, and AB). Now, in the 2020s, we are discovering that perhaps people can be classified into categories of bacterial environments, since we are learning that different entero-types have different food preferences. Some studies classify them in the following way:

ENTEROTYPES

Type	High Levels of Bacteria	Food Cravings
1	Bacteroides	proteins and animal fat (saturated)
2	Prevotella	starches; fruits and legumes
3	Ruminococcus	oils (unsaturated) and alcohol

Is this century offering us a new way to characterize ourselves based on our individual microbiomes? Have we found a new "biological fingerprint"? Is this not analogous with prakruti and the concept of three doshas or individual body-mind constitutions, and the ayurvedic princi-ples associated with diet and lifestyle?

Your microbial composition can be impacted or modified by genetic and environmental factors such as diet, hormones, toxins, carcinogen exposure, and your physical location.[23] What comes first, the chicken or the egg? Our inherited prakruti (the host) carries genetic characteris-tics, and the environment is a modifier or amplifier of our microbiome (the guest). How can the various types of prakruti adjust to or inte-grate the abundant variability of the microbiome? We have here three different factors or variables that require study. Perhaps addressing the question through envisaging different types of hosts, as per ayurvedic prakruti, will give us deeper understanding of these processes. This understanding could be of great benefit for the treatment of imbalances and ailments.

The multifaceted bionetwork crafted by the microbiota is constantly interrelating with us as its host. Our diet and the ecosystem are very relevant factors affecting the microbiota composition. However, despite the numerous approaches proposed to regulate our human microbiota using alimentary resources, we are still not reaching that goal.[24]

When we look at modernity's improvements to our lives, we must also consider the other side of the coin. We've seen the negative impact of, for example, rigorous usage of cleaning and disinfecting products, anti-microbial treatments (antibiotics), and harmful foods containing damaging additive and preservative components—all parts of industrialization that are badly affecting our microbiome. For example, alterations in the gut microbiota could be the cause of pathologies such as IBS, obesity and metabolic disorders, *Clostridium difficile* infection, pathogen colonization (e.g., *Enterococcus* resistant to vancomycin), allergic reactions and autoimmune diseases, and even neuropsychiatric disorders.[25]

It is important to keep in mind that when we take an antibiotic, it may eliminate the unwanted bacteria within us, but at the same time it may also destroy essential bacteria in our gut forever, since antibiotics have the effect of a cluster bomb. They are designed to destroy bacteria, and they do this by killing the intended target and inflicting collateral casualties, such as good bacteria, along the way. This causes deforestation of our good bacteria.[26] My stance is not against the use of antibiotics—they are lifesavers. But we need to learn how to use them in a safer way to prevent harm being done to our essential microbiota and, consequently, our balance. Ask yourself, when you are prescribed antibiotics, are you told about the side effects? Are you encouraged to replenish your intestinal flora after a course of them? The use of antibiotics has increased steadily over the past sixty years. The Pasteurian microbiological approach to disease commanded us to search for a pathogen. With illnesses such as IBS, mainstream medicine is following the same approach, blaming certain bacteria or viruses before considering that the real issue may be a systemic loss of healthy bacteria and thus a loss of their protective bodily functions. If you have taken antibiotics, help your gut by restoring that friendship.

In terms of quality food intake, another problem associated with our modern lifestyle is a powerful food industry and how it delivers food to us—and not only in relation to the reduction or absence of fiber in processed food. The scientific community is increasingly inquisitive about the ongoing addition of "innovative" artificial chemical molecules to our food and thus our health.[27] In the United States there are many opportunities to study the kinds of additives present in processed foods and to track their presence, and persistence, in any transformed product—and many studies have been conducted in this area.[28] As discussed earlier (see pages 128–29), processed foods with certain additives can cause inflammation in the lining of our gut, in the areas where food is absorbed.[29, 30]

Remember that your gut has little choice in accepting what you are providing (and only vomiting if necessary). Its role is not to determine if what you have eaten is digestible food or not. Instead, your gut might recognize the presence of artificial food ingredients, such as high-fructose corn syrup, as an unwelcome or problematic invader. Under such circumstances it may set off an inflammatory response in which our bodies are literally fending off these food additives as if they were an infection, since they are not chemically recognized as natural molecules. For example, most kinds of chocolate bars contain emulsifiers, which are additives used in food manufacturing to stabilize processed foods. Well, consider that the emulsifier is only there in the manufactured food to hold it together long enough to last the length of the supply chain, from the factory to the supermarket shelf and finally to your stomach. It is not there because it's nutritious. Your body is not begging for emulsifiers—quite the opposite. Some of these additives are used to allow a mix of fat and non-fat compounds to look fresh and stable in the supermarkets, despite the fact these additives can have other negative impacts on your efforts to maintain good health.

Are these additives affecting our bacteria? Could it be possible that a simple chocolate bar enhanced with additives changes our microbiome? The answer is yes. Several studies have shown these effects.[31] Eating healthy foods such as whole fruits, vegetables, and unprocessed meats can lower the metabolic stress placed upon your body.[32]

We are the first suppliers in the perpetual cycle of food nourishment. Consequently, we are the ones who must be clever and conscious enough to know what's going on; we cannot request that our gut tell us what to eat—although maybe we could if we had a real connection with our senses. The point here is for you to understand that you can do yourself a great service by awakening to the idea that it is time to address lifelong, everyday dietary habits that may be harmful and may be the cause of your extra weight or obesity.

Consider the imbalance caused by overgrowth of intestinal bacterial of the wrong kind (SIBO), populating the small intestine and leading to uncomfortable symptoms such as gas and diarrhea. SIBO can be evaluated by breath testing. Its risk is two to three times higher among obese people than among the non-obese. Studies have shown that blends of berberine, allicin, oregano, and neem extract can help to tackle methane-dominant SIBO when supported by a healthy diet rich in vegetables and whole foods to balance the microbiota.[33] Berberine (that is Indian barberry or *daruharidra* root and bark in ayurvedic medicine) stimulates enzymatic glucose metabolism, boosts insulin secretion, and suppresses adipogenesis and hepatic gluconeogenesis—events involving AMP-activated protein kinase (AMPK).

STRESS

I don't intend to cause you more stress when you are reading this section, but we must be honest with ourselves and take into account the implications of personal and social stress on our microbiome. So, what exactly do we know about the interplay between stress, the gut, and the brain?

The gut is home not to just 200 million neurons but also to hundreds of billions of bacteria that secretly influence our mood, energy level, appetite, memory, and personality.[34, 35] Stress is a major risk factor for several pathologies, including cardiovascular diseases, as a result of an increase in hormones such as cortisol and neurotransmitters such as adrenaline.[36, 37, 38]

In our bodies, everything is interconnected, so these conditions can change your gut, altering your microbiome distribution by turning it into a "butterfly cage" of distress and anxiety.[39, 40, 41, 42] Ayurveda understands that the more relaxed you are, the better you will be able to nourish your body, mind, and spirit. In our daily lives we are not just addressing digestion of material food.[43] Moment to moment, all kinds of influences are food for the body, the mind, and our consciousness. When eating, even if it is wholesome food, take the time to chew your food. This helps to start the digestive process by breaking down food into smaller pieces and stimulating the release of enzymes present in your saliva that combine with the food, giving signals to the rest of the body that it is time to pay attention to the digestive system.

TO MIND YOUR WEIGHT, MIND YOUR GUT, AND MIND YOUR MIND

Microbes make up 90 percent of all cells in the body, carrying a massive eight million strings of DNA in contrast to the 22,000 carried by our human cells. Based on recent epigenetic research, these bacterial genes may well be altered by our thoughts and belief systems.[44] The way we think and believe has been shown to modify the microbes in the gut, which in turn affect our body balance.

The process of digestion is surprisingly sophisticated. Breaking food down and making it into tiny little molecules that you can absorb and use to run your body is not an easy job, and you need a lot of metabolic power. Leaky gut syndrome is a good example to help us understand the mind-gut connection, this digestive condition that affects the lining of the intestines. Under normal conditions, the gaps in the intestinal walls allow water and nutrients to pass through into the bloodstream while keeping substances harmful to the bloodstream out. In leaky gut syndrome, these openings become wider, allowing food particles, bacteria, and toxins to enter directly into the bloodstream. A 2018 study stated that lack of balance in the gut microbiota can activate the body's immune response, causing an amplified intestinal permeability and gut inflammation.[45] Other studies suggest that leaky gut could participate in the process of neuroinflammation, inducing several neurodegenerative disorders such as anxiety and depression.[46, 47, 48]

THE GUT-BRAIN AXIS IN OBESITY

Several studies reveal that the variety of bacterial species within us and the quality of the exchanges among them are important factors for the development and maintenance of health among adults.[49] The trillions of microorganisms in our gut produce 95 percent of the serotonin, dopamine, and other brain chemicals that regulate our emotions, mood, and other mental and physical functions. Because stress can activate inflammation and increase gut permeability, researchers are trying to determine whether a leaky gut allows macromolecules and microorganisms to leave the gut and reach the brain, where they induce neuroinflammation. Novel data demonstrates a tight relation between obesity and gut microbiota in a large-scale Chinese population, which could offer potential targets for the prevention and treatment of obesity, with potential obesity-related biomarkers such as *Bacteroides caccae*, *Roseburia hominis*, and *Odoribacter splanchnicus*.[50]

The gut-brain axis is a bidirectional connection between the abdominal or enteric nervous system (ENS) and the CNS. That means that direct and indirect pathways exist between our brain activities—such as our thoughts and emotional centers in the brain—and the peripheral gut functions.[51] Recent neuroscientific studies describe the relevance of the microbiota in the development of our brain systems.[52]

Dietary fiber–derived SCFAs produced by the microbiome have been found to mediate interactions along the gut-brain axis through their impact on various communication channels that your gut and brain use to "talk" to each other, such as the vagus nerve, gut hormones, neurotransmitters, and the endocrine system. These SCFAs could play an important therapeutic role in giving some relief to cases of obesity that aren't associated with alcohol dependency.[53]

Scientific evidence shows that the microbiota-SCFA-brain axis mediates behavioral disorders induced by maternal obesity. Maternal obesity is associated with alteration of cognition and social engagement of children, and when the mother or offspring eats a high-fiber diet, this prevents behavioral disorders in the offspring, alleviating synaptic impairments and microglial maturation defects.[54]

We know now that every emotion manifesting in the brain will be echoed in the gut, and whatever is going on in the gut will be reflected in one way or another at the brain level.[55, 56, 57] Try to see yourself enjoying your meal after having a heated argument or receiving a bad piece of news. Remember, the main reason to keep a healthy gut is because it is the home of 60 to 80 percent of our immune system; and 90 percent of our neurotransmitters, the chemical messengers that help control mood, are controlling our digestive system.

If you have followed me until now, then you have terrific "gut" instincts.

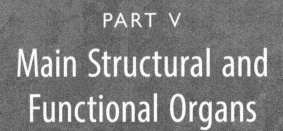

PART V

Main Structural and Functional Organs

Players in Your Bodily Imbalance

11

THE ADIPOSE TISSUE

The Visibly Guilty Actor

Ayurveda explains that the origin of all ill health and disease, including obesity, is the result of the lack of connection with our senses. It classifies diseases in different ways, and the examination of the patient is carried out using four, six, or eight types of evaluations. These ayurvedic concepts could offer us a very direct understanding of the relation between obesity and adipose tissue, fascia, and other tissues.

Let's visualize in the following chapters how this process occurs, starting with the study of the association between adipose tissue and fascia as two interacting "connective tissues."

THE ADIPOSE TISSUE
"The New Organ"

Even if some people dislike either the presence or absence of fat in their bodies, the fact is, our corporal lipids or fat tissues play several vital biological roles in our daily lives. The tasks they perform include providing food intake, a depot for the provision of energy, insulin sensitivity, preservation of temperature, formation of membranes or the lipid layer, biogenesis or conversion of lipids (i.e., cholesterol and fatty acids), production of chemical metabolic messengers, immune responses, having a role in inflammation (prostaglandins formation), and the production of vitamins.

The most conventional role attributed to the adipose tissue (AT) is storing spare energy in the form of fatty particles: When we eat, fat gets converted into triglycerides and fatty acids and stored in the adipose tissue, in cells called adipocytes. This is the most efficient system for storing energy in our bodies, since our fatty acids get released when the fuel is needed by our bodily functions. As an example, from the caloric point of view, and in terms of density, fat tissue represents eight times more calories per pound of weight compared to muscle. A healthy adult can have a total body weight made up of 15 to 25 percent adipose tissue, and in some people this proportion can be as high as 50 percent.

Fat storage and its distribution, our appetite, and our metabolism are regulated by several hormones produced by fat cells (leptins) and other organs, such as insulin, glucagon, adrenaline, noradrenaline, estrogens, androgens, and human growth hormone, to name a few. According to the immediate energy requirements of our bodies, the hormonal pathways can either encourage adipose tissue formation and storage—a process called lipogenesis—or start the release of fat from adipose tissue, a process called lipolysis.[1] For example, insulin is the hormone allowing the increased uptake of glucose (blood sugar) and its conversion into fatty acids for storage.

Main Types of Adipose Tissue/Fats

Let's first understand what we mean by adipose tissue and describe the main kinds. A fundamental property of adipose tissue is its high level of plasticity.

AT, also referred to as fat tissue or body fat, is found in several different places throughout the body and is fundamental for supporting energy homeostasis. It is composed of cells called adipocytes (the body's primary energy reservoir). They can be segmented into three cell types: white, brown, and beige adipocytes, which vary in function, color, structure, and body location.

White adipose tissue (WAT) is the most profuse kind of fat tissue in adult humans. WAT contains single large vesicles (vacuoles) that store lipids fabricated from the food we consume, via a mechanism called lipogenesis, which are then allocated within subcutaneous fat, visceral fat, and bone marrow fat.[2] WAT can be of two types: First, subcutaneous white adipose tissue (SWAT), found in the interspaces between the skin and underlying muscles of the whole body, and playing various roles, such as an insulation layer. The second type, called visceral white adipose tissue (VWAT), is the main type of adipose tissue used for energy storage, and it is mostly located throughout the abdominal cavity, surrounding vital organs such as the liver, intestines, kidneys, and the membrane, or peritoneum, that lines the outside of the abdominal organs. WAT is also present in the bone marrow adipose tissue (BMAT), the pericardium or membrane surrounding the heart, and as a kind of padding in other body areas such as the soles of the feet, eyeballs, and in some blood vessels.[3]

Contrasting with WAT, we also find brown adipose tissue (BAT), called brown adipocytes. BAT contains numerous small vacuoles that hold lipids and many "power stations" or mitochondria, giving that brown look to these fat cells. BAT's principal function is to oxidize lipids for heat production to keep us warm through a cellular mechanism branded "non-shivering thermogenesis."[4] BAT is principally situated on our backs, between the shoulders, along the upper half of the spine, and surrounding the kidneys. It is mainly active in the fetal period and when we are babies, and its size decreases gradually with age, but increases in cold settings. In our adult life, brown fat deposits can be situated surrounding the vertebrae, beyond the clavicles, in the upper back, and in the mediastinum, the central section of the thoracic space.

There is a third type of adipose tissue found in humans called beige adipose tissue (BeAT), which is disseminated throughout SWAT. It contains more mitochondria and performs more fatty acid oxidation than WAT tissues but accumulates less lipids.

Each type of adipose tissue and adipocyte releases different mixes of cell-signaling molecules, or adipokines; they allow highly regulated communication among the adipose tissue and other organs, to preserve metabolic energy balance.[5]

IF THE ADIPOSE TISSUE IS AN ENDOCRINE ORGAN, WHAT IS ITS RELATIONSHIP WITH OBESITY?

Several decades of research have made it evident that the adipose tissue is an important, metabolically active endocrine organ, for several reasons.

An endocrine organ produces hormones that are discharged directly into the blood and travel throughout the body tissues and organs. We know now that obesity is a disease because of its dysfunctional pathways that lead to an elevated body weight set point. An increased fat mass in an environment of obesity leads to chronic states of systemic low-grade inflammation. Normal adipose tissue consists of fat cells surrounded by a normal level of immune cells, including lymphocytes B and T, and macrophages.

There is real communication between fat tissue and other tissues in the body, making the adipose tissue an endocrine organ, so WAT in a normal state generates signals to multiple organs and the immune system, as was revealed in 1994 by Rudolph Leibel. He discovered that a hormone called leptin, secreted by fat tissue, signals to the brain regarding the body's fat stores, indicating whether there are sufficient energy reserves or if there's a state of negative energy balance and decreased energy stores. In fact, the endocrine organ of adipose tissue communicates with other vital organs such as the liver, protecting it from becoming a fatty liver, and preserves insulin sensitivity by storing fat in itself and not in the liver. It also protects the heart, muscles, kidneys, pancreas, vascular endothelium, and the immune system when it becomes depleted.[6] As a summary, AT is an endocrine and metabolic organ, producing numerous biologically active molecules called adipokines. These contribute to diverse functions, including food intake and satiety, modulation of energy balance, inflammatory response produced by visceral fat, and metabolism of steroid hormones—thus establishing direct communication with our brain and gut.

CAN WE TAP INTO THE DIFFERENT TYPES OF FAT FOR WEIGHT LOSS?

In general terms, ayurvedic pharmacology, or *dravyaguna sastra*, is the science that deals with the thought analysis of the properties, actions, and therapeutics of all the substances (*dravya*). Both food (*ahara*) and medicines (*aushadha*) are complex processes that will be discussed later, but basically, they relate to the qualities (gunas) of matter and taste.

Let me give you a brief picture of the process of becoming overweight or obese in modern medical terms:

In conditions of imbalance due to overeating and overnutrition, the healthy white tissue—under the influence of hormones such as ghrelin, or the "hunger hormone"—expands because of excess fat storage. Subsequently, the immune cells surrounding the adipocytes become more abundant and produce pro-inflammatory cytokines, causing adipocyte hypertrophy and stress. At some point, these cells under stress will burst, and then we have what is called a pro-inflammatory state, with recruitment of macrophages that promote inflammation exceeding that of cells that promote an anti-inflammatory response. More natural killer cells appear, and circulation decreases. There is less development of new blood vessels, more fibrosis, and low oxygen concentration (hypoxia), so less fat tissue is in contact with blood, and blood oxygen becomes abnormal.[7]

It is also well known that in response to food intake and other external pressures, the adipocytes can increase their size up to tenfold to store fat, but if more food is provided, another process can also happen: New and dormant cells will develop, and once they develop, they will be there forever, manifesting as an increase in our body size. If we try to lose weight, their contents may empty, but they will remain as cells.[8] Meanwhile, our

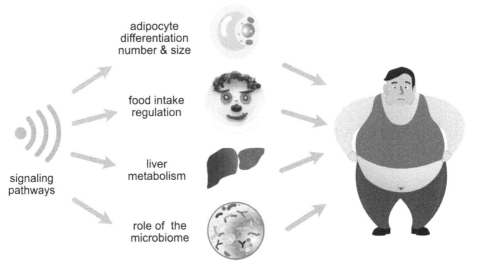

Fig. 11.1 Factors Influencing Your Individual Body Size

brain is going to protect them at whatever price, as well as the stores of fat, since they are vital for the brain's function and development.

FAT TISSUE
Endocrine Organ and Fascia

Regarding attempts to correlate fascia with the endocrine organ of adipose tissue, recent studies show that fascia can be converted into adipocytes or cells of the adipose tissue. It is something to be studied and understood in more detail. But under the guiding light of ayurveda, I would like to hypothesize that in a state of lack of awareness of the process of eating, digestion, and absorption, if there is not a presence of the self, then the feeling of satiety is not there.

When we are not actively participating in food intake and all the other digestive processes, the resulting effect is stress within the fascia network. Fascia, to keep its integrity, stability, and balance of the whole body, will try to compromise in the face of the external pressure of overeating conditions, which generate more fatty acid molecules that the body has to find a way to store. We are genetically predetermined to have a certain number of fat cells. As evolution shows us, after thousands of years of being exposed to cycles of seasons and other cyclical processes, we've learned to protect our bodies from dying of starvation by storing fat in our adipose organ, constituted by adipocytes.

Under pressure from the considerable accumulation of fat, the intelligent fascia feels obliged to generate or create more fat cells, in trying to assure the integrity of our body as a whole. These new fat cells will start integrating and storing all types of fat molecules, including lipids such as triglycerides and cholesterol, which dislike water. The consequence or problem created by this situation is that these new cells have memory of their existence—they were and are, by definition, part of the fascia network at origin—so they know about being recruited to fulfill the imbalance caused by our lack of connection of our real physiological needs, and now they would like to remain where they are. That is how the process of becoming overweight begins. It is easy to understand why, under conditions of morbid obesity, the fascia can no longer support the extreme excess of fat, and the tissues, including the fascia, collapse in a way that we can see it easily.

If a person becomes aware of their body imbalance and decides to address the issue, would like to reduce weight, and follows a diet or eats less, then during that process the lipocytes or fat cells will gradually empty themselves, a process that begins with the newcomers, moving all the way down to the cells that were programmed from the beginning of our lives. Yet while these newcomer cells may become empty now, they will remain within our tissues, always dormant—willing to become active and full again, ready to collaborate, always with the memory of experience.

If one really would like to address the relationship between our tissues and being overweight or obese, diet is a very important factor, but it's also essential to connect to the fascia's network and try to reprogram it in parallel to other aspects of lifestyle. Our regular daily life events are always linear based on repetitions or cycles of the process of overeating, which in today's society is more or less considered "normal."

So many times, scientists have asserted that certain phenomena did not exist because *they could not exist*. There are so many biomedical enigmas regarding how our bodies function at a molecular and cellular level, and at the same time so many preconceptions and taboos. Perhaps by surrendering to things we simply cannot figure out, we could relax the grip of our taboos. For my part, I have the deep impression that through practices such as meditation, relaxation, mindfulness, or whatever name we give to that introspective process of finding harmony within oneself, we are, in a very simple way, engaging in total communication with the fascia.

Manifestations from the mind are always linear, especially when eating food: "more or less," "I like, or I dislike." To create a proper level of perception of what one is eating, one has to develop a vertical observation, and within that verticality there is an inner observer.

If one would like to communicate with the whole fascia network, an acute sense of presence of the body's verticality (involving different levels or stages of this hierarchy or process) is required. This vertical communication could be possible through inner awareness and connection to our body-mind systems that are integrated by the fascia. The only infallible sensor we have is our body, not our mind. Unfortunately, the general pattern of the mind is to get lost in mental schemes, illusions, rationalizations, projections, etc. These are repetitive horizontal processes resulting from our identification with food (likes and dislikes) avidity, and so on. The way to start this dissociation from the "normal" pattern of the mind and connect to a more expansive version of ourselves is through real awareness of the fascia processes and their interconnection with the other systems in our bodies. Our minds and bodies could work together with the natural vertical processes as a new state of awareness. Under these circumstances, we could sense the changes from our efforts to rebalance our body-mind and go beyond repetitive horizontal associations with food, and life.

12

THE FASCIA

The "Fascia-nating" Invisible Living Strings

Our bodies can perform all kinds of physical feats such as running, skiing, or dancing. We celebrate our more than 600 muscles for their complex activities, but we do not give credit to fascia, most probably for lack of knowledge of what it does. For hundreds of years, medicine considered it an uninteresting filler tissue, and when medics were learning anatomy, they "dissolved" it away to better visualize the body organs they were studying without considering the important connection between our organs and fascia.

Today's understanding is different, and fascia is considered a main sensory organ in its own right, with some distinctive physical qualities that are still very much under-researched. We are going to look at its connection with other organ systems such as the lymph, gut, and body mass, including muscles, adipose tissue, and bones, and how imbalance in these interactions could be the cause of metabolic disorders such as obesity.

Let me describe fascia here, as many people are unaware of its existence, let alone its properties and function. Fascia can be defined as a huge network within a specialized thin sheath of fibrous or connective tissue that surrounds, supports, protects, and holds in place our organs, blood vessels, bones, nerve fibers, and muscles. It makes your body an absolute anatomic, functional continuum, capable of processing mechanic and metabolic communication and actions (physical force and effort), emotions and perceptions (reacting in the face of aggression), and other sensations.

In particular, fascia can be seen as a network of awareness within your body, protecting your balanced functional integrity from the very minor aspects of internal cellular activities and cellular and tissue interactions. For example, it connects muscle to skin and to all kinds of nerve endings, helping us to sense our bodies in space as well as what happens within. Since fascia is directly involved in all these processes as well as protecting your vital organs, it can have different compositions depending on the organ. For example, the fascia of skin and muscles has a particular structural constitution, composition, and elasticity designed to protect us externally as well as to shield our internal, more vital organs, while another type of fascia plays the role of supporting the organs within the different corporal cavities.[1] In other words, fascia is a system of integration; it is the network of awareness of our body since it has nerves that make it almost as sensitive as skin. The following diagram shows the different cells and tissues that originate from both mesodermal and ectodermal layers, which together comprise the fascial system:

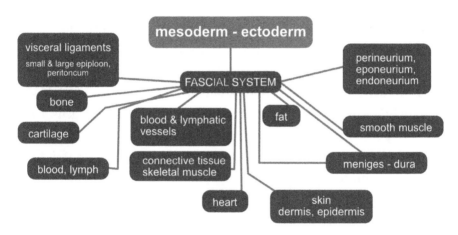

Fig. 12.1. Fascial System

UNDERSTANDING FASCIA

The fascial continuum involves both solid fascia and liquid fascia connecting our entire body with amazing dynamic and elastic properties. The new understanding of the fascia system is that fascia surrounds each of our forty trillion cells. We could visualize it as a kind of extracellular skeleton, an extension of the cell membrane that connects cells with every other cell membrane around them, in a similar way to how the intracellular skeleton communicates in the interior of cells. In other words, your internal fascia is everywhere; there is not a blood vessel, muscle, or organ that is not connected to or surrounded by it.

Fascia is one of the major types of supportive connective tissue, along with ligaments and tendons, all of which are mostly made up of stretchy packs of two proteins called collagen and elastin. These tissues are suspended in what is called the ground substance—a liquid, gelatinous goo—and their function is to keep us together and help us move around. Even among this supportive connective tissue, our ligaments and tendons mostly serve the metabolic role of transferring energy between muscles and bones by being strong and stretchy. Fascia does the same and more. For example, the connecting fascia in your foot that joins your heel to your toes also operates as a lubricant; it can be present between the muscle fibers within a muscle and also surrounding the whole muscle, helping to guarantee that your muscles can fully contract and at the same time avoid damage from friction when flexing.

Scientist are studying the different kinds of fascia to understand its many mechanical properties. In general, the stretchy collagen fibers and fascia are woven in mesh-like layers, but in some areas, these meshes are more tightly woven or contain more or different types of collagens. Fascia is also responsible for making organs and muscles slide against each other, and at the same time it is highly integrated with nerve endings, so it forms communication networks in the body. Fascia can stick together and can become a kind of glue: wherever fascia becomes stuck and glued, there is a lack of movement, and where there's no movement, there is the sensation of pain. It is not clear how many different types of fascial tissue exist, but fascia's ability to transfer from one state to another is truly incredible—it does so by changing its material properties and acting as a lubricant. When the tissue needs to be slick and slippery, it can basically liquefy, and if the tissue needs to be more rigid, it can take on a more gel-like form.[2]

As a summary, concerning fascia's behavior, there are three different views: The first is the thixotropic effect, which states that when stressed, fascia becomes more liquid, made so by the ground substance. The second view describes it as liquid crystal, similar to many solid crystals. When pressure is applied, an electrical charge moves throughout, and that charge movement could trigger the cells in the tissue to make or break down important components such as collagen. The third view points to mechanic sensors, special neural receptors sensing stretch or pressure. When activated they can tell muscle cells to relax, contract, constrain, or dilate blood vessels, and in that way move fluid around to adjust thickness.

Of course, more research is needed to determine which is the most accurate view, but the fact that fascia manages to transform from solid to liquid shows us that it is doing more than simply holding us together. It is interesting that, while it was considered for hundreds of years to be a filler, nowadays scientists think fascia may play all kinds of roles that remain poorly understood. These roles include providing an immune response or hormonal signal: since fascia surrounds all our organs, these signals cross our entire body and play a large functional part in all metabolic and cellular processes. Fascia is also one giant sensory organ that operates throughout our body and is filled with mechanic sensors. Its role in proprioception, or the ability to sense where our body parts are in space, is currently being studied. As well, fascia plays a possibly vital role in the skill of sensing what's going on inside our body, known as interoception.

Further, fascia enables contractibility, or the ability to contract or dilate blood vessels linked to the autonomic nervous system that unconsciously regulates internal organs' activities, including those of the gut, bladder, and secretory glands. Under certain conditions, fascia can also be the origin of non-fascia types of cells; even mechanical engineers are interested in fascia due to its biomechanical properties.

The workings of fascia may provide an explanation for various diseases and disorders, including psychological disorders—studies suggest that fascia plays a role in how we regulate our emotions and how we store trauma memories, since it sends our brain relevant information concerning the location of organs and condition of our body.[3] Fascia is also under study for its role in disorders such as fibromyalgia and chronic pain, due to the great number of pain receptors and the swelling of fascia (fasciitis), which could cause tenacious pain. Chronic pain is biochemical, but it is also psychological. Today's treatments need to address these two components and reconsider the real origins of pain.[4]

Concerning structure and function, we can infer that fascia produces intracellular, extracellular, and biomechanical responses in many body systems, and the stratification of collagen depends on where the fascia is found. Since every organ has a fascia wrapping, and these wrappings connect all structures in the human body, fascia gives our body its shape and support, and at the same time acts as a shock absorber due to its elasticity. For these reasons it is considered a "sliding" organ that regulates fluid flow in the extracellular matrix and is highly innervated. Fascia as a cellular tissue is nourishing, but it also requires nourishment. What metabolic role is played in terms of the kinds of molecules it is transporting? What happens when the fluids from the blood or the lymph, and everything they carry, are not flowing properly, and the relocation of byproducts or functional waste is accumulating? Do they then start to accumulate in the fascia?

It is quite logical to think that if there is proper flow, our cells, tissues, and organs are happy, healthy, and youthful. This is one of the main ayurvedic principles of balance. Unfortunately, this balance is rare nowadays; today's lifestyle challenges us all the time and we are not even conscious of it. Physically, we are not conscious of our posture, and we move without seeking alignment with ourselves. We all exist under the law of gravity, which is holding us here, but we are not really aware of what gravity permanently does to our physical body, including our fascia. Metabolically, in general, we are not necessarily conscious of what we eat. We are also not conscious of our breath. Yet all these external pressures to our different body systems affect the way we think. As a consequence, we become unbalanced and sick.

Another interesting observation from the ayurvedic scholars is the description of seven kinds of kalas (fascia) and their functions as mechanical supports but also as membranes with special roles.[5]

IS FASCIA THE GENESIS OF ADIPOSE TISSUE?

The adipose tissue as an "organ" and the described distinct types of adipocytes are integrated with the vascular, immune, neural, and extracellular connective tissue systems, playing many specific roles. Carobbio et al. described the several features of the variety of adipose tissue deposits, including their origins, cellular composition, plasticity, and capability of expansion under both balanced and unbalanced conditions, all of which are essential for maintaining proper metabolic function.[6]

However, when the adipose depots become disturbed as a consequence of continual fat or nutrient surplus, metabolic complications manifest, negatively affecting the proper roles and activities of the adipose tissue, which include its expandability and functional metabolic flexibility. In parallel, the global metabolic equilibrium processes are affected, such as thermoregulation by body weight (BWT). More studies seeking a better understanding of the three adipose tissues are required to develop curative methodologies for pathological conditions.[7]

We've described how the fascia system is a link between all body systems. The role of the fascia system and its connections with the nervous system and adipose tissue are still under scientific study, and embryological exploration could offer more evidence about the earlier configuration between the neuronal network and visceral fascia, from the tongue to the ending portion of the digestive tract. The results suggest that, firstly, fat cells (adipocytes) gradually emerge from the superficial fascia, which is able to provide the molecular precursors to induce spontaneous fat cell differentiation. Secondly, fascial adipocytes display distinct expressions of some proteins able to propel and break down fat, but a low response to catecholamines (adrenaline or noradrenaline). And lastly, a new population of white adipocytes originates from fascia.[8]

This last finding suggests a new understanding of the origin of adipocytes, and how the adipose tissue grows. Adipose precursor cells resident in fascia have been recognized, and these fascial preadipocytes make adipose cells to create primitive forms in superficial fascia.[9]

The understanding of the associate mechanisms between obesity and type 2 diabetes could be grounded in epidemiological evidence; however, the fundamental mechanism associating these two common, pandemic disorders is not clearly understood. Rather than obesity, malfunction of the adipose tissue's expandability due to genetic and environmental factors is hypothesized to be the central issue when trying to understand altered lipid accumulations.[10]

THE LYMPHATICS
....
The Hidden and Efficient Janitor

UNDERSTANDING THE LYMPHATIC SYSTEM
(RASA VAHA SROTAS)

Ayurvedic scientists considered the lymphatic system to be one of the most important body organ systems to be evaluated and treated. They studied its signs, symptoms, and functions, and described protocols for detoxification and nourishment. As well, they used longevity therapies called *rasayana* to treat the lymph, which they called rasa (from the Sanskrit root *ras* meaning "to go" or "continual flowing"); these therapies are still practiced today and have remained largely unchanged over the centuries. Rasa dhatu is considered the first tissue or dhatu channel carrying rasa, described as rasa vaha srotas, which includes plasma—the yellowish, fluid part of the blood that carries the blood cells—and lymphatic components.

Following the proper digestion of food, all the other body tissues (dhatus) are nourished by a healthy rasa dhatu, via channels carrying the lymph. Lymph can travel through all the subtle body channels due to its main content, the water element. Ayurveda described two types of channels in our body: *sthayi* or static tissues, and *asthayi rasa* or channels that carry the circulating nutrients for nourishment.

Let us consider ancient wisdom on the lymph and lymphatic system, while also drawing on the modern scientific exposition to improve our understanding and combine ayurvedic knowledge and modern science in a way that supports us in keeping our body systems in a state of balance and endurance. According to the ancient scholars, ingested food is fully digested with the support of agni. When it's finally assimilated in our body, it produces a milky-white fluid that forms in the small intestine during digestion, made of lymph fluid and fats, called lymph chyle (a mixture of lymph and chylomicrons) or rasa. This fluid can vary in its consistency depending on the type and quantity of foods eaten, the time of the food intake, and it forms the essence of the assimilated food. This lymphatic fluid is drained into the lymph channels and goes to the lymph nodes, where rasa is purified with support from the white cells of the immune system. The purified rasa, after traveling and being filtered through our approximately 600 lymphatic nodes, flows back to the heart or spleen, where it joins the blood system, continuing the journey of our digestion.

> *Humans are derived from the nutrient fluid (rasa) which*
> *should be protected prudently by the wise by keeping*
> *vigilance of foods, drinks, and regime.*
>
> Su. Sa. Su. 14/12

Biomedical scientists are now exploring the lymphatic system in more detail and are starting to appreciate its extensive role. They are developing instruments to measure its flow,[1] and they describe lymph—from the Latin *lympha*, meaning "connected to water"—as the colorless fluid or plasma containing immune cells, fats, proteins, and extra fluid, which flows through your lymph nodes, glands that are part of the lymphatic system.

The lymphatic and blood systems are our body's two main circulatory systems. The lymphatic system is an efficient, intricate, vital organ system that helps the blood, immune, and digestive systems, and whose functions are in some cases poorly understood even today. The lymph moves with the nerves, arteries, and veins, and by itself is twice the size of the arterial blood supply system. It is our body's biggest drain or channel filter, made of millions of tiny lymph vessels—channels structurally very similar to blood vessels, lined by endothelial cells, a thin layer of smooth muscle and adventitia. The lymphatic system contains around 500 to 700 lymph nodes distributed throughout the body. Its three main functions include, firstly, maintenance of blood volume balance and removal of cellular debris by redirecting extra fluid from the tissues to the central circulation, to compensate and regulate via a one-way network of vessels that drain lymph fluid from all over the body. Secondly, the lymphatic system helps the immune system fight infection, using surveillance by the lymphatic organs to identify and filter, via lymphocytes, all harmful microorganisms and toxicants. And thirdly, it helps the digestive system by transporting large food molecules, such as proteins and chyle (big fats), from the small intestine to the blood system, and delivering energy to the body in the form of fatty acids or other molecules.

For these reasons, it is very important to keep the lymphatic system unclogged. Just like the oil filter in your car, if it has not been changed or cleaned regularly, it will get dirty and clog up, decreasing its efficiency. The same situation can happen in our body systems, and will manifest first as swelling. Our lymph tissue is located in the following main body regions: the bone marrow, spleen, thymus gland, lymph nodes, adenoids, and tonsils. Other organs containing lymphatic tissue are the heart, lungs, intestines, liver, and skin. But the most significant locations of this lymphoid tissue are in the throat area; the intestinal area, where it is called Peyer's patches; and in the appendix, also known as the vermiform appendix.

HOW THE LYMPHATIC SYSTEM WORKS

Our lymphatic system regulates fluids, and filters harmful microorganisms from the blood by a tubular network via water motion or osmotic pressure, and muscular contractions, since it is not connected to the heart's pumping mechanism. Unlike the blood vessels that are connected by a network of capillaries allowing blood to flow as it circulates around the body, the lymphatic vessels do not allow backflow—the fluid only moves in one direction and is divided into superficial and deep lymphatic vessels. It only moves when our bodies move; in particular, the movement of the skeletal and muscular systems allows the lymph to flow. This one-way street begins with the tissues, where it collects watery liquid called interstitial fluid, then dumps it into the cardiovascular system at the other end; this process is responsible for draining up to 85 percent of this fluid, which originates from plasma filtration. The other 15 percent of the interstitial fluid remains behind in what is called the interstitial space, the narrow space between cells and tissues, where the lymphatic system is located. This process solves a problem, as our bloodstream certainly cannot continuously lose so much volume. Luckily, we have the lymphatic system, which collects and returns excess interstitial fluid to the bloodstream via the lymph capillaries, and this becomes lymph fluid. It enters the lymphatic vessels that pass by the lymph nodes, the places where macrophages destroy pathogens. Lastly, these vessels converge into large trunks known as the thoracic ducts, which drain into the heart, returning the lymph to circulation.

Our lymphatic capillaries can become two kinds of vessels: superficial vessels located just below the skin layer, collecting lymph from the superficial structures of the body; or deeper lymphatic vessels that carry lymph from internal organs, assisted by their allies the arteries, lending pressure to the lymphatics and thus allowing lymphatic flow to occur.

The cells that surround our lymphatic capillaries, known as endothelial cells, are connected in a very loose fashion. They form flaps that encourage the entry of fluid, proteins, and larger particles such as bacteria and other pathogens, and then prevent them from leaving. This is the normal journey for our fluids in the body, from the blood to the tissues, some to the lymphatics, and back to the blood. When our lymph vessels are congested, removed, or damaged, it can instigate a buildup of fluid, and this can cause swelling conditions known as lymphedema.

Recent findings tell us that along the inner digestive tract, we have what is called the lacteal lymphatic system, small finger-like projections playing the crucial role of absorbing compounds such as proteins, fats, as well as toxic products from the intestinal tract and into the lymph. If the outer membranes of our intestinal lining become aggravated, the gut-associated lymphoid tissue (GALT), which is the lymph around the gut, can get congested. Environmental toxins, fats, and undigested proteins like gluten and casein can overcharge the lymph and slowly congest the lymphatic system.[2]

Further, it is known that our gut is the place where most of the body's immune system resides, so if our lymph becomes congested due to factors such as stress or poor digestion, it will affect our beneficial intestinal microbiome, and then our entire lymphatic system can become congested. More recent discoveries show that our central nervous system also has a lymphatic drainage system called the glymphatic system, which supports healthy immunity, regulates inflammation, and modulates our emotional temperament.[3, 4]

AYURVEDIC INSIGHT

Can We Tap into the Power of the Lymphatic System for Weight Loss?

According to ayurveda, the described glymphatic system corresponds to one of the features of kapha dosha, termed *tarpaka kapha*, which has the function of literally draining toxins from the brain into the cerebral spinal fluid.[5] Under circumstances of imbalance due to congestion of the channels, a person's temperament could shift, brain recollection could be compromised, and the brain functions may become unclear. Among the causes of this imbalance, we can include continuous lack of sleep, cumulative impact of stress, weak digestion, and emotional trauma.

We know that when our lymphatic system is not working correctly, it causes swelling, which can be emotionally distressing, socially stigmatizing, and difficult to understand. In cases of weight gain or obesity, swelling may be a trauma issue.

Other studies have shown that obesity stimulates lymphatic irregularities, such as reduced initial lymphatic density, increased lymphatic leakiness, and other changes.[6] Moreover, the latest studies suggest that lack of regulation of the lymphatic system triggers the progress of multiple sclerosis (MS), encouraging obesity and insulin resistance.[7]

The relationship between obesity and type 2 diabetes is epidemiologically strong, but the underlying mechanisms have not yet been fully elucidated. One prevailing theory is that of adipose tissue expandability. This theory states that a malfunction in the capability for adipose tissue expansion (metabolic dysregulation)—rather than obesity by itself—is the key factor involving type 2 diabetes and the storage of excess calories in the subcutaneous adipose tissue.[8]

It is remarkable that ayurvedic scholars thousands of years ago understood the therapeutic value of addressing the fat tissue with thermic anti-obesity and antidiabetic approaches, which were described as part of the panchakarma protocols, such as *svedana* and *udvartana*—very common treatments in ayurvedic hospitals in India and abroad. These thermogenic regulator techniques have great potential for actively addressing obesity and require further investigation. Today's scientists are trying to target the regulators of thermogenic adipose tissue—composed of beige and brown adipocytes—in order to seek the restoration of its functionality and energetic distribution. We will be covering these very interesting protocols in another section (see pages 252–55).

Obesity predisposes individuals toward several chronic diseases. Total adiposity and BMI are deeply interrelated with cardiovascular and metabolic ailments that endanger our populations. You should consider that your waist measurement, more than your BMI, may be a better indicator of cardiovascular disease predisposition. Proper metabolic phenotyping of obese people will be very helpful for comprehension, prevention, and treatment of this condition, opening new avenues for addressing physiological imbalances such as cardiovascular and metabolic diseases.[9]

If you are feeling "chubby" or "weighty" and you visit your doctor for a general blood test, they could eventually tell you that within your lipid profile, LDL cholesterol, or lipoprotein (a), for example, is above the standard or normal value. The next step is a seemingly guaranteed prescription of drugs, such as statins, to bring it down and thus prevent a cardiovascular condition. Why opt to bring down your lipid profile to the standard values with medications that have side effects, when alterations to your lifestyle and diet could achieve the same result without medication? If we leave aside the question of the real normal value of cholesterol, or how we define those standards, we still must ask ourselves: Why is there a cholesterol imbalance in the first place? Could the high cholesterol be connected to defective drainage of the lymphatic system? Could the causes for that ineffectiveness be external and internal stress?

Well, according to ayurveda, a sluggish immunity, as well as a deficient process of waste elimination in which poor agni, digestion, and elimination of unwanted metabolites create potential ama, are the chief causes of unhealthy aging and early deterioration.

Ayurveda also described the use of adaptogen herbs such as brahmi (*Bacopa monnieri* Linn.), manjistha (*Rubia cordifolia*), and ginger root (*Zingiber officinale*) to remove toxins, detoxifying the lymphatic system and balancing the three doshas. These herbs also help support the immune system, and they have antimicrobial, anti-inflammatory, antipyretic, and antioxidant properties. In conjunction with the use of these herbs, it is crucial to adopt an anti-inflammatory diet based on wholesome products such as fresh fruits, vegetables, whole grains, healthy fats, and spices, in order to facilitate proper flushing of lymphatic fluids and increase the elimination of ama. Also relevant is the role of stress and the way we respond to it, which affects the lymphatic flow as well as our life flow. Let's allow flow (vayu) in our lives to boost an active rasa.

We previously described that the main drainage system we have in our bodies is the lymphatic system. It is comparable to the drains in your home, and blood is like the taps on your sink, or your toilet's flushing mechanism. If the drains in your home get clogged, you will not only need to clean the taps but also the drains themselves. If we do not regularly clean the bodily system properly (allowing vyana vayu movements), it can end up clogged for months or even years, and the process of detoxification will get disturbed, making it harder to conduct waste elimination. The loss of efficiency will end up negatively affecting our well-being and longevity.[10]

Now that we know about the links between congested brain lymph, immunity, mood disposition, and inflammatory concerns that relate to both our body and mind, we can ask ourselves about the association with our long-term cognitive function, and what can be done to maintain proper flow. Well, if we would like to keep the lymph fluid flowing, it is recommended that we drink sufficient water; limit exposure to wireless radiation; avoid cow dairy products, for mucus production; wear comfortable clothes, so as to avoid unnecessary pressure; maintain good food quality; reduce unnecessary chemical load; and process our emotions, thus eliminating chemical and mental toxins.

I describe, in appendix 3, a protocol that is supportive of the activation of the lymphatic system: body self-massage. At all ages, we need to detoxify our bodies in a dynamic way, but especially when we start aging. At this point in our lives, we require more efficient elimination of toxins for our body-mind well-being, optimal health, and longevity.

THE VAGUS NERVE

······································

The Master of Ceremonies

OUR CHANCE TO WANDER AND RELAX!

The Western scientific community has acknowledged a body-mind connection for some time, and it was notably discussed by Charles Darwin in 1872. Darwin described the gastric vagus nerve as an essential part of our PSNS and called it the "nerve of emotion."[1] Ancient Eastern civilizations have had the knowledge of this connection for thousands of years and have succeeded in developing some great techniques to help modulate the mind through the body and vice versa. This occurs via our extraordinary nervous system made of more than one hundred billion nerve cells, which releases data from the brain to the rest of the body, then accepts the data that returns again.

The vagus nerve is one of the most important integrated controls for bidirectional communication between the brain and body organ systems. It is also called cranial nerve X or the tenth cranial nerve, the most complex and longest of the twelve pairs of cranial nerves. The pair arises from the CNS in the cranium (brain stem), and travels bidirectionally to the sacral region, carrying 80 percent of the PSNS functions. In simple words, it runs from the brain through the face and thorax to the abdomen, and the "cables" or nerves are a mix of PSNS fibers.[2] Perhaps you've heard a mention of the vagus nerve but are not aware of its functions and how vital it is for our lives—so let me tell you about it. The following information will be very helpful to you for connecting the dots between the gut, metabolic disorders, and other body-mind imbalances.

The name *vagus* comes from the Latin *vaga* and means the "wandering nerve," which describes its wide distribution throughout the body, regulating essential internal organ functions. After weaving its way through your body, it ultimately ends up in your cranium, passing through your neck and branching off past the outer edge of your ear. This wandering, long cranial nerve forms the link between the CNS and the body, supplying nerves to major visceral organs such as the GIT, heart, and lungs. It exercises control of a vast array of involuntary body processes such as digestion, heart rate, and respiratory rate, as well as affecting the narrowing and widening of the blood vessels, or vasomotor activities; certain reflex actions such as swallowing, coughing, sneezing, and vomiting; and other actions that include hearing, speaking, tasting, bladder movement, orgasms, and fertility.

The vagus nerve plays a key role in communication between the gut and brain, an integral part of the gut-brain axis, which also involves another essential player: the gut bacteria. In discussing this interaction, we consider the gut bacteria, the vagus nerve, and the central nervous system as they monitor metabolic processes. Notably, approximately 80 percent of the nerve fibers or afferent fibers of the vagus nerve are responsible for transmitting signals from the gut to the brain, rather than the reverse. The vagus nerve is a real vagabond! The other 20 percent of fibers send information down into the body. The sensory fibers of the vagus nerve detect in real time information from the liver, pancreas, gallbladder, and small intestine, based on the presence of molecules called metabolites—that is, the hormones and enzymes that participate in the breakdown of any food that one has consumed.[3, 4]

But perhaps are we forgetting something in this whole process? Does this "vagabond" vagus nerve pass via the heart in the direction of the brain? And what connections, implications, and potential imbalances could result?

We human beings form an emotional or sensitive brain long before we create a logical or rational one—and before we acquire either, we have a beating heart. The heart has been viewed as the source of emotion, courage, and wisdom for centuries. I believe that the vagus system is the connecting cord or hormone highway of our emotions, allowing a flood through our body's various systems in the form of hormones and neural messages. We all know the physical meaning of phrases such as "having a broken heart," "going with your gut," and "feeling a flutter in the stomach." Each of these represent the ways emotions manifest in different parts of our bodies. The reason for these sensations is simple: our stomachs, guts, and hearts all contain within their cells' membranes tiny structures formed from proteins called neuroreceptors, which are designed to accept information and become activated by chemicals on the outside of the cell, known as neurotransmitters.

Innovative studies, mostly unfamiliar outside the fields of psychophysiology and neurocardiology, show that beyond its vital role as a sustaining life pump, the heart is also a gateway to a source of insight and intelligence that we can call upon. In this way, we connect to enhanced creative and intuitive capacities that are vital for a balanced body-mind, improving the rapport between our inner and outer selves and providing us a healthy life filled with serenity and joy.

Studies have looked at how stressful emotions affect the activity in the autonomic nervous system (ANS) and the hormonal and immune systems, as well as the effects of emotions such as appreciation, compassion, and care. Results show a consistent association with heart rate variability or heart rhythms, which stand out as the most dynamic and reflective indicators of one's emotional state and, therefore, one's stress and cognitive processes. Stressful or draining emotions, such as being overwhelmed or frustrated, lead to increased disorder in the higher-level brain centers and ANS. This disorder is then reflected in the heart rhythms, adversely affecting the function of virtually all bodily systems.

How does the heart work? Nowadays, we understand that it has its own independent, complex nervous system known as "the brain in the heart," and studies have indicated that the heart communicates with our brain and body in four ways:

- ▼ biologically, or biochemically, via hormones and neurotransmitters
- ▼ electrochemically, or neurologically, across the transmission of nerve impulses

▼ gravitationally, or biophysically, via pressure waves

▼ magnetically, or energetically, through electromagnetic field exchanges

A properly functioning vagus nerve permits us to approach the areas of the brain accountable for creativity, higher cognition, and multifaceted decision making. If our vagus nerve is imbalanced, we mostly have access to the parts of our brain that control primal instincts such as fear and fight-or-flight response, via our sympathetic system. Consequently, a healthy vagus nerve is essential for leadership and decision making. However, the functioning of the vagus nerve can be impacted by conditions such as stress, anxiety, and poor lifestyle, which may include lack of exercise, overwork, improper nutrition and sleep, and habits such as smoking and drinking alcohol. When we engage in such behaviors, we cannot function to the best of our ability. If we do not "digest and rest," the body-mind connection becomes susceptible to a variety of ailments, including digestive disorders, obesity, diabetes, cardiovascular disorders, hypertension, chronic inflammation, kidney malfunction, infertility, Parkinson's disease, and many other dysfunctions linked with anxiety and depression.

The signals from the vagus nerve come mostly from outside stimuli—in other words, they are 80 percent afferent. They carry information from the heart and other internal organs to the brain, telling the brain what they are sensing, such as temperature. Signals from the "heart brain" are redirected to brain areas such as the medulla, hypothalamus, thalamus, amygdala, and the cerebral cortex, showing us that the heart sends more signals to the brain than the other way around.[5]

The vagus nerve also brings information from other internal organs, signaling between our brain, liver, GIT, and heart. For instance, its altered function can affect the stomach's muscular movements, causing gastroparesis, or can trigger fainting from low blood pressure (vasovagal syncope) in some individuals. In other words, the stomach and the heart are related, and stomach issues can mimic or cause heart issues such as palpitations and chest pain.

In parallel, a functional relationship between the gut microbiome and the heart circadian rhythm—known as cardiac vagal nerve activity (CVA)—has been demonstrated. Twenty-four-hour CVA was evaluated for adult female participants, and their stool samples were analyzed to investigate CVA's connection with gut microbiome diversity. The results indicated that CVA is associated with gut microbiome patterns in women.[6]

Despite the fact that we don't currently have a deeper scientific understanding or explanation for how and why heart activity affects mental clarity, creativity, emotional balance, intuition, and personal effectiveness, it is nevertheless clear that we are not observing a simple pump. Instead, the heart is an information processing center with its own functional brain, the heart brain. This system communicates with and influences the cranial brain via the nervous system, hormonal system, and other pathways, and its effects on brain function, as well as most of the body's major organs, play a critical role in our body, mind, and emotional experiences, impacting the quality of our lives.

Today's mainstream medicine is developing internal, implantable electroceutical devices that discharge electric impulses to hack the vagus nerve, trying to increase its activity to aid with body imbalances such as migraines, headaches, depression, and epilepsy. These interesting passive devices could be quite invasive and lead to side effects, and their effectiveness is still under study.[7]

STIMULATING THE VAGUS NERVE
Yoga and Ayurvedic Protocols

Unlike such modern approaches, ayurveda offers natural ways to stimulate the vagus nerve with protocols such as breathing exercises (pranayama); meditation; yoga; diets tailored for your gut; exercise, particularly long walks; and massages that focus on acupressure or marma points, some of which are described at the end of this chapter (see pages 174–76). Let us address one of these techniques here, with a short description that you can practice— and through which you'll observe the role of one of the powerful yoga and ayurvedic practices, strengthening the vagus nerve via breathing techniques.

You can control your own breathing consciously and affect the PSNS. This is one of the most effective ways to stimulate the vagus nerve and has positively impacted millions of people around the world for thousands of years. For example, when you are in stress mode, your breathing is modified; typically, you are breathing in slowly but breathing out very shallowly, and mostly through your mouth. The following exercise may help if, at nighttime, you are trying to sleep and have difficulty, or if you'd just like to calm your nervous system down.

🌿 Breathing Exercise

First, slowly breathe in for four seconds, through the nose. Take a pause for two seconds, and then slowly breathe out for six seconds. That will decrease your breathing rate, aiding relaxation and improving vagal nerve tone. Just by doing this for a few minutes, you'll calm down the nervous system, feel more relaxed, and most probably fall asleep easily.

When you practice this simple breathing exercise, or a more detailed pranayama, your breathing and heart rate slow down. The vagus nerve can collect signals from the various body organs, and then, when your body realizes that things are calmer and more restful, it will pass on this message to the brain. Your brain then listens and allows you to digest physical and mental impressions, enabling you to relax and rest.

Some studies show that regular practice of pranayama activates the vagus nerve, which has been shown to significantly relieve depression, decrease the release of cortisol, and reduce anxiety. It also improves deep sleep and hormones that contribute to well-being.[9]

Due to the activation of the vagus nerve, you can experience benefits after regular practice of pranayama, enjoying outcomes such as stress resilience, enhanced immunity, happiness, creativity, and better relationship with yourself and the others—all of which are very helpful to one's ability to handle challenging situations.[10]

Despite today's understanding of all the above, the vagus nerve is a continued subject of study.[11, 12] Even with all these investigations, the body continues to surprise us with its subtle ways and functions in relation to love and compassion, sense of connection, intuition, and our mental and physical well-being. All these factors are integral parts of a balanced life, and they are incentivized and better connected if we keep our vagus nerve properly nurtured.

CAN WE TAP INTO THE POWER OF THE
VAGUS NERVE FOR WEIGHT LOSS?

There is limited knowledge available on the role of the vagus nerve in regulating metabolism and weight loss, and controlling diabetes. However, a recent study shows that the vagus nerve senses the states of insulin resistance, stimulating beta cell proliferation in the pancreas by producing a chemical or neurotransmitter called acetylcholine. In states of insulin resistance, when an individual is experiencing what is called metabolic syndrome, there is an increased demand on the body to produce insulin. The vagus nerve then gets stimulated, and it causes the beta cells to produce insulin so they can proliferate. It was also observed that individuals who have vagus nerve stimulation induced by vagus nerve stimulation (VNS) artificial devices, as a treatment for their epilepsy and depression, saw the side effect of unintentional weight gain. This shows that the vagus nerve potentially plays a role in weight management or weight regulation.[13]

Due to the global rise in obesity, there is a growing demand for efficacious, safe, and accessible treatments. Neuromodulation interventions such as deep brain stimulation (DBS), transcranial magnetic stimulation (TMS), transcranial direct current stimulation (tDCS), percutaneous neurostimulation (PENS), vagus nerve stimulation (VNS), and gastric electrical stimulation (GES), have all been proposed as novel therapies. However, a systematic review sought to examine the safety and efficacy of neuromodulation therapies in reducing body weight in patients with obesity in sixty clinical trials found that none of these treatments induced a striking reduction of body weight due to the complexity and multifactorial nature of obesity.[14]

PRACTICES FOR METABOLISM STIMULATION
BY ACTIVATING YOUR VAGUS NERVE

It is possible to rewire ourselves and reduce stress, induce parasympathetic activation, and encourage our metabolism in a number of ways, without involving external devices. These practices include:

breathing: responsible for helping the lungs to fill up fully and to relax

meditation: balances and rests your body-mind system and increases the activities of the genes responsible for self-regulation and healing

cold water therapy: cold showers or washing your face with cold water, which activates what is call the mammalian dive reflex, a fight-or-flight instinct

hot/cold therapy: skin, being our largest organ, responds to alternating hot and cold showers as a stimulant and can have its tactile sensitivity activated via therapeutic touch or simply touch alone

gargling: stimulates the vagus nerve since it assists the throat muscles

singing and chanting: benefit vagus tone by prolonging the exhale and thus allowing the nervous system to relax. Singing also allows us to express the joys of our heart

pranayama or vocalization: variety of breathing exercises such as humming the bumblebee sound, and *ujjayi* ("victorious breath"), are examples of beneficial breath control practices to stimulate vagal tone. Devotional sounds often come from Sanskrit mantras such as *hum*, *om*, and many others that you can investigate.

social interaction: opening our emotional capacity and sensitivity, especially when it is based on positivity and feeling safe amid love, compassion, gratitude, and kindness

laughing: diaphragm and belly laugh movements to increase vagal tone, releasing tension, increasing lifespan, and allowing people to create long-lasting bonds.

Further, we might use yoga postures (asanas), such as cat-cow (*marjaryasana*) and downward-facing dog (*adho mukha svanasana*), to promote both tone and the stretching and lengthening of muscles involved in these asanas. The sun salutation (*surya namaskar*) is also beneficial. Yoga, tai chi, and qigong equally help you to correct body postures that perhaps are putting harmful tension on the spinal cord. We can utilize exercise and long walks to stimulate the vagal tone, preferably in nature, which allows clean breathing and keeps us away from electronic devices for a while! We might seek out massage or work on acupressure or marma points, which are excellent detox activities because they open the lymphatic channels, also stimulating the vagus nerve. And of course, we can pay attention to nutrition and food, incorporating a high-fiber diet and intermittent fasting.

Now you know that the vagus nerve works as a superhighway of information from the brain to the body and from the body to the brain, an expressway we can always reach. By following the above recommendations, you can aid its work by moving from the fight-or-flight sympathetic state that our society's pressures place on us, to a *digest and relax* parasympathetic state. Take these gentle invitations to participate in an interesting dance between the two nervous systems, while increasing your vagal tone and thus connecting to a more balanced body-mind state within yourself.

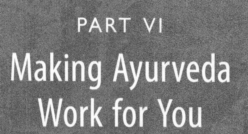

PART VI

Making Ayurveda
Work for You

Rebalance via Proper Food and Diet

15

BEYOND SIMPLY EATING LESS

....

Acquiring an Ayurvedic Mastery
of Food and Nutrition

THE FOODS THAT ARE ALWAYS WELCOME

Ayurveda describes three pillars for promotion of health:

ahara: intake of a balanced diet
nidra: complete and sound sleep
bramacharya: morally guided celibacy

Damage or destruction of any pillar leads to the damage or destruction of health. Since our ayurvedic goal is to restore your metabolic body-mind balance, let me introduce central concepts and basic practical information about food intake, nutrition, and diet that will help you address imbalances in a natural way. There are three ayurvedic factors for proper body-mind well-being:

pathya: nourishing food intake
agni: resilient digestive fire
apathya: food alertness for wrong food intake

We are going to consider how these factors, properly applied, support you in achieving body-mind well-being in a natural way.

Pathya: The Role of Proper Food for a Balanced Diet

Ayurveda is supremely clear about how food, environment, lifestyle, and habits influence not only physical health but also our thinking and feeling functions, and has recommended pathya—a healthy, balanced, wholesome diet—as the base for a balanced body and mind. The value of pathya, as opposed to an unhealthy or unwholesome diet (apathya), is neatly described by Sushruta when he says:

> The body is made up of diet. A patient who follows a
> healthy diet doesn't need medicine as much as a patient
> who doesn't follow a wholesome diet.
>
> Su. Sū. 1/25

In other words, a person who eats healthy food doesn't need medicine because their body is in a state of equilibrium. Yet in truth, the patient who doesn't follow a wholesome diet doesn't need medicine either, because medicine can be ineffective in an unhealthy body. This concept has usually been attributed to Hippocrates, commonly seen as the father of medicine, even though ayurvedic scholars conveyed this long before his existence. Hippocrates is often quoted as saying, "Let food be thy medicine and medicine be thy food." The perpetuation of an imbalanced diet or overeating creates imbalances of the mind that gradually manifest in different forms, including becoming overweight or obese. Balance can be achieved when physical, mental, and spiritual qualities are organized according to the principles of dynamic balance, as opposed to imbalance or inertia. However, balance has to come from within, as we will be exploring here.

CASE STUDY

Apathya

A good illustration of apathya is the case of Didier, a fifty-two-year-old man, overweight, and a smoker with vitiligo (skin patches due to loss of the melanin pigmentation normally produced by melanocytes) caused by an autoimmune disorder. After an ayurvedic evaluation of his prakruti (vata-pitta) and vikruti (kapha-vata), and discussing in detail his dietary regime, it was quite clear that he was very keen on milk products, especially mature cheeses. His tongue was coated white/green, a clear sign of ama accumulation, and his skin patches were mostly in the elbows, back of the neck, and knees. I recommended a tailored diet, including removing milk products since they were not conducive or wholesome to his body/mind constitution, together with lifestyle changes. He described that it was impossible to live without eating cheeses or other milk products. However, he agreed to have a go for a period of one month. On his next visit his skin was less itchy and inflamed, and his tongue was less coated (due to both less cheese intake and the use of a copper tongue cleaner). Didier could see that his milk and cheese consumption was likely the basis of his apathya. He largely maintained the tailored diet and lifestyle changes, and his condition cleared up over several months, with the occasional appearance of small white pigmentations when he experienced lapses from his tailored diet.

ORGANIC INTELLIGENCE
How Ayurveda Classifies Food Items

We start our examination of food by describing the basic principles of wholesome food, based on the ayurvedic concepts of constitution, quality, action, and taste. We do this so as to integrate wholesome food knowledge with modern nutritional concepts of diet and lifestyle that we know work to support body-mind balance.

Ayurveda assesses foods based on three group classifications:

1. **constituents:** the five elements, or panchamahabhutas
2. **the twenty gunas:** the qualities of matter
3. **tastes:** the six different flavors, or rasas

Ayurveda's unchanging purpose is to restore your body-mind balance. I will illustrate the usage and meanings of ayurvedic terms with everyday examples to make them easier for you.

The Five Constituents of Food
The ayurvedic view of the five elements (panchamahabhutas) can be put to practical use for your food consumption by characterizing the nutritive components as earthy, watery, fiery, airy, and spacious in the following manner (Ca. Su. 25/5–50):

THE FIVE CONSTITUENTS OF FOOD

	Earthy	Watery	Fiery	Airy	Spacious
Types of Food (examples)	vegetables, grains, animal materials	milk, buttermilk, fruit juices, soups, ghee	ginger, chilies jalapeños, cayenne/black pepper	air as food for bodily metabolic processes	allow blending transformation of the other four elements.
Some Digestive Effects	sensation of solidity, grounding, heaviness	moistening, pleasantness, liquefaction, softness	heat, spiciness, warmth, transformation	lightness, cleansing, assimilation	hollowness, post-digestion, lightness

Additionally, ayurveda categorizes foods in a similar way to the classifications of foods we have in today's world.

Gunas: The Qualities of Matter

Modern physics and chemistry describe the three fundamental phases or states of matter as solid, liquid, and gas. The properties of matter include measurable traits such as: substances, density, color, mass, volume, length, malleability, melting point, hardness, odor, temperature, and others.

Ayurveda uses an ingenuous and effective way to look within and around us through the specific qualities of matter, recognizing twenty fundamental qualities—expressed as ten qualities and their mirror opposites as described in the below table.

"Like increases like" is an essential ayurvedic principle, expressing that the elemental qualities already present in our prakruti type will be increased by similar qualities present in our food intake (ahara) and the environmental conditions we experience. As a result, we tend to build up an imbalance due to an excess of one quality or another. By contrast, a food intake prioritizing opposite qualities will support and balance your vikruti.[1]

The following table represents the ayurvedic connection between our food items when classified into twenty gunas and their impact according to our prakruti tendencies.

GUNAS AND THE BODY

Sanskrit Name	Guna (Property)	Mahabhutas (Constitution of Elements)	Body Outcomes	V	P	K
Guru	Heavy	earth, water	induces bulking; heavy to digest	↓	↑	
Laghu	Light	space, air	bulk-reducing; easy to digest	↑	↓	
Shita	Cold	water, air	cooling; induces nourishment	↑	↓	↑
Ushna	Hot	fire	sweating; energy flow, appetite, increases agni	↓	↑	↓
Snigdha	Unctuous	water	moist; supports body tissue nutrition	↓	↑	
Ruksha	Dry	air, fire	dryness; decreases fluids, fat, weight	↑	↓	
Manda	Dull	earth	slow; reduces movement and digestion	↓	↑	
Tikshna	Sharp	fire	acuity; appetite and increases agni	↓	↑	↓
Shira	Immobile	earth	stability, firm; produces muscles, fat, bones	↓	↓	↑
Chala	Mobile	air, water	motion, action	↑	↑	↓
Mrudu	Soft	space	unstiffening	↓	↑	↑
Kathina	Hard	earth	rigidity, rough	↑	↓	↓
Vishada	Clear	space	clearing; diffuses flow circulation	↓	↓	↓
Picchila	Sticky	water	adhering, coating; induces bulking	↓	↓	↑
Shlakshna	Smooth	space	softness	↓	↓	↑
Khara	Coarse	air, fire	roughness	↑	↓	
Sthula	Gross	earth	obstructing; induces bulking, obesity	↓	↑	

Key: ↑ = increases; ↓ = decreases; V = vata; P = pitta; K = kapha
(As. Hr. Su. 1/18; Ca. Su. 26/65)

GUNAS AND THE BODY (cont.)

Sanskrit Name	Guna (Property)	Mahabhutas (Constitution of Elements)	Body Outcomes	V	P	K
Sukshma	Subtle	air, space	piercing; creates lightness	↑	↑	↓
Sandra	Dense	water, earth	solidifying; produces stability and strength	↓	↑	
Drava	Liquid	water	fluidity; supports body exchanges	↓	↑	↑

Key: ↑ = increases; ↓ = decreases; V = vata; P = pitta; K = kapha
(As. Hr. Su. 1/18; Ca. Su. 26/65)

Our Senses: Taste and Its Six Flavors

I keep repeating in this book, as I repeat to all my patients, the following ayurvedic teaching: "The origin of all diseases is the lack of connection with our senses." If we would like to move away from body-mind imbalances, it is essential to understand and connect to this notion, and it requires an awareness of the five senses we often neglect and take for granted.

The sensory quality of food is evaluated by humans using their five senses:

gustatory sense (taste): registered by the tongue's taste buds and the soft palate

olfactory sense (smell): in the nose and nasal passages/membranes/linings

visual sense (sight): visual receptors located in the eye apparatus

hearing sense (earing): ear sensorial structures translating vibrations into sound

touch sense (skin): specialized neurons on the surface of our hands and skin

Our mind, its senses, and our dense physical body are deeply interconnected. The aim of our various body senses is to "feed the fire" correctly. In other words, to stimulate all the mechanisms that ultimately create body secretions associated with the digestive fire (agni), to allow the variety of foods present on our plate to be properly burned. To keep a body-mind balance, our senses need to be operating in such a way that we are feeding the digestive fire at regular intervals, and not in an erratic way.

THE SIX TASTES OF FOOD AND YOUR PRAKRUTI

The tongue is a mirror of the body. It registers six taste bud groupings.

TASTES AND THEIR DOMINANT ELEMENTS

Sanskrit	Taste	Element
Madhura	Sweet	Earth and Water
Amla	Sour	Earth and Fire
Lavana	Salty	Water and Fire
Katu	Pungent	Fire and Air
Tikta	Bitter	Air and Ether
Kashaya	Astringent	Air and Earth

The tongue is the only organ that is both inner and outer to the body. One of the tools of the ayurvedic practitioner is the analysis of the tongue and its correlation with the state of the various organs in the body. In ayurveda, when something is out of balance within the oral cavity or tongue, this corresponds to some imbalance or illness in your system.

SIX TASTES AND THEIR TASTE BUD GROUPINGS

Sanskrit	Flavor	Location on Tongue
Madhura	Sweet	front tip
Amla	Sour	front left, front right
Lavana	Salty	back left, back right
Katu	Pungent	front center
Tikta	Bitter	middle left, middle right
Kashaya	Astringent	back center

The deep study by ayurvedic scholars of internal organs and their functions allowed them to map the organs onto the tongue, and even correlate organ and taste bud locations with areas of the tongue. These profound concepts are still under study by both ayurvedic and modern scholars.[2]

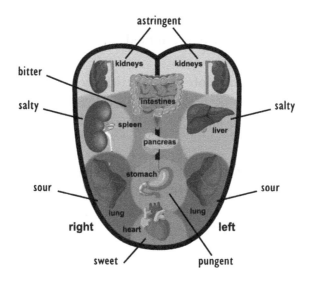

Fig. 15.1. Ayurvedic Mapping of Body Organs to the Tongue

Regarding the relationship between taste preferences and the different ayurvedic constitutions, let me present to you the metabolic implications of body imbalances, stemming from a lack of understanding or application of basic physiological and biochemical principles.

▼ Earthy or kapha-prevalent individuals have a tendency to crave foods with the tastes of sweet, sour, and salty tastes. The strong cooling and metabolic effects of sweet, or neutral, tastes can worsen their prakruti.

▼ Fiery or pitta-prevalent individuals have a tendency to desire foods with sour, salty, and pungent tastes. The energetic heating and metabolic effects of sourness, or acidity, can aggravate their prakruti.

▼ Airy or vata-prevalent individuals tend to enjoy foods whose tastes are pungent, bitter, and astringent. The strong cooling and metabolic effects of pungent, or alkaline, tastes can disturb their prakruti.

Incorporating the six tastes into your daily meals by diversifying your choices of foods is the start to your journey to reaching a better state of health. Then, the pleasure of food will become a regular and welcome part of your daily life, gradually helping you reach and maintain balance. When paying attention to your body and food content, you will start feeling the diverse tastes and will begin attuning to them. You will soon be able to sense the difference between foods that resonate with your dosha and foods that don't.

The ayurvedic principle of "like increases like and opposites decrease" is pertinent here. The three doshas can be balanced either by increasing or decreasing their intrinsic qualities:

EACH DOSHA NOURISHED BY DIFFERENT TASTES AND NEUTRALIZED BY THEIR OPPOSITE

	Kapha	Pitta	Vata
Taste	pungent, bitter, astringent	sweet, bitter, astringent	sweet, sour, salty
Properties	warm and dry	cool, fresh	moist, smooth, warm
Neutralizes	cool, sweet prakruti nature	hot, sour, pungent prakruti nature	dry, cold, bitter, mobile prakruti nature

In modern terms, we can say that when we sample the environment through our sense of taste, this sensory modality guides us to identify and consume nutrients while avoiding indigestible materials, through the approximately 5,000 taste buds present on the tongue and in the oral cavity. Modern medicine recognizes that diverse sensory inputs tickle our taste bud receptors and classifies the so-called "basic" six tastes as sweet, pungent, sour, salty, bitter, and astringent.

Stimulation of taste bud receptors initiates biological reflexes that prepare the gut for absorption of foods—releasing digestive enzymes, initiating peristalsis, and increasing mesenteric flow. It also signals other organs to make digestive adjustments, such as insulin release, sympathetic activation of brown adipose tissue, and increased heart rate. Collectively, these reflexes, which are triggered by the anticipatory sight, smell, and taste of food, and are further enhanced by chewing and swallowing the food, prepare our gut for the best processing of our ingested foods. This process is called cephalic phase response (CPR). Taste is often confused with flavor, the combined sensory experience of olfaction (smell) and gustation (taste from the tongue).[3]

Why does your mouth feel like it is on fire when you eat a very spicy pepper? Well, when you eat a spicy chili pepper your mouth feels like it is burning because your brain actually thinks it is burning. The heat-sensitive receptors are activated; your body thinks it is in contact with a dangerous heat source and reacts accordingly. You start sweating and your heart beats faster. The peppers have provoked the same fight-or-flight response that your body engages to respond to most dangers. Certain compounds in spicy foods activate sensory neurons called polymodal nociceptors. We have them all over our body, including in the mouth and nose—the same receptors that are activated by extreme heat. However, you know that foods have different levels of spiciness depending on the types of compounds involved.[4] For example, capsaicin and piperine found in black pepper (*Piper nigrum*) and chili peppers (*Capsicum annuum*) are composed of larger, heavier molecules called alkylamides, which largely stay in your mouth. The opposite occurs when you eat something containing menthol. The cool, minty compound triggers your cold receptors. As another example, horseradish, mustard, and wasabi are made up of smaller molecules called isothiocyanates that easily float up into your sinuses. This is the reason why chili peppers burn your mouth and wasabi burns your nose.

Current studies are looking at how our genes play a role in taste preferences for spicy food or other tastes,[5] to help corroborate the role of our individual constitutions or doshas, as per the ayurvedic explanations, and to better support us in eating balancing foods.[6]

The taste, smell, and visual appearance of a complete food product essentially set within us a way to naturally recognize and accept every kind of food we are eating, creating a thoughtful, deeper appreciation. We all know that the taste sensation of drinking fruit juice or a fruit or vegetable smoothie is not the same as eating the actual fruit or vegetable. When we eat solid foods, chewing with our teeth breaks down the foodstuffs, and they are dissolved by saliva. Taste, flavor, and texture are perceived during chewing and will contribute to our appreciation of each particular food. When drinking a smoothie, we also get a flavor, but it will pass very quickly through our digestive system. Also, the individual flavors of a fruit or a vegetable by itself, with all its constituents, including complex fiber for the work of our microbiome, play a very important role in selecting and recognizing nutritive food.

A balanced food intake should include all six tastes tailored to your body-mind prakruti, to nourish your doshas. What are your likes and dislikes: sweet and sour flavors? Salty and spicy foods? Or maybe you enjoy bitter and astringent flavors? Are you able to recognize the tastes in the food you eat daily?

A food's taste derives from its biochemical constitution or inner elemental composition. All types of natural foods we ingest display the five elements in different proportions. Some foods could have nearly negligible amounts of one or more tastes, and many other foods can be a blend of two or more predominant tastes if we are savoring them properly.

What could be the impact on our body's prakruti when we eat foods that are rich in one particular taste? Can they affect our metabolism and cause us congestion or even disease? Two simple examples of the concept of "like increases like" provide the answer: First, foods that are overpowering in earth and water elements (kapha), such as heavy dairy products, will induce mucus production in your body—this is the case for the kapha-type constitution in particular, and is expressed as congested sinuses, among other symptoms. Second, foods predominant in heat, like hot peppers, are only suitable in small amounts for pitta-type people since these foods would increase one's fire constitution even more.

EXAMPLES OF SPICE AND VEGETABLE TASTES

Spice	Sweet	Sour	Salty	Astringent	Pungent	Bitter
Basil	+				+	+
Bell Pepper	+					+
Black Pepper					+	
Cardamom	+				+	
Cayenne					+	
Chili Pepper					+	
Cilantro			+		+	
Cinnamon	+			+	+	
Cloves	+				+	+
Coriander	+				+	+
Cumin					+	+
Garlic	+			+		+
Green Mango	+	+				
Fenugreek	+			+	+	+
Onion					+	
Sea Salt			+			
Turmeric				+	+	+

These concepts are very easy to understand, but regrettably, modern medicine rarely applies them. It is worth noting here that simply recognizing these concepts is a step toward rebalancing without becoming dependent on medications or making drastic lifestyle changes. It also costs nothing, other than your time, to take this first step. That is what I call a cost-effective health system. Let me use two more cases to illustrate the effect that the qualities of various foods or types of diet can have on your body-mind.

INVITATION TO DISCOVER YOUR OPTIMAL PERSONAL TASTES FOR BODY-MIND REBALANCING

Imagine you have a strong cold with a heavy mucus cough. Are you ready to go out and have a big ice cream or a double-cream pastry outdoors on a cold evening? No—instead, I think we all naturally know that nothing could be more helpful than drinking some warming, sharp, dry ginger tea, or using spearmint to open your respiratory airways. Or you might wish to rest for a while under hot, dry sunlight.

Next, imagine you are in hot and dry weather. Perhaps you feel your body becoming hot and dry as well. Would you like to have a warm coffee or tea under the hot sun? Or would you prefer to drink a cooling coconut water or iced tea, or take a nap in the shade, or walk in cool, humid moonlight? Again, our natural common sense knows how to address the conditions of heat and dryness.

If you integrate the concept of guna, or quality, with the concept of "like increases like," you will recognize that to correct diet and lifestyle imbalances, you need to aim for opposites.

When we are aware of an excess, our natural instinct is to decrease the "like" around us. In this way, those qualities present in you provide the intelligence needed to reestablish balance through lifestyle and food intake. However, don't flip to the other extreme and try to diminish your exposure to the various tastes. Ayurveda's ancient knowledge understood that people whose diets are dominated by only one taste are putting their health at risk. The reason is pretty simple: when our body tissues are not nourished properly, insufficiencies become obvious sooner or later, gradually manifesting as weak immune system activity. We can become more susceptible to imbalances affecting our physical or mental health. Imagine somebody living on a food program based on processed sugars or other "bad" food; the result is an open invitation to diabetes or other pathologies, including obesity. On the other hand, individuals whose food intake embraces the six tastes are better equipped to have flourishing bodies and strong natural resistance as a result of a balanced diet.

It is important to mention that some of the tastes are only required in small amounts to satisfy and balance our body-mind system; more is not always better.

Now that we've analyzed in some detail the role and participation of the sense of taste in our food intake, let's cover in a more general way the participation of the other five senses, to appreciate their importance in supporting our connection with food. This will help motivate us to practice proper intake to achieve body balance. Our six senses hold the memory of our well-being in connection with food.

HOW OUR OTHER FIVE SENSES CONNECT WITH FOOD

Smell

Odors or aromas are part of the flavor experience during food consumption, through a process known as retronasal olfaction. In the presence of food, olfactory signals can be perceived before consumption, and stimulate appetite in anticipation of food intake. Studies have demonstrated that odors trigger appetite specifically for food products we already know. From a nutrition perspective, changes in or loss of olfactory capability mostly impact food enjoyment and can, but do not automatically, lead to changes in dietary patterns. Smell is also a reliable way through which social interaction can occur among us. It is known that olfactory loss is associated with depressive symptoms, as the absence of smell can have a more general impact on quality of life and well-being.[7] Evaluation by ultrasound scans of fetuses' facial expressions showed their reaction to specific flavors. Aromas from the mother's diet are present in the amniotic fluid and reach the chemosensory receptors. The taste buds can detect taste-related chemicals from fourteen weeks' gestation, and odor molecules can be sensed from twenty-four weeks' gestation.[8] Ayurveda recommends enjoying cooking for yourself or your loved ones, to trigger the olfactory nerves into giving you the desire to taste food that has a mouthwatering smell.

Vision

We can understand one of the factors in obesity if we take a closer look at the potential role of vision and question the impact of our increasing digital exposure to images of desirable foods—what is frequently identified as "gastroporn" or "food porn." Digital interfaces unintentionally exacerbate our desire for food and can create what we call "visual hunger."[9]

There is a growing body of cognitive neuroscience research proving the profound effect that viewing such images can have on neural activity, physiological and psychological responses, and visual attention, especially in the "hungry" brain in which technology plays a crucial role in informing our decisions, whether conscious or automatic.[10] On a personal note, I remember what my parents used to say when we were served food on our plates: "Your eyes cannot be bigger than your stomach." I also came to understand the importance of combining food items' colors for visual activation of the appetite.

Sound

Even the ear participates in the process of digestion, since sound has a physiological effect. We all know the feeling of working in a room where somebody is cooking. The sounds of chopping, mixing, and frying are far more than a simple distraction and are music to your gut. They ignite the digestive fire within you, and your mind might wonder when food will be ready. Additionally, an example of the role of hearing is how the sound of chewing food will provide evidence on whether a product is fresh or stale.

Touch

Touch is fundamental to your health and well-being. It is remarkable how many cultures in Asia, Africa, and Mesoamerica love eating food with their hands, or traditional implements such as chopsticks. Many people view eating with hands as unhygienic, primitive, and nauseating; however, eating food with our hands is associated with the body, psyche, and soul. There is logic behind the Indian routine of eating with fingers.[11] Most probably you know the feeling of licking your fingers after eating a delicious fruit. Consider also that you may not wish to eat your dinner with your hands—unless it is pizza. Who eats pizza with a knife and fork?

Our Sixth Sense: The Microbiome?

The human brain constantly receives input from the stomach and intestines. These sensations are intuitively fused into decision making during daily life, as "gut feelings," yet we still know very little about how the brain processes our gut signals. Trying to understand the neural processes that govern the human gut-brain connection is very challenging due to the inaccessibility of our body's interior.[12] However, we know that food perception does not just depend on one individual sense but appears to be the result of multisensory cellular intelligence and integration of unimodal signals.[13] Recent reviews show that gut bacteria influence mood and emotions, stressing their connection with a range of psychiatric disorders.[14, 15, 16]

CURRENT SCIENCES

Biochemical Categorization of Food Items

Current science understands a nutrient as a food substance used in our body to sustain growth, for vital activities such as maintenance and repair, and to provide energy. Our bodies comprise an enormous diversity of biological molecules and require the intake of foods containing certain vital compounds, from water to amino acids, fats, carbohydrates, vitamins, and minerals. The breaking down, absorption, and utilization of food by the body is fundamental for nourishment and is facilitated by these digestive processes. However, most of the molecules in food, while metabolized or integrated into the body, are not necessarily crucial.[17] For example, if you decide to eradicate carbs from your regular diet, their lack would not necessarily cause sickness even if they were replaced with other kinds of nourishment able to fulfill your normal caloric body requirements.

Basically, the fundamental nutrients essential for well-being are categorized as follows:

Macronutrients: Carbs (glucose), proteins (amino acids), and lipids or fats (triglycerides, cholesterol) account for the bulk of our food intake, requiring the presence of specific enzymes and cofactors to become accessible for cellular absorption and functionality.

Fats, or Lipids: We've already discussed in detail fat classifications and roles. I would like to add that your diet requires essential fatty acids (FAs) omega-3 and omega-6, which are vital to the care of all your cell membranes and linked to the prevention of degenerative brain conditions. These FAs are present in foods like nuts, seeds, and fatty fish. Sadly, long-term intake of other fats, such as trans fats, compromises your body-mind balance.

Proteins: These are large molecules composed of twenty different building blocks called amino acids, and have different combinations according to their many vital biological functions. They can be essential (required in our diet), or nonessential. One of their roles is to be components of neurotransmitters—chemical messengers carrying signals between neurons and affecting mood, sleep, attentiveness, and body weight. These neurotransmitters are part of the reason why you feel more alert after a protein-rich meal or feel calm after eating a large plate of pasta. Foods can stimulate brain cells to release mood-altering neurotransmitters such as serotonin—of which 95 percent is supplied by your gut bacteria—as well as norepinephrine and dopamine.

Micronutrients or Cofactors: Vitamins and minerals are chemical elements needed in trace amounts for the normal function of all your body organs and are made available by our digestive system via different mechanisms. For example, the brain requires a steady supply of antioxidants, present in fruits and vegetables, to support the brain in reducing free radicals that destroy brain cells. This enables your brain to work well for a longer period. Also, vitamins such as B_6, B_{12}, and B_9 (folic acid) protect your brain from becoming prone to brain disease and mental decline. Trace amounts of the minerals iron, copper, zinc, and sodium are essential for a healthy body and cognitive functions.

Water: The most essential element is needed to rehydrate, which occurs by drinking fluids and eating foods that contain water, vital for all our cellular and tissular requirements. A grown-up individual is almost

60 percent water, which we release through breathing, sweating, digestive processes, and urinary elimination.

Carbs: These are sugars, starches, and fibers found in fruits, vegetables, grains, and milk products. Starches consist of very large chains of glucose molecules linked together, which eventually get broken down by enzymatic actions into smaller groupings and finally into single molecules of glucose, or blood sugar, which is absorbed into the bloodstream. Carbs can also be small molecules like the lactose in milk or natural fructose in fruits. Glucose is the only fuel our brain accepts despite the fact we get different kinds of sugars from our diet. Although your brain represents only about 2 percent of your body weight, it uses up to 20 percent of your energy resources. Selecting a varied diet of wholesome foods is an essential tenet of ayurveda. Let's discuss how the choice of good-quality food has a direct and long-lasting effect on our brain and body.

THE POWER AND ROLE OF CARBOHYDRATES

Because carbs are among the different kind of foods that are generally blamed as the main cause of obesity and being overweight, let me discuss certain relevant aspects of them. While most nutritional labels group all carbohydrates into a single total carb count, the ratio of the sugar content and fiber subgroups to the whole amount affects how our body and brain will respond to them.

For example, white bread undergoes very rapid breakdown and intestinal absorption, and causes quick release of molecules of glucose (sugar), raising blood glucose levels higher and more quickly than most other foods. Thus, white bread is a high-glycemic food. White bread carbs are metabolized very quickly, and blood sugar from this source is rapidly depleted, altering your attention span and mood.

Meanwhile, oats, grains, and legumes, aside from providing minerals and vitamins, have a high fiber content and more complex carbs. For that reason, they are broken down and absorbed more slowly, so the molecule of glucose moves gradually into the bloodstream over a longer period of time.

DOES COLOR MATTER?

Power of Brown Carbs and Why to Learn to Love Them

What does it mean to switch to "brown" carbs? This basically involves eating brown cereals like brown rice, whole grain brown bread, and whole grain pasta, and choosing unpeeled potatoes over mashed, fried, or other processed forms. The ingestion of refined carbs is unnatural and invites the body to respond by increasing insulin production. Natural brown carbs contain more dietary fiber than their "white" equivalents. The fiber in our diet can be either soluble, as found in beans, fruits, vegetables, whole grain rice, psyllium husk, and oat bran; or insoluble, as with wheat bran and cellulose. We cannot digest fiber to use as an energetic substrate; instead, fiber provides the food substratum for our microbiome.

For many years it has been well known that soluble fiber lowers blood cholesterol levels. There are three grams of fiber found in one bowl of oat bran cereal or oatmeal, and clinical studies examining soluble oat bran supplements have shown them to lower blood cholesterol levels by as much as 23 percent. Several other studies demonstrated that eating oats after a high-fat meal kept arteries clearer and open in healthy volunteers. Findings suggest that fiber could be more significant than saturated fat in decreasing the risk factors of heart disease. Those eating higher fiber content had lower levels of insulin, blood pressure, and blood cholesterol, as well as less obesity, cancer, and diabetes.[18, 19]

OTHER MATTERS OF INQUIRY

Regarding macronutrients, our body enzymes permit their conversion into other components or substances, according to our body-mind necessities. Our bodies have systems of adaptation or metabolic interconversion via numerous enzymatic chains of reactions, well-known pathways, and biochemical cycles, by which our fats and amino acids can be converted into glucose, and vice versa.[20]

The amount of carbs, proteins, and fats you should be consuming, and the combinations in which you should ingest them, is a topic under continuous discussion by best-selling diet authors. However, their recommendations are striking in their divergence, from too much protein to too little, no meat versus a diet rich in meat, and so on. Some nutritional experts are big proponents of low-fat, low-protein, high-carbohydrate diets. Others encourage just the opposite: foods high in protein and fat but low in carbs. Still others emphasize minerals and vitamins. The issue always remains, however: Can these one-size-fits-all dietary requirements be effective across a population of hundreds of millions of prakrutis, each of which has its own individual dietary and nutritional needs? The clear answer ayurveda gives is "no." Perhaps the inability of these one-size-fits-all diets to distinguish among the needs of prospective dieters is one reason why they fall away as quickly as they rise in prominence. It is intriguing that despite the thousands of years since the classic ayurvedic texts were written, ayurvedic understanding of digestion and cellular interaction is consistent with the modern description of intercellular uptake and release of molecules, only using a different vocabulary.

Today's lifestyle opens many questions about how to create a properly balanced food intake, due to widespread confusion on multiple issues. People lack knowledge of the diverse biochemical composition of nutrients and their metabolic pathways that govern the conversion and interaction of different qualities and actions of food molecules. We may feel overwhelmed by the vast amount, complexity, multiplicity, and discrepancies of scientific literature. There is a lack of understanding regarding when and how nutrient combinations are required.

The big food industry, the agribusiness sector, and nutritional "influencers" on social media create misconstructions, predispositions, and biases relating to labeling or marketing of products. Our existing natural foodstuffs are combined with novel, combined, manufactured, synthetic compounds whose potential harm we must recognize.

Let's now explore how to enhance our nutrients according to ayurvedic principles, before examining in further detail the crucial ayurvedic concepts of agni and ama.

ENHANCING AND TREATING
DIFFERENT TYPES OF NUTRIENTS
....
The Prakruti of Food

The ayurvedic classics gave the following food intake instructions for better digestion and assimilation (*ahara vidhi vidhana*):

▼ Food should be taken hot and unctuous to facilitate digestion.
▼ Eat in adequate amounts, and don't eat again until the previous food intake has been digested.
▼ Eat foods with similar potency (*virya*) together. Avoid combining hot and cold foods simultaneously.
▼ Do not eat too fast or too slow.
▼ Avoid excessive talking or laughing when eating; focus your attention on the food.
▼ Avoid eating with anxiety, grief, fear, anger, or pain.
▼ Don't fall into sedentary habits.
▼ Don't eat late at night.

INTRINSIC QUALITIES

The physical aspects of a substance or product are described as intrinsic attributes. Food has a prakruti, a very important factor to pay attention to when making a personalized diet to support metabolic body-mind rebalancing. According to ayurveda, the taste of food (rasa) results from the predominance of basic qualities (gunas) or molecular particles that are part of the food's composition, present in different proportions and forming its diverse tastes.

Ayurvedic scholars' recommendations include:

1. Methods of preparation (*karana*): The way you cook your food can prevent potential intrinsic adverse effects for your body-mind constitution; although, be aware that certain methods of cooking harm the inner qualities and properties of food.
2. Food combinations (*samyoga*) are paramount. We must be intentional

about what we "link together," and avoid unwholesome combinations of nutrients carrying opposing qualities. Every food has its own intrinsic taste (rasa), energetic qualities of cooling or heating (virya), and a post-digestive outcome (*vipaka*). If two or more foods holding different post-digestive effects are mixed, then agni can become overloaded, affecting our cascades of enzymatic reactions, causing incompatibilities that generate ama and could be the cause of body imbalances in the long term.

3. We must consider amount (*rashi*). It is recommended that we ingest a mix of solid foods and liquid, in three parts: one-third of the stomach's volume should be filled with food, and the other two-thirds should be filled with water and air, respectively. Sound advice, since our gastric secretions and enzymes require space, one of the five elements, in order to properly mix with food and allow proper action of the digestive fire (agni).

4. It's important to pay attention to habitat and foods grown nearby (*desha*). Eat local, fresh foods that are exposed to the same climate as you are, and nourished by the same settings, instead of eating exotic foods.

5. Food consumption time (kala) is key. Processing food entails a robust agni, so try to have a light and lively breakfast, then eat your largest meal at midday, the time when agni is strongest. Have a small dinner two hours or more before going to bed.

6. Be aware of consumer physiological and mental state (*upayogasamastha*). It is essential to calm your mind and collect your senses before eating. The digestive metabolic processes will be altered if you are feeling under stress.

7. Acknowledge seasonal period (*ruta*). Always adjust food consumption to fit the present season. Eat more salads and fruits during summer, even if you are a kapha type. In spring, boost your consumption of kapha-decreasing foods; when summer arrives, eat more fresh foods, and be careful to avoid heat-producing foods. During the cold season, consume more vata-reducing foods.

8. Recognize the importance of moderation and awareness. Have respect for whatever you are eating.

Let me give you a couple of examples related to our food intake and potential aliments. Our diet can quickly modify the configuration of the microbiome. For example, Western diets high in meat products, providing nutrients such as choline and carnitine, can instigate certain gut bacteria to produce trimethylamine (TMA). TMA is absorbed into the bloodstream and then oxidized in the liver to form trimethylamine-N-oxide (TMAO). It has been suggested that high levels of TMAO contribute to cardiovascular diseases by affecting the cholesterol metabolism and its transportation, foam cell formation, and platelet aggregation.

Another example is dysbiosis. It arises when the delicate and elaborate ecology of microbial communities is disturbed either by internal or external factors. A disturbed microbiome is characterized by the overgrowth of one or more of the diverse microbial colonies. When fiber intake is reduced, gut bacteria may disturb the cardiovascular system (CVS) and cause disease, since the richest source of food for gut bacteria is fiber from diet. Reducing it can lead to a diminished bacterial production of butyrate (a short chain fatty acid). This alteration could trigger local inflammation and dysbiosis in the gut lining. The consequence will be a weakened function of the gut barrier, with the possible leakage of bacterial toxins such as lipopolysaccharides into the bloodstream, affecting the CVS.

Ayurvedic scholars have devised tables of foods to eat based on your body prakruti, the qualities that each taste holds, and the influence it will have on your doshas.[21] To discover which diet is more suitable for you, remember to come back to the evaluation included earlier in this book and the score defining your individual prakruti constitution (see pages 271–77). Take into consideration that the following food descriptions correspond to adaptations from the ayurvedic scholars' texts by contemporary ayurvedic practitioners, since some of these food items did not exist in India during the time of the original scholars.

AGNI: AYURVEDA AND FOOD CONVERSION AND DIGESTION

Agni in Sanskrit means "fire," a crucial life-supporting element accountable for all metabolic functions, including ingestion, digestion, absorption, and assimilation of food. Charaka said agni is the base (*mool*) of life (Ca. Chi. 15/4). Sushruta described agni as the root of our being; the root of our life, body, mind, and senses (As. Hr. Ni. 12/1).

Fire is one of the five elements (panchamahabhutas), and agni is one of its manifestations. Its attributes are represented as hot, sharp, light, penetrating, spreading, luminous, subtle, and clear. Of course, agni is not real fire, but it is the digestive fire that breaks the chemical bonds in the various foods we eat, making them small enough to allow essential elements and nutrients to pass through our gastrointestinal tract (GIT) in order to reach all cells. Our body-mind psychobiological functions respond according to this digestive fire, so a vigorous agni supports a healthy body and mind, whereas depleted agni compromises them.

Ayurvedic scholars defined up to forty different agni, their bodily locations, and their specific physiological functions, all without the tools of today's biomedical technology. They even described the digestive agni of the cellular membrane (*pilu agni*) as well as the agni inside the cell in the nuclear membrane (ancestral or genetic *pithara agni*). All body cells require fire (energy) to power the many mechanisms that keep them alive and functional, therefore metabolic functions lean on the quality and quantity of accessible agni. In the process of understanding metabolic imbalances associated with conditions of being overweight or obese, we will be using the term *agni* in a broad sense—the collective digestive fires.

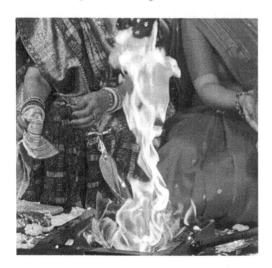

Fig. 15.2. Our Inner and Outer Metabolic Fire

Roles of Agni

The major command of our bodies is to fulfill the requirement of every single cell for energy derived from fats, carbs, or proteins. For that reason, the mother of all agni is considered the digestive or gastric fire, named jataragni. Ayurvedic ancient texts described it as located in the stomach and small intestine or duodenum, and as being the chief authority supervising all the other sorts of "micro agni" present in the various body systems. As noted on page 32, Charaka described agni as being divided into thirteen types.

Why does jataragni act like the chief power source supplying energy to the various agni? Because jataragni provides energy from the intracellular components to all body tissues, and through them to the entire body. All types of agni depend directly on their quality and quantity. At a physical level, jataragni is responsible for the processes of digestion, absorption, assimilation, transformation, and governing cellular intelligence, including cellular selectivity. Jataragni is also involved in gastric mucus secretion, peristalsis, opening of the pyloric valve, stimuli from the hunger center in the brain, and secretion of the various gastric and intestinal enzymes. Equally, it is in control of the formation of urine, feces, and sweat, all of which neutralize potential toxins (ama). Ayurveda reveals that we can trace most disease back to a disturbance in the digestive system, and if all systems are working in harmony, they keep us in a state of balance, assuring good nutritional restoration and cellular communication. All these roles permit us to have power, stability, and vitality, as well as sustaining our body temperature.

Jataragni, at the mind level, supports our sensory perception, intelligence, discrimination, mental clarity, and eagerness for life—joy, laughter, confidence, affection, contentment, and courage. In this way it sustains resilience, vigor, and endurance.

Functional Alterations of Jataragni

When foodstuffs or mental impressions are not well digested, the unprocessed issues create dysfunction in our cellular metabolism. Charaka has mentioned that the seven tissues (dhatus) that support the body contain their own jataragni, and by their own jataragni they digest and convert the materials provided to them to make their own constituents for assimilation and sustenance (Ca. Su. 28/15). When the condition of jataragni or digestive fire becomes disturbed, it is unable to process food adequately. In that case, toxins can linger in the body as physical or mental undigested materials, eventually becoming deleterious if toxins are not eliminated. This is what ayurveda calls ama. The process of apoptosis, a cellular mechanism by which cells shut down as a result of disturbance of the extracellular space through which cells communicate, is an example of how ama can affect cellular, tissular, and systemic functions. How?

Well, if ama keeps building up and recirculating in our body, it will ultimately end up stuck in our digestive channels, vessels, or arteries, structures designed to carry the small units of wholesome food to the body instead of clogging it with ama deposits. Many studies, including research conducted in the UK, show that these unmetabolized accumulations from physical or mental stress could be one of the main causes of conditions such as arterial blockages, generating physical and mental imbalances.[22] Even a disturbed digestion after eating high-quality foods could make you as sick as eating a poor-quality diet; both induce depletion of jataragni and result in ama accumulation. We will be discussing ama in detail, but here is a short introductory list of signs and symptoms of ama production and accumulation in our body-mind systems:

▾ abnormal vata flow, indigestion or poor appetite, congestion of body channels
▾ stagnation of energy flow, fatigue
▾ heaviness, feeling of filthiness, sexual weakness
▾ coated tongue, lack of taste or spoiled taste in the mouth
▾ mental confusion, sickness, disease

Perhaps you can see an association between the doshas and jataragni, and you are asking yourself: are agni and pitta the same? Well, that was and remains a subject of discussion, and theories have their own importance.[23, 24] As stated by Sushruta: there is no existence of any other agni in the body without pitta (Su. Sū. 21/9). Though they have similar properties and actions, they are not analogous.

I suggest you try to see how you relate to one of the four types of jataragni in the second table below. Most of us feel inclined to identify with one or more of them. Unfortunately, today's lifestyle pressures from processed foods, social media, and other factors make it more difficult to keep up a stable metabolism in relation to your individual constitution. The following factors are the main examples of these lifestyle problems:

NEGATIVE IMPACTS OF MODERN EATING HABITS

Food Intake/Diet	Physiological/Mental	Environmental
undereating, eating at wrong times	emotive stress such as anxiety, fear	social media, screen exposure
leftover or unsuitable food blends	suppression of natural urges	unusual weather (damp or too cold)
overeating, late meals, wrong fasting periods, wrong water intake	excess alcohol, smoking, drug use	night shift, changing schedules
extremely dry or cold food	excess worries	unsettled

There are four common types of imbalanced jataragni, with different relationships to our constitutional types (prakruti) and varying consequences for physical or mental ama in our body-mind system.

TYPES OF METABOLISM: JATARAGNI AND ITS MANIFESTATIONS

	Metabolism	Inner Fire	Health
Sama Agni	Balanced	balanced doshas	stable health: excellent GIT, immunity, mind functions

TYPES OF METABOLISM:
JATARAGNI AND ITS MANIFESTATIONS (cont.)

	Metabolism	Inner Fire	Health
Vishama Agni	Irregular	irregular; vata associated; on/off digestive fire that cannot digest food completely	appetite/digestion, gasses, constipation, abdominal pain, flux, heaviness, guts gurgling, dry mouth, receding gums, cracking joints, sciatica, low back pain, muscle spasm, restlessness, anxiety, insecurity, mental fluctuations
Tikshna Agni	Fast Metabolism	sharp; pitta associated; an overly intense digestive fire that can burn food, preventing complete digestion	intense, strong appetite; following digestion: dry lips/throat/palate, heartburn, hot flashes, strong desires for sweets; hyperacidity, gastritis, hypoglycemia, colitis, diarrhea, dysentery, liver pain, nausea, vomiting, inflammatory states; anger, hate, envy, judgment
Manda Agni	Slow Metabolism	dull; kapha associated; a digestive fire that burns often at low temperature, giving partial digestion	dull/heavy: fast to gain weight, sluggish digestion, gut heaviness, cold, congestion, cough, oversalivation, craving hot/sharp/dry/spicy foods; allergies, nausea, mucus, edema, obesity, diabetes, hypertension, lethargy, extreme sleep, clammy skin, body weakness, attachment, greed

Advice for Managing Your Agni

> *Strength, health, longevity, and vital breath are dependent*
> *upon the power of digestion, including metabolism. When*
> *supplied with fuel in the form of food and drink, this power*
> *of digestion is sustained; it dwindles when deprived of it.*

CA. SU. 28/342

Eating your food in a conscious way for quality and quantity is the secret for a good inner fire. An unwholesome diet, an unsupportive lifestyle, and unresolved emotions can easily impede agni by diminishing its strength and consistency. Learning to use your body's agni properly is the main path toward rebalancing of your body-mind.

Fuel your fire regularly, especially when there are signs of hunger. For that, you need to eat your food at optimum physiological times; this is the best way to keep your agni healthy, fostering good digestive processes and resulting in good immunity.

Long periods of bad digestion result from persistent overeating or even a lack of interest in food. These manifestations show that your body-mind state is heading in the wrong direction, into disorder, and is affecting your agni.

The physical manifestations of disturbed agni are clearly observable by obvious disorders such as obesity, gastric ulcers, and fainting spells. Even mental impacts can be identified, though their manifestations may take longer to appear. The best approach to these conditions is to first eliminate ama, returning the power of agni to a normal, functional level. Then treatment is implemented to counter the amplification of the disturbed dosha.

Ayurveda takes the profound view that a depleted agni, or low internal fire, is the root cause of our many physical and mental pathologies. After several years studying agni, I now grasp that agni is something more than just a simple digestive fire. It is like an advanced intelligence allowing us the possibility to live freely from sorrows triggered by our physical or mental fluctuations.

Learn to ignore the external burdens around you, and instead listen to the language of your gut! I have the chance to be a daily witness to the importance of agni and the gut, thanks to my clients, and so I suggest to you that in order to reestablish your body-mind health, it is paramount to protect your inner fire. Agni is the principle that functions through the metabolic processes to transform food and sensations into consciousness.

FOOD SUPPORTING
YOUR PREDOMINANT DOSHA

Tables presenting in detail the different types of foods that each person should eat according to their preponderant dosha are included in appendix 2. These recommended foods will help to keep you in a state of balance or to rebalance your doshas based on your predominant dosha. Very strong imbalances will need a more personalized program.

I am not suggesting you follow a particular type of diet, such as eating or avoiding meat or becoming vegetarian or vegan. I am very respectful of those issues, since I deeply agree with the ayurvedic principle that your diet has to be tailored to your individual constitution. It took me a while to abandon my belief that I had a deep understanding of diets after three intense years researching vegetarian diets, which I did as part of my academic degrees in biomedical science at medical institutions.[25, 26]

FOOD COMBINING

Here is a brief description of three other important ayurvedic metabolic indicators known as virya, vipaka, and *prabhava*, for the purpose of rebalancing in case of incorrect food combinations.

> **virya:** the potency or energy of a substance and the secondary action of an ingested substance experienced after taste, with heating or cooling energy considered its chief potencies
> **vipaka:** final, post-digestive effect of food, a process that happens in the colon, influencing our eliminations (sweat, urine, and feces); described as sweet, sour, and pungent

prabhava: special dynamic efficacy, a substance efficacy that cannot be easily explained based on its energy, taste, and post-digestive effects; an exception to the rule

While it is true that a person's agni largely determines how well or how poorly food is digested, food combinations are also of great importance. When two or more foods having different tastes, energies, and post-digestive effects are combined, agni can become overloaded, inhibiting the enzymatic system, resulting in the creation of undigested food "toxins." Yet if these same foods are eaten separately, they may well stimulate agni, be digested more quickly, and even help to burn ama. Similarly, compatible combinations enhance assimilation. Poor food combining can produce indigestion, fermentation, putrefaction, and gas formation, and if prolonged, can lead to toxemia and disease. For example, eating bananas with cold milk can diminish agni, affect the microbiome, produce "toxins," and cause sinus congestion, cold, cough, and allergies. As another example, milk and melons should not be eaten together. Both are cooling, but milk is laxative, whereas melon is diuretic. Milk requires more time for digestion. Additionally, the stomach acid needed to digest the melon causes the milk to curdle, so ayurveda advises against taking milk with sour foods. Concerning fruits, avoid combining fruits by eating fruit by itself. Fruit combinations could become sour and potentially indigestible in the GIT when mixed together.

FOOD FOR YOUR MIND SETUP
Truth (Sattva), Action (Rajas), and Inertia (Tamas)

Qualities of the mind = qualities of the body.

Food dependency is a factor that requires physical and psychological support if you would like to address your body imbalance properly. All of us, in one way or another, know the role nourishment has played in our lives in relation to our physical activities and temperament. Perhaps you recall phases in your life when you were very hungry, or sought calming external pressures by overeating, or celebrated your happiness with a delicious meal; or maybe you remember celebrations or parties when you knew you'd gone beyond the limit of food or drink you would normally tolerate. On the other hand, perhaps you have been incapable of eating a meal because you were feeling irritated, unhappy, or disappointed; or you may have decided to compensate your irritation by overeating, or oversleeping, leading to a state of lethargy that can contribute to weight gain. What better examples than to feel your body's desperate need for food after a long morning at work, or those negative emotions informing your body that now is—or isn't—the right time to eat? Your body very cleverly decides to tell you to eat or not eat in these situations, according to your agni level. Psychoneuroimmunology shows us how our temperament and moods of happiness, stress, or anger felt in these moments will play a central role in our immune system—for example, disturbing your body-mind balancing processes by increasing the accumulation of body fat and activating inflammation.

Ayurvedic texts state that all diseases originate at the subtle, psychic level, and from there they influence the physiology of a person. If an imbalanced mental state continues, it will manifest as an imbalance or disease at the physical body level. Ayurveda holds that a good appetite indicates a well-functioning agni; so, the quantity and type of food you eat should be chosen accordingly. However, we must understand the difference between feeling hunger and appetite. The feeling of hunger is an authorization to eat, while appetite must be delimited according to your real needs.

Based on guna characteristics, ayurveda describes various foods as light (sattva), rich or passionate (rajas), or sluggish or dull (tamas). Again, take into consideration that the following food descriptions correspond to adaptations from the ayurvedic scholars' texts by contemporary ayurvedic practitioners; conditions were different in the original scholars' time, and some of these food items did not exist in India in ancient times.

Foods with Light Quality (Sattva)

A sattvic diet essentially consists of wholesome foods represented by agricultural products that have been naturally grown and processed. When eaten in the right quantities, they will not cause body-mind imbalances.

Such foods include fresh organic fruits, vegetables, whole grains, beans, plant-based oils, natural sugars such as honey and molasses, and spices like basil, cinnamon, coriander, ginger, and turmeric.

Foods with Rich or Passionate Quality (Rajas)

The word *rajasic* derives from the word *raja*, a Hindi word of Sanskrit origin meaning "king" or "prince." Rajasic food's effect on the body-mind stimulates the person beyond normal capacity and capability, energizing almost all body systems, so eating rajasic food in moderate amounts provides energy and drives us toward stimulating activity and creativity.

According to ayurveda, some of the most common rajasic foods are fruits like sour apples, banana, guava, and tamarind; vegetables including potatoes, cauliflower, broccoli, spinach, and winter squash; grains such as millet, corn, and buckwheat; and beans like red beans, yellow dal, and mung beans. Animal-origin foods include dairy products, and fish, shrimp, or chicken. Very spicy foods as well as sour, salty, hot, and dry foods are considered the most rajasic. If eaten in excess or in an imbalanced way, they could leave a person feeling restless, overwhelmed, tense, or aggressive and domineering—effects that disrupt the body-mind balance.

To handle the continual demands from the external world, we require sensible support from these passionate energies, so eat them according to your daily life activities. For example, an individual who does heavy physical labor every day cannot afford to eat like a person with a sedentary life. Our passion and potential have to be kept up to a certain level. Despite that, in order to maintain balance, our diet cannot consist of only passionate foods; it mostly requires foods of a sattvic quality.

Foods with Sluggish or Dull Quality (Tamas)

The foods that ancient ayurvedic texts consider tamasic comprise meats like lamb and beef; dairy products such as mature cheeses; vegetables like garlic, onion, and pumpkin; and some grains and spore-born organisms such as mushrooms.

Today, tamasic foods also include modern, unwholesome foods—"junk foods" such as heavy pastries and cakes, canned and frozen foods, meat products that have been stored or treated, dry milk, grains that cause dryness, leftovers, stale food, overcooked food, processed food, strong alcoholic drinks, and medicines with side effects. Some of the foods included in today's tamasic group have high nutritional value but are potentially harmful. For example, meat may be packed with hormones and antibiotics. Some foods taste and look as fresh as if they were natural but are carrying chemical additives from intensive industrial production processes. Studies show that after exposure to highly palatable, energy-dense, and nutrient-poor junk food in the womb and through breast milk, brain reward pathways become desensitized to these foods; in the same way that drug addicts need ever-increasing doses of drugs to achieve the desired high, the theory goes that these children will need more junk food.[27, 28]

Also, the subject of tamasic food needs to be tackled carefully, as the effects of these foods vary according to what you have been eating since childhood—such as familiar foods that your body recognizes and metabolizes well according to your individual constitution and history. The writings on tamasic food state that these items decrease the body's ability to remove toxins, viruses, and harmful bacteria and yeasts, such as those causing inflammation and long-term disruption of proper performance of the immune system. Foods that once were sattvic can turn into tamasic foods as a result of overeating, reheating, or eating leftovers or stale foods. Since tamasic foods eaten alone or in large amounts require so much energy to digest, they are considered inappropriate and unwholesome because they make people feel lazy, inefficient, and slow. The natural biological state of the mind is to be creative and productive, but tamasic foods bring stagnation in movement, physical activity, and thinking, leading to body-mind imbalances; thus, these foods tend to cause disease and distress. The final result of eating sluggish tamasic food is weight gain, cravings, lethargy, and obesity; and with these troubles come strong mood swings, insecurity, pessimism, and irritability. As a result, the person who moves to a tamasic condition is quickly tired, may be unable to deal with others in a peaceful way, and often longs for prolonged sleep.

The light at the end of this dark tunnel of consuming tamasic food, as with everything, is found in these three precepts: moderation, moderation, and moderation! We know from experience that tamasic qualities come in handy during phases of strong physical pain and stress, such as from bitter cold weather or physically strenuous work. In such situations tamasic food helps to briefly dull the senses, giving your body the space to repair itself, thus providing stability and restored drive. But, under normal conditions, keep tamasic foods at bay.

Remember the most general prakruti traits for the three body constitutions:

vata: anxious and tends to lose weight
pitta: prone to anger and preoccupation
kapha: tends to sleep excessively and, as a result, gains weight

Our nature and behavior are a complex interplay among all three doshas (prakruti) and qualities (triguna) in fluctuating degrees. Defining the body's prakruti traits in a brief way can distort the information since we are the result of a combination, in different proportions, of three doshas, according to our parents' DNA. Equally, ayurveda perceives manas prakruti as characterized by sattva, rajas, and tamas—not only rajasic, and not only tamasic. Some people display conduct that is more rajasic with a significant influence of sattvic guna; in others it is rajasic with a significant influence of tamasic guna.

My final recommendation, based on my understanding of the ayurvedic scholarly texts and from my practice, is that if you are seeking to rebalance your body weight, you need to consume mainly sattvic foods, adding a quota of some rajasic and tamasic foods in order to obtain the energy, stability, and strength to support an active lifestyle that keeps you inspired and perseverant. Note that today's nutritional trend is to recommend sattvic diets. This approach is increasingly common, irrespective of any ayurvedic influence on nutritionists, so perhaps we are relearning the ancient wisdom of ayurveda subconsciously.

The key is that you should plan what you eat, be active in organizing your food, and be mindful of the parameters you should use to select your food.

16

AYURVEDA AND DIET

··

Dietary Advice for Your Rebalancing Journey

We all know that the eventual outcome of many diets is often weight gain, so finding a truly balanced, personalized diet is the key to understanding and addressing individual conditions, which so many people are currently trying to address with drugs. If we consider the pharmacological management of weight with anti-obesity medications (AOMs), we observe a long history filled with numerous disappointments, often delivering insufficient efficacy and dubious safety even when the drugs are associated with diet. One of the multifactorial reasons in the case of obesity has been the restricted translational research value of animal models to predict metabolic and cardiovascular safety, since patients' lifestyles frequently create risk of circulatory conditions, and comorbidities complicate the safe assessment of drugs. Thus, our distressed society could greatly benefit from a clear, scientific ayurvedic description of how our bodies and minds interrelate with food. We need proper information and awareness regarding the nutritional and metabolic aspects of imbalanced conditions such as being overweight or obese. How do we obtain such understanding?

Well, we do so by integrating the profound knowledge of ayurveda with today's biomedical tools, to get a proper vision of the physiological, biochemical, and psychological aspects of obesity. Ayurveda explains that a good digestive/gastric fire or agni in the GIT is the main gateway through which nutrients enter the tissues and then pass into our cells to maintain life functions, thus avoiding the formation and accumulation of ama or undigested food components.

Diet (ahara) is the cause of the birth, maintenance, and destruction of all forms of life on this earth.

Su. Sa. Sū. 46/3

Ayurvedic literature describes five types of nutritional disorders:

▼ Quantitative dietary deficiency: insufficient food causing undernutrition or starvation
▼ Qualitative dietary deficiency: malnutrition through lack of essential nutrients or certain food combinations upsetting the normal functioning of the gastric secretions, interfering with the state of our doshas and creating ama
▼ Qualitative and quantitative overnutrition: emotional overeating, and other issues creating conditions such as obesity, high cholesterol, hypertension, heart attack, or paralysis
▼ Toxins in food: certain nutrients causing toxemia, leading to digestive disorders
▼ Foods unsuitable to our bodies: affecting natural resistance, causing disease

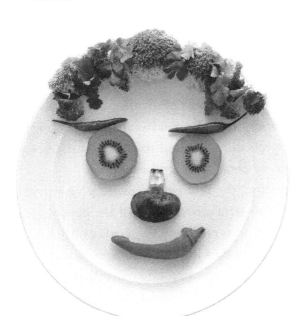

Fig. 16.1. A Happy Plate Makes for a Happy Body-Mind.

There is a common denominator in all the above factors, and it is stress levels and the production of ama. Over time, elevated levels of stress lead to consistent release of stress hormones, and changes in metabolic functioning, which are also associated with accumulation or storage of body fat and obesity.

MAINSTREAM INFORMATION ON DIET AND NUTRITIONAL CONCEPTS

The modern medical system has been altering its views on diet based on a combination of scientific research, food and industrial agricultural alimentary studies and their interests, and media manipulation, all with the impact of harm and cost to our citizens.

To expand your vision, I provide here some scientific endnotes in case you would like to explore such diet information from the "four food groups" to the "food pyramid" and "my plate,"[1, 2, 3] Mediterranean diets,[4, 5, 6, 7] the intake of egg, butter, margarine, and so on,[8] and the vilification of dietary fat.[9, 10, 11, 12, 13]

It is fascinating that modern scientific research is describing the digestive processes such as intercellular uptake, molecular release, and cellular communication in ways that validate the knowledge conveyed by the classic ayurvedic texts a few thousand years ago; the two paradigms are separated only by different vocabularies. Fortunately, in the days of the ayurvedic texts, food industry misinformation didn't exist, so ayurvedic scholars were able to summarize these processes by saying: "What we take in is what we become," or, "You are what you eat." In other words, those many centuries of Indian trial and error allowed them to find ways to address health through diet, understanding that what we ingest and digest becomes our strength, and what we cannot digest becomes our vulnerability, manifesting sooner or later in the form of physical or mental imbalances.

MAINSTREAM DIETS AND YOU!

Here, I am not suggesting or providing detailed information about different types of diets, such as low-carb, paleo, gluten-free, vegan, Mediterranean, carnivore, and so on, since far more important than these diets is you, and how you approach your daily diet.[14, 15] We are not just an impression or result of what we eat; it is about when, how, how much, and what state of mind you are in during the process of food intake. Once you understand your constitution and the potential imbalances between your prakruti and vikruti, you can adapt your lifestyle to gain a proper body-mind connection. Only through this knowledge and acceptance of your potential imbalance will you truly know what kind of foods and diet are right for you, and with this understanding and motivation assume responsibility for yourself. Ayurveda invites you to develop an inner awareness about your dietary habits and potential mistakes to be corrected. A well-rounded understanding of the individual is the real key to finding a truly balanced diet.

Of course, there are many other aspects we can take into consideration; I will not go into depth given the innumerable different ideas of diets and approaches from media promotors, (and behind them the food industry), "diet gurus," movie stars, and others, with a number of them lacking adequate scientific support.[16]

A diet or lifestyle needs to be supported by trustworthy research, so the well-rounded ayurvedic approach to a balanced diet and lifestyle, tried and tested by billions of people over thousands of years, is the best scientific support. In the previous chapter addressing food, we discussed the essential role of agni, or digestive fire, in keeping a state of balance. Let's now investigate how to optimize our nutrients by analyzing in more detail the very important ayurvedic concept and role of ama.

COMPLICATIONS DUE TO IMPROPER DIETARY HABITS
Undigested Food (Ama)

Improper diet is the cause of illness.

Su. Sa. Sū. 46/3

The Sanskrit word *ama* can be translated as "undigested," "uncooked," "unripe," "raw," or "immature." Essentially, ama is a form of unmetabolized waste that the body cannot use. In all our cellular metabolic processes, including digestion, molecules and compounds are formed that our bodies cannot process and that we need to remove. This is a principal reason why we must pay special attention to avoiding overeating. Ama formation in small amounts is a normal part of the digestive process, and under ordinary conditions of strong agni or metabolic fire, ama will be efficiently eliminated. However, when we eat in excess, our body systems cannot clear these components that trigger conditions such as weak agni; then, we risk entering into a vicious and self-perpetuating cycle. The origins and causes of ama formation were very well studied by the ayurvedic scholars, particularly as they related to conditions such as extra weight, obesity, and other pathologies.

Our bodies are made up of over 200 different cell types forming different tissues. Under balanced circumstances, every type of cell in your body specializes in accomplishing a particular function, usually by being part of a specific tissue and communicating to neighboring cells via complex sugars combined with proteins coating the surfaces of the cells. This is a part of the beautiful, continual process of maintaining equilibrium, which we call inner intelligence. In the dynamic realm of cells, intelligent communication must flow. Ama blocks that flow of communication at the level of our circulatory systems, a topic I explored as a medical scientist for many years.

When ama is located in the digestive tract, it is fairly easy to clear, but once it extends into the deeper tissues, it becomes far more difficult to eliminate. Ama that accumulates in other tissues inevitably obstructs the channels of the body and disturbs tissular nutrition by preventing nutrients from being delivered efficiently to the cells, and waste from being discharged efficiently from the body. For instance, heavy metals may accumulate due to environmental exposure and obesity, or ama in the form of oxidized LDL molecules may block blood circulation and communication in the arterial walls through its accumulation—creating what is known as "bad cholesterol." These accumulated "bad" or "wasted" LDL in the wrong tissues inhibit arterial flow and cellular communication, and even weaken the immune response.[17]

Removing the ama generated by the constant attack of several environmental pollutants, which either combine with our natural bodily molecules or undergo bioaccumulation in our tissues, is a big challenge.[18] Ayurvedic practices are valuable when seeking successful environmental ama removal. These type of ama pollutants affect our cellular intelligence and are strongly associated with a wide variety of body-mind imbalances that can manifest as chronic pathologies if they are not addressed in time.

Formation of Ama

Ama is noticeable in the human organism under two different conditions: by accumulation in our body tissues, disturbing physiological processes, and by accumulation or interference in our mind, presenting as changes in our rational manners and processes.

Ayurveda describes ama as the result of a deviation that cannot be tolerated, between the individual and nature. When that harmony is lost, a physical or mental disease can arise.

> *Ama has got the capacity to vitiate the tridoshas due to its various properties.*
>
> CA. SA. VI. 2/11–12

Ayurveda gives special value to these three fundamental causes of disease: First, *asatmendriyartha samyoga* refers to incorrect, improper, or excessive utilization of the sense organs of vision, sound, smell, taste, and touch. This incorrect contact of the senses with their objects results in an overstimulation or deficiency of sensory activity that harms the body-mind balance—for example, overindulgence in a bad diet.[19, 20, 21] Extreme indulgence, or hyperactivity, in physical or mental activities results in an increase of vata, triggering the release of neurotransmitters and endocrine regulators that will start all the metabolic and transformational actions of pitta, causing structural changes at the cellular level that represent the involvement of kapha.

Second, *prajnaparadha* translates as "mistake of the intellect" and refers to wrong actions performed by an individual deliberately as a result of any poor decision made by the mind. In today's medical terms, these wrongful actions from a disconnected mind lead to emotional stress conditions, causing imbalances in physiology that affect different natural biological pathways. This results in the subsequent release of certain neurotransmitters, such as catecholamines, increasing the uptake of endogenous and exogenous lipids such as LDL, which affects the physiological balance of dosha homeostasis.[22, 23]

Third, *parinama* is a Sanskrit term that stands for any unfavorable or abrupt changes in climatic conditions that could hamper the stability of doshas. It means that the cause of disease is being out of harmony with the rhythms and cycles of nature and has to do with two types of time: seasonal variations of our constitution or doshas, and a predominance of doshas that is appropriate to a person's age. Seasonal and age-related variations cause vitiation of the doshas: vata gathering during the summer and vitiating in the rainy season, pitta gathering in the rainy season and vitiating in fall, and kapha gathering in the cold season and vitiating in spring.[24] With regard to age, kapha leads in childhood, pitta in middle age, and vata in old age.

It is important to become aware of these cycles and adapt your lifestyle appropriately to avoid creating discordance through tridosha imbalance. Our chronobiological rhythms were well known to the classical ayurvedic scholars. Here, I cite scientific studies illustrating particular body-mind disturbances caused by perennial disrespect of our biorhythms.[25, 26, 27]

Signs and Symptoms of Ama

A simple example of ama is when vata, the dosha of motion, feels disturbed, and its fluidity is not normal due to blockages by the element of kapha that cause indigestion. In such cases, your body will manifest symptoms that may include gas, bloating, constipation, or even mental confusion and physical exhaustion. It is similar to how, if you do not regularly apply oil to your bicycle chain rings, chain, and cogs, they will become rusty. The same happens in your body when channels are blocked. For example, the formation of plaque at an arterial level causes strength deficiency, a lethargic feeling, or heaviness, as a result of deposits of fatty substances, cellular waste products, calcium, and other components.

Ama and Obesity

What you eat absolutely does matter, and your choices of foods for every meal or snack are either promoting imbalance and disease in your body or promoting improved health—depending on your digestive fire (agni), the time of day when you decide to eat, the quality and quantity of what you are eating, and your frame of mind. These are all the most common potential factors leading to the accumulation of ama, or unassimilated metabolic byproducts.

The diet should be made up of all the six tastes, and
according to their properties diet again can be of
two types: heavy or light to digest.

SU. SA. SŪ. 46/525

Ask yourself: are the foods I am eating day in and day out associated with my condition of being overweight or obese, or suffering from anxiety or brain fog? Let's be honest and realistic—you are already aware that poor quality foods, bad habits, certain medications, and negative impressions contribute to the prevalence of obesity and associated disorders such as diabetes, heart disease, high blood pressure, irritable bowel syndrome, celiac disease, autoimmune diseases, cancer, and even mental health disorders. These troubles all have a common denominator: formation and accumulation of undigested or unmetabolized products (ama) in your body. This is an area that has not been explored properly in modern efforts to manage excess weight and obesity.

Dietary choices are a complete and complex circuit that can affect your body's portfolio of stocks and savings. Let us imagine you would like to eat the types of food (potential ama) to fuel your digestive fire (agni). Now, let's look at your options: you can accumulate riches in the form of robust health by eating the right healthy foods, which is like putting money into your bank account and spending in a balanced way (since your agni will be functioning efficiently); or you can consume unwholesome foods, which is like making purchases on credit—it might feel good now, but eventually it will drain your healthy bank balance. The ingestion of unwholesome foods will end up draining your agni (energy bank account), producing ama (debt), and causing body-mind inequities. Building ama is a very bad investment because it drains your savings account and stocks until you find yourself in debt.

Of course, there is always an underlying reason why we feel the way we do. Every effect has a cause. We have to remember that ama can alter our body-mind system in two different ways: ama manifests in a material sense by accumulating in your bodily tissues, but it is equally able to manifest through accumulation or interference at the level of your mind, causing mental imbalances such as obesity. Individuals living with obesity often struggle with depression and other mental health disorders, on top of their physical challenges. A recent study showed that adults with excess weight had a 55 percent higher risk of developing depression over their lifetime, and that individuals with depression had a 58 percent increased risk of obesity.[28]

Ayurveda also refers to the process of gathering mental ama as mistakes of the intellect, senses, and time. Mistakes of the intellect begin when a person sees what is harmful as useful, or they do not eat according to their level of hunger or digestive power. Mistakes of the senses arise through sensory desire, which is often seen in cases of overeating. Mistakes of time include not eating according to the seasons. These mistakes lead to poor diet, wrong eating habits, overeating, unnecessary cravings, and unhealthy routines. These results in turn lead to aggravation of the vata, pitta, and kapha doshas, imbalance within the channels of the body, and weak or dull digestive fire (agni), which can lead to accumulation of more ama.

AYURVEDIC RECOMMENDATIONS
TO KEEP AMA AWAY

Food for the Body–What, When, and Where?

The functions of diet (food) are: instantly satisfying, gives strength/energy, and maintains body functions, vitality, memory, and agni, increasing longevity.

Su. Sa. Ci. 24/68

Ayurveda recommends the following, regardless of your predominant body-mind constitution: eat only after full digestion of the previous meal. Please do not eat because it is "mealtime;" eat when you are really hungry (except for late at night).

What we call Western culture has developed in us a very strong tendency to eat far too much. If you eat again before the previous meal has been fully digested, then you are forcing the body to simultaneously deal with the arrival of fresh food while still handling the half-digested food from the previous meal. Also, for example, if you had a late breakfast, how can you expect that your body will be able to digest and assimilate a full lunch at midday? Eating when the previous meal is half-digested invites the production and secretion of enzymes and other factors present in the digestive juices, and in the long run this situation alters the normal balance of secretions by the internal organs that support your digestion. The final impact of this type of behavior is the encouraging of the doshas to become vitiated, or impaired; thus, you are building up body-mind disturbances. At the physical body level, typical examples of such imbalances include fermentation of food substances, decrease of enzymatic secretions, and flatulence.

Furthermore, if you feel hungry after a part of the day when you were under stress, or when you experience depression or anxiety, then eat well, but preferably not too much, to avoid wearying your GIT with a large amount of food to digest. Always respect your three meals per day in terms of proper times and quantities. In that way, you can attain a true hunger state. To achieve it, abstain from unnecessary snacks between meals, or have only a very small snack, if unavoidable. Wrong food intakes can be one of the causes of mental imbalances manifesting as bad moods, weariness, fatigue, and depression, all of which originate from ama production at the physical and mental levels.

Eating with Awareness: What You Ended Up Swallowing

Ayurvedic scholars described in detail the importance of the actions of swallowing, salivation, propulsion of food, respiration, and digestion of food (Ca. Ci. 28/6; Su. Ni. 1:13).

Become conscious of how important it is to take time before each meal to really appreciate the food you are going to eat. Aroma, taste, flavor, color, and a relaxing atmosphere add another dimension to the nutritional value of your meal. How often do you eat in front of screens, at your desk while managing documents or emails, or even while standing up or walking along the streets in a hurry? Do you think that is the way your body will appreciate food and get a sense of being nourished? Are you surprised if, later on, your body struggles to assimilate hurriedly ingested food? Realize how important is to take the time to chew your food.

We've discussed how all these factors send signals to the brain and will induce the release of secretions, from the salivary level to gastric juices and enzymes, ensuring they play their roles in breaking down your food and allowing absorption and assimilation. The feelings of appetite and satiety involve complex interactions between hormones from the gastrointestinal tract to the hypothalamus, and subsequent feedback. Within the hypothalamus are specific regions where hormones interact in producing sensations of appetite and satiety, leading to food consumption or a feeling of fullness.[29]

Best Ways to Decrease Ama

You can prevent ama formation by eating foods according to your prakruti and vikruti, and by abstaining from ingestion of foods until the previous meal is digested by your agni. Avoid erratic eating habits so that you are not kindling your agni all the time. Only eat when hungry, and not for the sake of eating. In balance, we should feel hungry at regular mealtimes, according to the physiological body rhythms, but this is not always the case, and we should exercise restraint so as not to overeat. Perhaps it will take time to connect with these rhythms, especially if you have been eating erratically. For example, after deciding to have a small dinner, it is probable that your body will really feel the need for breakfast the day after. Also don't skip lunch, and especially avoid eating a large dinner. Don't overindulge in food, especially processed, heavy, fat, fried, sugary and rich, or conflicting foods. Keep away from stale or contaminated foods such as those that are packaged or long-frozen; instead, choose fresh foods.

Abstain from eating cold meals or drinking ice-cold water or drinks during your meal. When eating, remove distractions that prevent you paying full attention to the meal, such as media screens, or situations that cause you to eat too fast. Reduce emotional tension and stressful conditions in your life to cultivate a supportive state of mind. And of course, you should incorporate physical activities and exercise.

You can cleanse the digestive tract according to your prakruti by using specific spices or herbal preparations. Drink hot water and lemon in the morning, or spices such as ginger. And it's possible to reactivate your metabolic fire (agni) and reduce your ama by implementing a strict diet, initially with liquid meals, moving progressively to solid food. Further, a supervised detox program or panchakarma can decrease ama, and excess kapha, pitta, and vata. Remove ama with ayurvedic herbal recipes or by using a gentle detoxification herbal formula like *triphala*, described in chapter 17.[30, 31, 32]

Remember, our bodies were not designed or destined to become toxic dumps. However, inadequate food ingestion, overstress, and chemical contaminants—present in the air we breathe, the water we drink or wash with, and the foods we eat—are endlessly creating metabolic byproducts that can lead to a toxic scenario in our bodies. You need to flush them out of your system on a regular basis. Ayurveda offers you all the above protocols to use before this potential toxic buildup manifests as a strong body imbalance. The older we become, the less capable our body's mechanisms for eliminating impurities tend to be, so we need periodic cleansing. As always, I recommend that you discuss these matters with your doctor or a qualified ayurvedic practitioner before taking any steps.

ROLE OF KAPHA ON MANAS PRAKRUTI
Ending Body Weight Imbalance Cycle

It's no secret that the balance between eating (energy in) and burning off those calories (energy out) is why your weight goes up and down. If you take in more than you burn, you gain weight—sometimes right away. However, it presupposes the intention of changing your mental setup, and with it your habits, those that got you into an imbalanced state.

We've already covered your mental constitution (manas prakruti) based on the components of sattva, rajas, and tamas, which explain the different mental types relevant to body and mind imbalances, allowing us to better understand your own condition—whether sattvic (knowledge/purity), rajasic (movement/activity), or tamasic (inertia/heaviness).

As a result of the ayurvedic evaluation and analysis of your body-mind processes by the prakruti, vikruti, and manas prakruti evaluations (see pages 271–87), you now have substantial information on the way you function and the way you interact with others. This new attitude invites you to live in search of awareness by observing your daily life habits and routines and accepting them without judging them. Recognizing our wrong habits is the first step toward change.

Body imbalances, including obesity, have a direct connection to our biology and are closely related to our biochemistry and physiology. We live under the rule of neurotransmitters that generate feelings and dispositions toward satiation, hunger, pleasure, or even our sense of short-term happiness; and we can gradually learn to observe these states.

I will briefly summarize the ways in which mainstream medicine's understanding of diet agrees with the ayurvedic understanding. Then I will take you one step further, showing you examples of tailored food and diet advice based on your manas prakruti, to complement the food and diet recommendations you already have based on your body prakruti and actual vikruti state.

DIETARY INTAKE AND YOUR BODY
Mind Setup for Obesity

The typical American diet is shortening the lives of the country's population: nearly 900 deaths a day are linked to poor diet. Nutrition and diets in the United States are in crisis. The Covid-19 pandemic highlighted the problem, with much worse outcomes for people with obesity and other diet-related diseases. In fact, obesity is not the only collateral effect associated with diets that include overprocessed foods. Recent research shows that eating overprocessed foods such as soft drinks, flavored cereals, and frozen foods leads to a faster decline in cognitive results like memory, verbal fluency, and executive function, and may contribute to a higher risk of developing dementia.[33, 34]

We have to think outside the box. The American diet is deadly; eating wholesome foods is vital to nourishing and treating your physical health and preventing significant imbalances of your body-mind-consciousness triumvirate. The foods that maintain equilibrium in your body tissues are the ones considered natural or wholesome; they lead to the balanced growth of living beings. Unnatural or unwholesome foods cause diseases through accumulation of ama. Earlier, we addressed in detail how wholesome or unwholesome food constituents bring about opposite effects depending on variations in quality, quantity, process of preparation, time of ingestion, body constitution, age of the individual, potential disease stage, and environment.

To assure your body-mind balance, the above factors need to be incorporated when tailoring a diet based on your prakruti, manas prakruti, and individual condition, without making so many restrictions that it becomes challenging to live.

Unfortunately, if we are honest, whether we're of average weight, or overweight or obese, we all eat without being hungry. Most of the time, we do so simply because of the time of the day, or because our senses are attracted to the taste, appearance, or smell of something. Or we may eat due to our family and educational habits or based on our understanding of nutrition.

As a result of not necessarily knowing the right way of eating, we potentially contribute to the decline of our mental health, increasing the push toward extra weight, obesity, and collateral manifestations such as anxiety, loss of focus, sleeplessness, fatigue, brain fog, or even severe mental issues. If you are also taking a mixture of drugs—perhaps antidepressants, or drugs for hypertension or to reduce cholesterol—their side effects are also impacting your body-mind-consciousness triad, causing the formation of more ama or undigested particles, the underlying cause of many health issues.

DIGESTION STAGES OF FOOD INTAKE FOR BODY AND MIND PRAKRUTI CONSTITUTIONS

All bodily systems are necessarily interconnected for proper function, but you can sense which ones feel more disturbed under conditions of obesity.

Vata: All body movement functions are controlled by vata, including all sensory and motor functions of the nervous system. A vata-type physiology achieves proper digestion thanks to the large intestine, as well as the kidneys and bladder, all under regulation of the brain that provides communication and organization of the bodily functions. In obesity, the principal vata manifestation is dryness. In terms of digestion, a dry colon leading to constipation is a manifestation of poor functioning.

Pitta: Digesting or metabolizing ingested food for correct biological transformation and generation of body heat, metabolic energy, and promoting relaxing and gentle impressions to keep under control the natural, vibrant role of pitta. Since the small intestine is the main pitta organ, in obesity all digestive processes are affected, including regulation of assimilation, hunger, and thirst. This involves all internal organs like the heart, liver, spleen, and gallbladder, causing, for example, alteration of bile production and the digestion of fats.

Kapha: The kapha-type physiology is responsible for digestion of proteins, fats, and carbohydrates, via its main organs, the stomach and pancreas. Abnormal ingestion of food manifests clearly in relation to digestive kapha functions. Since kapha is the slowest and steadiest of all three doshas, an imbalanced lifestyle and diet combined with hereditary traits will instigate a visible imbalance manifesting as obesity, due to metabolic dysfunction in the processing of fats.

Let's go one step deeper into the understanding of how ama could affect our ponderal weight and become the cause of so many disturbances.

Even before reflecting on the role of food, ayurveda teaches us that poor digestion (low agni) is the primary cause of most diseases and that imbalance affects our bodies and minds.

> *It is obvious that the body elements cannot be*
> *nourished and developed when food is not properly*
> *digested by agni.*

CA. CI. 15/5

Ama, generated from undigested food in the digestive tract, is the source of gastrointestinal disorders. An inefficient digestive tract is unable to process food intake, generating ama.

Ama subsequently leaks from the gastrointestinal tract into other body systems and settles in vulnerable or fragile places, including our nervous system. The ancient ayurvedic scholars called these defective tissular or organ spaces *khavaigunya*: places where doshas settle and initiate subsequent pathologies. We all have an Achilles' heel or vulnerable area in our bodies susceptible to emotional or physical lesions. Inherited disorders or unhealthful lifestyle choices can also be the cause of khavaigunya. This ayurvedic conception of weakness is analogous to the concept of a weak immune system in mainstream medicine. It is well known that everyone has an immune system that is sensitive to conditions such as weather and food, as well as emotions.

CASE STUDY
Khavaigunya

We all have personal physiological vulnerabilities, which Ayurveda calls khavaigunya, meaning "weak space" or "defective part of the body," generally caused by genetic defects, previous injuries, or illness. Let me give you the example of Theresa. She came to me for a consultation, having been unable to sort out her problem of recurrent episodes of left shoulder pain at the clavicula level, as a result of a serious car accident, and having visited several health practitioners. During her first visit I understood there were unresolved emotions associated with the accident—in my judgment manifesting as strong tensions and muscular spasms in that area from sitting in a car, watching films involving car accidents, or when experiencing flashbacks. I explained to Theresa how our tissues have memory at the level of the fascia and sometimes the memory of such a major physical trauma may become trapped in the fascia. As a major component of her treatment protocol, I suggested for her to practice relaxation techniques and pranayamas, which she adopted and continued to practice regularly. She returned two years later, that time for another medical issue, and described that by using these techniques she was able to find release from her spasms and pain despite that the vulnerability or "weak space" was still there.

The strength of agni—digestive fire that plays the role of biochemical energy used to break down, metabolize, absorb, and assimilate nutrients without creating much waste—determines a person's appetite. Agni regulates digestion, absorption, and metabolism of nutrients to transform them into part of our functional cellular structures.

Agni turns food molecules into energetic molecules in service of the whole organism. If your agni is weak, the processes of digestion, absorption, and metabolism of nutrients will be improper, leading to poor nourishment and then ama generation. Under these conditions, your ama will eventually start disturbing your cellular functions, creating all kinds of tissue alterations and dysfunctions that will affect your metabolic processes on various levels, from the digestive system up through the nervous system. These problems will manifest in your metabolic functions, creating body-mind imbalances.

Let me be crystal clear: What you eat absolutely does matter.

The kind of food you eat each time you have a meal or snack is either causing disease, building disease in your body, or reversing disease and improving health, depending on your individual constitution, digestive power, and factors such as what, when, and how much you eat. Try to eat the type of foods that correspond to your prakruti, so your intake will be a sorce of positive energy currency you are putting in a kind of body savings account, and giving you strength by reducing ama accumulation. Nothing could be better than depositing noble savings in your body. Are you the kind of person who becomes sick as a result of making continuous deposits into the illness account by accumulating toxins, while always withdrawing from the well-being savings account? If that's the case, then it's time to change!

NURTURING YOUR BODY AND MIND
ACCORDING TO YOUR TYPE OF OBESITY

Tailoring Your Diet for Your Unbalanced Body-Mind: Obesity as a Kapha Disorder

Food is one of the major pleasures in our lives and essential for our existence. Under normal metabolic circumstances, when we are hungry and eat food, we acquire materials and energy from nature that our gastric system processes into cellular-intelligent energy (ATP), which we integrate into our body tissues and organs to ensure their functioning. In cases of energy excess (calories), they can be stored, up to certain limits, in specialized organs like the liver and muscles, as fat. If the excess of energy becomes overwhelming, the processed energy gets converted into fat, migrating either to the adipose tissue or to other tissues for storage. When the pressure is too high, the process becomes repetitive, translating into a person putting on extra weight, becoming overweight or, as is under study, developing different kinds of obesity.[35]

From the ayurvedic point of view, when considering obesity, I've described it as a disorder where the gastric fire (jathara agni) is high and dhatu agni is low. That is to say, overweight and obese people have strong appetites and slow metabolisms, and imbalance arises from inappropriate food intake. Since they tend to eat enough, but what they consume is not processed fully, their unburned fire (calories) turns into an excess of kapha in the system, along with low agni. In all body constitutions, when kapha dosha increases, which relates to unprocessed or unburned calories, it causes an imbalance resulting in weight gain and the development of obesity (sthoulya), which has more serious implications for individuals with kapha prakruti and kapha vikruti.

Ideally, your food intake should build, provide energy to, and repair the cells in your body-mind organism. Thanks to the subtle dynamism of your body tissues and the various systems described earlier, the food you eat also influences your sensations and reactions. We have the tendency to forget that just as food influences your physiological digestive processes, it also plays an influential role in your mental processes. Let me present to you some dietary recommendations for dual-prakruti (vata-kapha and pitta-kapha), and kapha-predominant prakruti.

If you choose to have a certified ayurvedic practitioner or diet consultant tailor a diet for your body weight imbalance, they may in some cases propose a diet that does not look like the one you need to support the condition of, for example, an increased kapha. Possibly this initial prescribed diet is intended to reduce a particular symptom or dosha related to your disorder or to the kinds of medications you are taking. For instance, consider that you can be predominantly kapha but at the same time be a dual-doshic type such as vata-kapha or pitta-kapha. You will follow the prescribed diet until the symptoms of your disorder decrease, and then you will return to the diet fully corresponding to your body-mind constitution. Let's discuss this in more detail.

Diet for Vata-Kapha Dosha Types

Digestion plays a major role in our health. A vata-kapha dual-doshic type needs to pay attention to which doshic propensity is most prevalent in their digestion or if it is a close combination of both dosha. When addressing agni, vata digestion is called vishama agni or irregular digestion, whereas kapha digestion is called manda agni or slow digestion. For this reason, a vata-kapha person will frequently have slow agni or manda agni.

Vata appetite and digestion are erratic, while kapha qualities have a dampening effect on both, making vata-kapha dosha appetite and digestion either erratic or weak. In other words, vata-kapha people have an imbalanced digestion, often feel bloated, and have a tendency toward constipation.

Well-Being Tips for Vata-Kapha Types

In terms of taste (rasa), the tastes that are pacifying to vata are aggravating to kapha and vice versa; vata and kapha are not pacified by any of the same tastes, making for confusing dietary advice. But since vata-kapha dosha wishes for warmth more than anything, hot or warming tastes like sour, salty, and pungent are better than cold or cooling tastes like sweet, bitter, and astringent. Remember that sweet tastes are most aggravating to kapha dosha, and bitter and astringent tastes are most aggravating to vata dosha, so moderate intake and the seasonal period are very important in determining which foods are best for your dual dosha. A kapha-reducing diet is suggested for the spring and winter seasons, and a vata-reducing diet is recommended for the fall and summer seasons. Lunch is the most important meal of the day. Eat a light breakfast so lunch is not hampered, then have a small dinner.

Vata-kapha types need to keep balancing their constantly changing state with sufficient warmth, easiness, and awareness. Regular warm meals to keep the digestive fire (agni) ignited, regular yoga, and maintaining the discipline of daily routines are the prerequisites for attaining a healthy body-mind balance.

Advice on Vata-Kapha/Kapha-Vata Dosha Diet Plan

If this is your personal type, you are under the influence of the gunas of vata as well as the gunas for kapha. In addition to the lists of food for the vata-kapha and kapha-vata dual doshas, you'll also need to look at the tables of food recommendations for vata as well as kapha included on pages 288–90, 293–96 and make a plan that corresponds to your needs and goals. If doing so seems too complicated, see a professional, qualified practitioner for an accurate food plan.

My recommendations for this type are, first, moderation; second, plenty of fresh and seasonal wholesome, nutritive foods. Vegetables should be seasoned with a wide range of spices and should mainly be fresh and home-cooked to support food digestibility, as well as to avoid more weight gain and to keep the mind grounded.

Body Nurturing: Food Intake/Diet for Kapha-Vata/Vata-Kapha Doshas

vegetables: green beans, asparagus, peas, beets, mustard greens, okra, onion, zucchini, parsnips, radishes, spinach, yellow squash, watercress

fruits: low-sugar fruits such as apricot, pears, berries, cherries, lemon, lime, peaches, melon, raisins (soaked), tamarind, tangerine; avoid fruit juices

grains: barley, oat, millet, quinoa, buckwheat, basmati rice; preferably whole grains

beans: adzuki beans, lentils (red or brown), split mung beans, yellow split peas

meat: white meat is easier to digest

nuts/seeds: coconut, pumpkin seeds, sunflower seeds, sesame seeds

dairy: ghee, goat's milk, butter

oils: ghee, sunflower, almond, flax oil, and sesame oil with moderate intake.

sweeteners: honey (raw and uncooked), dates

spices: allspice, anise, asafetida, bay leaf, black pepper, caraway, cardamom, cilantro, cinnamon, cloves, coriander, cumin, dill leaves, garlic (cooked), ginger, mace, marjoram, mint, mustard seeds, nutmeg, oregano, paprika, parsley, peppermint, rosemary, saffron, sage, savory, star anise, thyme, turmeric; avoid spicy foods

teas: ginger, lemon balm, lemongrass, peppermint, basil, chamomile, cinnamon, cloves, chicory, elderflower, eucalyptus, raspberry leaves, rose flower, sage

snacks: These should be limited during the day and avoided altogether after dinner.

herbal support: Use triphala before bed to aid in digestion, elimination, and detoxification.

Mind Nurturing

To be promoted: truth, harmony, fearlessness, patience, courage, self-acceptance.

To be discouraged: confusion, lack of direction, blues, grief, unhappiness.

Diet for Pitta-Kapha Dosha

Since digestion plays a major role in our health, a pitta-kapha dual-doshic type needs to pay attention to which doshic propensity is most prevalent in their digestion or if it is a close blend of both doshas. When addressing agni, pitta digestion is called *tikshna agni* or strong digestive power and appetite, whereas kapha digestion is called *manda agni* or slow digestion. For this reason, a pitta-kapha person will frequently have a strong agni despite the dampening drift effect of kapha. Usually, individuals with the pitta-kapha or kapha-pitta constitution keep a very strong agni (digestive fire) and can tolerate nearly all kinds of foods until around middle age. As a result of this strength, an inclination toward an unhealthy lifestyle—such as overeating, too little exercise, and indulgence—results in a tendency to become overweight or obese and to develop skin diseases later in life, since the kapha side enjoys retaining "toxins" that get absorbed by the body. For that reason, monitoring and maintaining a balanced agni is important for pitta-kapha types, allowing them to avoid formation and accumulation of ama, liquids retention, and risk of intoxications.

In terms of managing a pitta-kapha diet according to the seasons, keep on a pitta-pacifying regimen during the late spring and summer seasons, particularly if the weather is hot. During the cooler times of year such as fall, winter, and early spring, and especially if the weather is cool and damp, adopt a kapha-pacifying regimen. Always remember that awareness, an active life, and moderation are the best moves if you want to improve your body weight and mental state. For that reason, a regular, dynamic, and powerful exercise program, a meditation practice, and healthy eating are all strongly recommended.

Advice on Kapha-Pitta/Pitta-Kapha Dosha Diet Plan

In general, follow a stricter kapha-reducing diet in the winter and early spring, and a stricter pitta-reducing diet in the late spring and summer. Remember that pitta is hot by nature and kapha is cold, so it is better to ingest warm, cooked foods that are nonetheless cold in terms of their nature seasons. Since you will be under the influence of the gunas of both pitta and kapha, you need to look at the tables of food recommendations for pitta as well as kapha (see pages 288–96) and plan a program that corresponds to your needs and goals. If it is too complicated for you, I suggest you speak with a qualified practitioner for a professional food plan.

Eat and drink foods and beverages with bitter and astringent tastes since they are cooling for pitta, lightening for kapha, and drying for both doshas.

Body Nurturing: Food Intake/Diet for Kapha-Pitta/Pitta-Kapha Dosha

vegetables: celery, leafy greens, green beans, and other watery vegetables (zucchini, squash, melons, and gourds) can be eaten freely. However, raw salad leaves are good in warm weather but could aggravate kapha if taken in cold weather, so it's better to cook your vegetables in cold seasons. Vegetables that are not too starchy are good for pitta-kapha.

fruits: apples, blueberries, pomegranates, pears. Avoid very sweet or overly sour fruits and juices.

grains: barley, whole wheat, wild rice, quinoa, and oats with bran. They pacify pitta and kapha.

beans: green moong dal and pink or yellow lentils

meat: lean, easy-to-digest protein such as fish and chicken.

nuts/seeds: sunflower, pumpkin, and sesame seeds.

dairy: Avoid yogurt as it aggravates both pitta and kapha. Instead, low-fat, fresh buttermilk can be used during the daytime to feed your microbiome.

oils: olive, soybean oil, and ghee in moderation will balance pitta without aggravating kapha.

snacks: fruits, sprouts, roasted seeds (sunflower, pumpkin, etc.)

spices: fennel, coriander, garlic, curry leaves, mint, cumin. Turmeric and fenugreek seeds are recommended in small quantities due to their hot properties; their bitterness will not aggravate pitta and will appease kapha when used in the right proportions. Use black pepper, long peppers, and fresh ginger if kapha gets aggravated—which causes white coating on the tongue, mucus production, lack of appetite, and lethargy.

liquids: Drink water according to the season, for thirst and hydration needs. Cooling drinks and herbal teas are good during hot seasons. Avoid alcohol, coffee, and cold beverages.

Mind Nurturing

To be promoted: forgiveness, serenity, friendship, kindness, devotion.

To be discouraged: attachment, possessiveness, greed.

Kapha Dosha–Predominant Obesity

If your prakruti corresponds to a predominantly kapha dosha type, you need to be more attentive and rigorous concerning your food intake. By all means enjoy your food, but also be smart about the times you eat, food combinations, quantities, and quality.[36] Use the food recommendation table for kapha type included here, and for your constitution (see pages 288–96). In that way you can always keep healthy despite a ponderal weight above what it is considered normal.

Mind Nurturing

To be promoted: courage, flexibility, independence, disengagement.
To be discouraged: deep confusion, nothingness.

SUMMARY

Your personal diet is unique, and the guidelines in this chapter are meant to reflect that, serving as a model for vata-kapha/kapha-vata, pitta-kapha/kapha-pitta, and kapha-predominant types, as well as reference for vata- and pitta-predominant types since we all have a kapha dosha component within our body-mind triumvirate. You can also use these guideline tables at your own discretion, timing your meals and selecting the right foods according to the more well-defined or preponderant dosha; however, contradictions may occur. In any case, all the included ayurvedic recommendations can point you in the right direction. Just make sure to include a wide variety of these foods, using the information provided in the vata, pitta, and kapha tables of food recommendation included in this book (see appendix 2).

We present here many pieces of advice and recommendations for your body type, but take into consideration that obesity does not always mean ill health. Even mainstream genetics researchers and doctors affirm that we can be obese but remain healthy,[37, 38] a concept that ayurveda understood thousands of years ago when it described prakruti, vikruti, and manas prakruti. There is no blame or shame, just a body frame, body makeup, or an external anatomy to be cared for by a balanced mind in search of awareness. Ultimately, what ayurveda always emphasizes is the importance of lifestyle and nutrition in keeping us healthy, using a range of natural foods available in our personal surroundings. Basically, avoid consumption of heavily processed and refined foods containing endocrine disruptors, as these foods are known to raise ama levels, increasing the risk of chronic lifestyle diseases. Endocrine disruptors, such as nanoplastics, are present in all our tissues from brain to sperm cells.[39]

You can improve your body-mind well-being with what you eat. Please, come back to Nature!

THE FUTURE OF
AYURVEDIC MODALITIES IN
THE AGE OF EPIDEMIC IMBALANCES

Visualizing the Whole Picture and Taking Action

REBALANCING THROUGH AYURVEDA

Prevention and Management of Body-Mind Imbalances

Integration of All Body Systems:
The Issues Are within the Tissues

The previous chapters introduced and analyzed the main body-mind organ systems associated with body weight and gut dysfunction through the lens of modern scientific knowledge and ayurvedic comprehension of the anatomical, physiological, and metabolic functions of our body systems. I offered a general vision of how each works under normal circumstances and how ayurveda understands these systems and processes. At the same time, when possible, I gave specific scientific explanations of potential body-mind dysfunctions associated with being overweight or obese and other pathologies.

I start this section on integration using my favorite saying that concerns problems in our body-mind organ systems: "The issues are within the tissues." When ayurveda and Western medicine each address the physical body in terms of its organ systems, the perceptions of the two sciences are distinct from one another. Let's first describe the importance of terminology here. A body system is a group of organs and tissues that work together to achieve vital functions in the body, and an organ is considered a self-contained group of cellular tissues that accomplishes a specific function in the body.

Based on that definition, Western scientists describe eleven organ systems as follows:

skeletal: provides structure, support, and movement; protects organs; makes blood cells

muscular: allows movement, helps to circulate blood, and protects vital organs

endocrine: guides growth, metabolism, and reproduction via several hormones

cardiovascular/circulatory: manages blood flow around the body via the heart, arteries, and veins

respiratory: moves fresh oxygen into our body while eliminating carbon dioxide as waste

digestive: breaks down, absorbs, and converts food via secretions and enzymatic reactions for energy

urinary/renal: provides filtration of blood, producing urine eliminated as waste

reproductive: produces, matures, nourishes, and stores ovulum and sperm cells

integumentary: handles heat regulation, sensory aspects, protection (via hair, skin, and nails), and waste removal

immune: a complex network that defends the body against all kinds of pathogens

nervous: a signal transmitter-receiver-coordinator that operates via the brain and through nerves including the vagus nerve

Under normal conditions, all teams of these organ systems work in synchronicity, and each one of them is trying to regulate their own entropy. However, to understand the various functions of whole organ systems, our analytical minds require descriptions of the parts, dissected and subdivided, to properly grasp their processes and to comprehend their roles and functions.

In succinct and general ayurvedic terminology, we can say that the Western classification of eleven organ systems corresponds to the following seven organ systems (as you may recall from pages 28–29):

rasa (plasma): the circulatory system
rakta (blood): the circulatory system
mamsa (muscle): the muscular system
meda (fat): the adipose tissue system
asthi (bone): the skeletal system
majja (bone marrow): the immune system
shukra (generative): the reproductive system

We have to take into consideration that ayurvedic scholars analyzed the human body according to its anatomical and physiological functions based on their descriptions of these seven major organ systems, as well as their tissues or derivates that connected to and built on one another.

Since our main matter of interest is the kapha component of fat or adipose tissue, both in terms of body type and functionality, ayurveda states that the organ systems and their tissues sustained by kapha dosha are plasma (rasa), muscle (mamsa), fat (meda), bone marrow (majja dhatu), and reproductive tissue (shukra). Remember that they also gave consideration to the organs of secretion (malas) in the forms of sweat (sveda), urine (mutra), and feces (purisha).

For the purposes of an integrative approach and a better understanding of the origins, expansion, significance, and general impact of kapha resulting from an obesity imbalance in our body organ systems, the kapha component has been considered by modern medicine and ayurveda as a tissular organ existing mainly at the level of the adipose tissue, visceral organs, skeletal muscle, and bones. However, if we include state-of-the-art scientific reports based on the specific roles of these body components, we could consider five "new" organ systems. By integrating them with the other eleven organ systems, they could provide us a clearer view of the ongoing processes involved in body weight imbalance, and at the same time allow us to bring together the conceptual knowledge of both sciences:

adipose: vital "new" metabolic organ involved in the control of whole-body energy homeostasis

lymphatic: "sewerage system" that operates via lymph fluid, removing fluids and protecting the body

excretory: bastion and balance of the GIT, which removes body wastes, excess water, and salts

fascia: web supporting all cells and organs that transmits, perceives, and coordinates mobility

microbiome: helps digestion, controls the immune system, and destroys harmful bacteria

My perception is that, among the sixteen body organ systems, our nervous system, via the long vagus nerve—also known as the vagal nerves, the main nerves of our parasympathetic nervous system (PSNS) that relaxes your body after periods of stress or danger—plays the role of chief or master of ceremonies.

The PSNS is a network of nerves that, along with relaxing us after challenging periods, helps to run life-sustaining processes such as digestion during times when we feel calm and safe. The PSNS helps to control our body response during times of rest by balancing our sympathetic nervous system (SNS), which controls our body's fight-or-fight response. The vagus nerve supports the running of life-sustaining functions, as a brain modulator of all the other organ systems, with the active participation of the fascia system. Here, I will briefly describe its involvement with the various systems.

In the digestive system, the vagus nerve is the vast expressway that conveys all digestion-related data from our gut to our central nervous system, with reverse transportation of metabolites, small molecules and small proteins that can travel all the way to the brain. It also regulates appetite by boosting the rate of digestion, diverting energy to support the digestion of food.

The adipose system lacks direct innervation from the vagus nerve but regulates inflammation throughout the body, including inflammation associated with obesity, and could be a modifier of obesity.

Within the endocrine system, the vagus nerve, among many other roles, participates in the process of synthesis and release of insulin by the pancreas, in that way supporting the process of breakdown of sugars, and allowing your cells to use them to maintain glucose homeostasis.

Regarding the lymphatic system, although the vagus nerve does not innervate the lymphoid organs directly, it does play a role in the neuroimmune axis and can be stimulated in a variety of ways, including breathing and meditation.

Through the immune system's responses both adaptive and innate involving the lymph and lymphatic system, the brain can know what's going on in the gut. Our immunity, in a silent way, is connected to our emotional responses, even playing a role in mood regulation. For instance, the intuitive line of communication when one is nervous or anxious can be transmitted to the gut as tummy aches via the vagus nerve.

Within the nervous system, the vagus nerve influences sensory activity in your eyes as they shrink or constrict their pupils, controlling how much light enters. It is involved in the production of tears, and the production of mucus and saliva by your nose and mouth, respectively, as well as in supporting digestion and breathing in times of rest.

The cardiovascular/circulatory system partly relies on the vagus nerve to regulate cardiac beat-to-beat function by lowering your pumping force and heart rate variability (HRV), maintaining a physiological homeostasis. Epidemiological data shows that the resting heart rate, as a measure of vagus nerve function, predicts mortality.

In the pulmonary system, the vagus nerve tightens air passage muscles and eventually reduces the extent of work your lungs do during times of pause.

As well, the vagus nerve could stimulate bone growth in the skeletal system through osteoclasts, special cells that degrade bone to initiate normal bone remodeling, and mediate bone loss in pathological conditions by increasing bone resorption.[1]

The vagus nerve aids the integumentary system by delivering somatic sensation information for the skin behind the ear, the external part of the ear canal, and certain areas of the throat. It also supplies visceral sensation information to the larynx, esophagus, lungs, trachea, heart, and digestive tract.

Further, it assists the reproductive system by innervation to the ovaries and distal colon. It also participates in sexual arousal.

In the urinary or renal system, stimulation of the vagus nerve can turn on the PSNS, improving renal flow and participating in cases of inflammation.

Regarding the microbiome, it is known that the subdiaphragmatic vagus nerve assists as a major modulator pathway between the brain and gut microbiota, playing a crosstalk role associated with depression.

The vagus nerve also plays a crucial role in the brain-gut-microbiota axis. It can detect microbiota metabolites through its afferents, transferring this gut information to the central nervous system.[2]

We've discussed in detail the significance ayurveda gives to diet and nutrition in keeping a body-mind balance. Its recommendations require planning and selection of foods, and choosing a certain lifestyle, according to your personal constitution or prakruti. When we take into consideration the above functions, we can understand why it is possible to carry on with a "wrong" lifestyle that affects our existence by compromising the vagus nerve's roles, creating a cascade of complications. Fortunately, the vagal function, as part of the PSNS, can be reactivated and bring back body balance, reestablishing health; but it requires our awareness and desire for active participation. Consider the informal descriptions of bacterial activity as "rest and digest" and "feed and breed."

I now would like to consider another aspect that relates to active, conscious participation. One of the best collaborators with the master of ceremonies is a quite invisible structural matrix or web with an inner intelligence, functioning as the body's keeper of our balance: the "fascianating" fascia. In a deeper context, I see fascia as a pulsating matrix organ supervising the tuning and retuning of the tissues and organs of our body's organ systems, due to its active and dynamic structure. This starts with trying to keep our bodies in a certain normal condition and progresses up to the several functions of our various organ systems, either at a structural or metabolic level.

But what is meant by connection with the vagus nerve and the fascia? Well, due to the continual external pressures of daily life, most of us become unaware of or disengaged from our bodily sensations.

When we look at introspective activities such as relaxation or meditation—pillars of the ayurvedic medical approach to sorting out body-mind imbalances—other avenues become possible, avenues that perhaps are there waiting for our participation.

During the process of meditation, if the active meditator gradually manages, with the support of the vagus nerve, to surrender to the external influences and pressures of the outer world, calming down and resting all the organ systems, a shift of perception can take place. Then, the meditator in that state of relaxation or alleviated tension comes into contact with what we could call an observer, a higher mind, or even a superior intelligence. In that state, the observer begins to perceive and connect to body misalignments or tensions, such as traumas or pain; and unconsciously, possibly by being present with these specific observations, the body can start to unwind these trauma impacts and pains. What is the invisible but perceptible unwinding net that is operating on the meditator? It is nothing other than the fascia, gathering and undertaking a collective integration, helping us let go of previously acquired impressions by giving us a structural, functional, and metabolic realignment, rebalancing our original nature and, in short, reconnecting us. When experiencing active meditation, the presence of an observer within, every aspect of our existence changes to what I will call a calm, multi-dimensional reality, which results from fascia integrating or reconnecting with other body organ systems—a condition that some practitioners of meditation call connecting to their deeper self or heart.

We only use 5 to 10 percent of our DNA sequence for building our bodies, codifying proteins to allow body functionality; the rest remains dormant and is called "junk DNA" by scientists. Is it possible that during the process of meditation, and thanks to the role of the vagus nerve and fascia integration, we will get in contact with the other 90 to 95 percent of DNA that is locked up, unraveling it and potentially finding deeper levels of perception of ourselves? A closer link to our fascia via meditative practice of observation could mean a more attentive connection to our twisted tissues and pains, relaxing our neuromuscular, circulatory, and digestive systems, among others. This may help us to resolve these issues by ourselves instead of depending on pharmaceutical drugs, such as painkillers or anti-inflammatories. Perhaps the 98–99 percent of "junk" DNA in our bodies is not so useless as we believe at the moment and could still be engaged in some fashion with our essential DNA, relaying confidential messages that we are unable to decrypt due to our lack of technological tools or understanding of their role. Why does our intelligent body safeguard all our DNA with various nuclear proteins and our nuclear membrane? Are they there to be used for unknown mechanisms of our consciousness that we do not really understand? In any case, if by chance there is some junk, then we will need a janitor to put the house in order.

When you clean your house or apartment, you find dust around, and also some rubbish, if you don't do it frequently. Well, the same happens with our body organ systems, as a result of wear and tear, poor nutrition and diet habits, normal metabolic reactions to toxicity from junk food, or other reasons. If, for example, we experiment either with a short fasting period or detox, or even eating less and at the proper biological times, then we support the rebalancing of our organ systems through these simple processes. Fortunately, our bodies have a brilliant sweeper or janitor that is fairly invisible to the eyes: the lymphatic system. This janitor is working all day long, but mostly operates in the dark hours of sleep as it regulates our immune system processes.

Remember that the lymphatic system relies on the proper functioning of the fascia in supporting and activating muscles and joints to sustain movement, such as through pressure changes during breathing and skeletal muscle contraction. If your body is physically active during the day, the lymphatic system plays the active role of janitor by transferring the hazardous or toxic components to the lymphatic ganglions all through the day. And during our sleep, the immune system will be processing and ditching most of the transported alien bacteria, foreign antigens, and exosomes— tiny extracellular vesicles containing cell constituents secreted by all cells, such as proteins, unhealthy fats, and lipoproteins. The left side of the body is the dominant lymphatic side. Ancient knowledge tells us that sleeping on the left side facilitates and gives more time to your body when it comes to draining and filtering toxins, lymph fluid, and waste through the lymph nodes and thoracic duct. Sleeping on the right side of your body could make the activity of your lymphatic system more sluggish.

As you can see, the dance continues again, involving each of the sixteen organ systems. Maybe this integrative analysis of all organ systems sounds like a plot out of a science fiction book, or a Star Trek episode from when I was a young man; but now it is, for me, real. Hopefully this integration process that supports the role of calming down, relaxing, and meditating will one day be properly studied and understood, and ultimately validated as supportive of body-mind rebalancing.

ACTIVE AYURVEDIC MODALITIES FOR REDUCING WEIGHT

🖋 *Daily Routine (Dinacharya): The Key to Good Health*

As an exercise, try the following steps in your daily routine. These steps are essential to making changes in body, mind, and consciousness:

- ▾ Wake up early in the morning to dissipate kapha.
- ▾ Connect to something superior to you before leaving bed.
- ▾ Clean the face, mouth, and eyes.
- ▾ Scrape your tongue to remove toxins (ama).
- ▾ Clean your teeth with natural toothpaste.
- ▾ Drink a glass of water first thing in the morning to cleanse.
- ▾ Promote evacuation (bowel movement) with a supplement such as triphala powder.
- ▾ Gargle or chew using warm sesame oil, neem oil, or sesame seeds.
- ▾ Use nasal drops (*nasya*), such as *anu thailam* oil.
- ▾ Use oil drops in the ears (*karna purana*).
- ▾ Apply oil to the body with a body massage (*abhyanga*)—for example, warm sesame oil for kapha. Ayurveda has an oil for every condition and every doshic combination—sesame is recommended for all constitutions,

however, there are other oils for vata and pitta predominants or doshic combinations.

▼ Get regular exercise: For kapha people, exercise daily to half your capacity, until sweat forms on the forehead, armpits, and spine. Do twelve sun salutations, and try yoga postures such as the bridge, peacock, palm tree, and lion. Vigorous "hot" exercises can include jumping, jogging, and running in the early morning. Please consult your physician before starting a new exercise routine.

▼ Pranayama: For kapha people, after exercising, sit and do one hundred *bhastrika* deep breathing exercises.

▼ Practice meditation.

▼ Eat breakfast.

Seasonal Regimen (Ritucharya)

Time is movement, and chronological time is based upon the movement of our planet. Our biological time is ruled by the movements of the three doshas according to chronological time—for example physical digestion, respiration, elimination, and psychological time governed by the movement of our thoughts. Each geographical area has slightly different seasons, so these protocols are suggested on a seasonal basis. Our doshas have the tendency to accumulate, aggravate, and pacify during the various seasons, so ayurveda's preventive and curative approach involves pacification (samana) of the doshas, and purification (*sodhana*) treatments to eliminate toxins from the body as a prophylactic measure for seasonal disorders.

Yoga

Yoga is the system of postures (asanas) and breathing techniques (pranayamas) codified by Patanjali (1–5 BCE), to support our compulsory mind in restraining itself from focusing on external objects, or past or future experiences, with the intention of grasping a present state of consciousness. Today, millions of people use yoga for body constitution, spiritual, or mental reasons to improve their quality of life. Yoga helps all types of people, and when combined with healthy eating, it can help reduce BMI.[3]

Some similar principles between yoga and ayurveda:

▾ nonviolence (*ahimsa*)
▾ repressing of the thoughts or actions (*yama*)
▾ non-stealing (*satya*)
▾ non-accumulation (*aparigraha*)
▾ purity (*soucha*)
▾ contentment (*santosha*)
▾ self-study (*swadhyaya*)

Particular examples of different yoga forms include hatha, a combination or series of basic asanas focused on breath-controlled exercises (pranayama). The yoga imparted in the West is mostly modifications or styles of hatha. Iyengar, another option, is a precise type of yoga, attentive to finding the right alignment and time in a pose. You might also try vinyasa, which involves synchronizing the breath with a continuous routine of a series of poses; ashtanga, which links movement and breath, and has practitioners perform the poses in an exact order; power yoga, a higher-intensity variety based on achieving rapid fitness; or bikram, also known as "hot yoga," twenty-six challenging poses performed in a room at 104 degrees Fahrenheit.

Some asanas (poses) are mountain pose (*tadasana*), halfway rotation (*ardha katichakrasana*), waist rotation pose (*katichakrasana*), standing forward bend (*uttanasana*), child pose (*balasana*), cat-cow pose (chakravakasana), downward-facing dog (adho mukha svanasana), sun salutation (surya namaskar). In one way or another, all of them promote good posture, flexibility, leg and abdominal strength, improved circulation, activation of the digestive track, reducing stress and anxiety. A sequence of asanas can be followed by corpse pose (savasana), which allows rest, relaxing the full body into the floor.

Several yoga asanas aim to clear the lymphatic system and thereby boost the immune system in removing infections and reducing inflammation in the body. Exercise and yoga relieve strains in different body areas. For example, a dehydrated, stiff, weak, and rigid fascia network or lymph can be activated by exercise, yoga, and hydration of the connective tissue.

LYMPHATIC FLOW

Some Recommendations to Activate Its Circulation

Do not strain. When practicing yoga, you should be increasing lymph flow through postures and breathing; improving general well-being including flexibility, strength, and balance; and reducing stress and pain.[4] Remember, the lymphatic system does not have its own pump.[5]

Regarding the effects of yoga on circulation, poses like side bends, twists, forward folds, and inversions boost lymph flow and activate the fascia and vagus nerve by altering your body tissues in relation to gravity, since the movement of lymph is affected by gravity. This occurs when your head is below your heart.

FASCIA

Recommendations to Stimulate It

Since yoga is one example of an exercise or body practice that works on our fascial network at the same time as our lymphatic flow, let me give you some practical recommendations for performing yoga. First, drink water. Fascia works at its best when well hydrated. Second, incorporate a range of unusual movements into your daily life and physical activities. These new movements help to keep the water moving and flowing to those key areas. Another option is to walk or run barefoot, using more minimal footwear at home. Third, if you get a mild injury and would like to address your body fascia manually, do not target the area of pain directly, but rather the surrounding muscle tissue, avoiding any bony areas. When you sense a release, that is the stage at which you could gently work deeper into the area. Fourth, in general, avoid areas like the lower spine and instead focus on tight or restricted muscles. And lastly, practice relaxation and meditation; it could help you to relieve tension in the fascia and increase mobility in proprioception. For example, begin contracting the muscles in the area where you feel tension, and then allow them to relax as much as you can. If possible, meditate prior to starting your daily activities, even for ten or fifteen minutes, focusing on each part of the body. It will help you to address life's physical and mental activities with greater focus, increase the body-mind awareness, and reduce the likelihood of injuries causing by easing tension.

As usual, please speak with your physician, physical therapist, or a certified yoga instructor before starting any practice.

Breathing Exercises (Pranayama)

Prana is considered the vital force or refined essence of movement without which life cannot occur. It is the current of tissular intelligence that controls cellular communication, sensory perception, motor responses, and all subtle electrical impulses of the body.

Pranayama, "control of the life energy" or "extension of the prana or breath," is a form of breathing exercises within yoga. Pranayama uses various techniques that regulate and restrain breath, helping to control the mind and improve the quality of perception and awareness. Since our thoughts come and go like clouds in a windy sky, a conscious breathing practice like pranayama (see page 173) can serve as an anchor.[6]

We take breathing for granted because it is an automatic process, most of the time. However, when breathing becomes disturbed or altered, such as by physical factors or mental stress, it becomes very noticeable. By making instructed changes to our routine breathing patterns, we can actively participate in these alterations. Pranayama does not require special equipment, only your body, and can be practiced wherever you are. However, you should seek proper instruction on practicing pranayama, as altering breathing patterns can do harm if the alterations are inappropriate for you. Successful application of pranayama exercises will see effective results right away—it will create body organ system connections, and observance of the mind, and, in the long term, reduction of weight and BMI, as well as pulmonary rehabilitation for the prevention and management of related conditions such as COVID-19.[7, 8, 9]

Meditation as Body-Mind Exercise

Meditation was most probably originally developed to help deepen understanding of the sacred, mystical forces of life. Ayurvedic physicians practiced it, and advised it for balancing mind and body and for expanding self-awareness and cultivation of your intrinsic state of balance. Today's meditation styles are commonly used for relaxation and stress reduction and are considered a type of body-mind complementary medicine.

Meditation, conducted correctly, helps you bypass restless chattering, and permeates deeper levels of consciousness. It creates a significant gradual shift, rewiring the brain to reason and function differently and produce a deep state of relaxation and a tranquil mind, allowing a clearer perception of your food dependencies and other weakness by bringing you back to your real self. The meditative technique identified today as "mindfulness" has even been shown to have a beneficial effect on genetic expression with the process of aging, promoting a healthy microbiome, which in turn boosts the overall immune system and supports your body balance in general.[10, 11] A very recent study performed on Buddhist monks found evidence that frequent deep meditation could help synchronize the gut microbiome and reduce the possibility of physical and mental ill health. The monks' enriched gut microbiota boost their immune systems, reducing the risk of cardiovascular disease and psychosomatic conditions such as depression and anxiety, and increasing their well-being.[12]

⬤ Meditation Exercises for Different Prakruti Types

In the state of restful awareness created through meditation, your heart rate and breath will slow down, and your body will drop the levels of production of the stress hormones cortisol and adrenaline, while increasing the production of neurotransmitters that improve your health, like endorphins, dopamine, serotonin, and oxytocin.

Try the following meditation recommendations depending on your main prakruti:

Vata: Focus on a light source that isn't bright, to calm emotions.

Pitta: Focus on spatial expansion or outer awareness, with compassion.

Kapha: Meditate on the limitless and the shapeless.

*Peace can be reached through meditation on the knowledge that
dreams give. Peace can also be reached through concentration
upon that which is dearest to the heart.*

PATANJALI

We've been reviewing various ayurvedic physical methods to tackle, in
a general way, the condition of being overweight. Many patients coming to
me seek a better understanding of the ayurvedic modalities. They want to
"know" the process and how it works, in ayurvedic terms. For that reason,
let me introduce this process to you in a more detailed way.

Panchakarma: Purification Treatments

In Sanskrit, panchakarma means "five actions," and this is a broad set
of ayurvedic detox procedures useful for eliminating body-mind toxins.
The detox provokes the removal of accumulated irregular metabolic waste
(ama), both internally and externally, to reestablish balance of your organ
systems. If your body or mind are not removing undigested materials, toxic
physical components (microorganisms, synthetic chemicals, xenobiotics,
drugs, etc.), and undigested mental experiences (repetitive intrusions or
thoughts), then these products—both physical and mental ama—will
accumulate over time and manifest as conditions such as being overweight
or obese. Under ordinary circumstances, your body has a natural ability
to efficiently process and remove waste materials by means of the normal
metabolic processes. This is true even when your constitution is in a state
of mild imbalance. However, when constitutional imbalances become
more severe, it leads to the accumulation of toxins throughout the body,
which results in prakruti imbalances, manifests as vikruti, and potentially
generates illness.

This ama gathered at the cellular level of your body's organ systems
needs to be entirely discharged from the body. Regarding detox, some
health consultants recommend periodic detoxes using various protocols,
which may go to extremes that cause depletion of minerals, vitamins, and
calories. Instead of being beneficial, these kinds of depletions could induce
severe cravings, loss of lean muscle mass, hormonal imbalances, mental dis-

orders, and other issues. Other health consultants believe that it is totally pointless to cleanse, because our GIT completely rebuilds its cellular coating continuously and the body has a natural detoxification system. That perception that we do not need to detoxify our bodies is incorrect, in my opinion, based on my decades of research and clinical experience. The efficacy of the ayurvedic process of body detoxification or cleansing has been applied for centuries, and its efficacy is well demonstrated. The ayurvedic scholar Sushruta described these medical procedures in detail in the *Sushruta Samhita*.[13, 14] It is true that our bodies have a natural detoxification system in place, but today's lifestyle places continuous pressure upon our bodies through the accumulation of toxins from the polluted air we breathe, the unhealthy food and medications we ingest, and the incessant strains we face in today's world. For these reasons, we have to keep trying to remove those physical, mental, and emotional toxins resulting from conscious or unconscious traumas.

It is interesting that we consider it critical to check and regularly change the oil in our cars, but we don't apply the same concern to our own body organ systems. Doing so involves tailored protocols. These detoxification protocols that tackle each of the disturbed constitutions (doshas) are:

- ▾ **purgation/laxative therapy:** the best treatment for removal of excess pitta
- ▾ **emesis:** the finest therapy for elimination of excess kapha (mucus)
- ▾ **enema:** the best treatment for elimination of excess vata
- ▾ **bloodletting:** either by blood donation or applying leeches, for excess pitta
- ▾ **nasal cleansing:** inhalation using medicinal oils to remove kapha from the head

In a panchakarma detox program, each step of the detox is tailored to your predicament.

Mainstream medicine finds it easy to accept the idea that metabolic byproducts are physical substances that can be harmful to the body, but it is far more difficult to concede that some kinds of emotions or thoughts

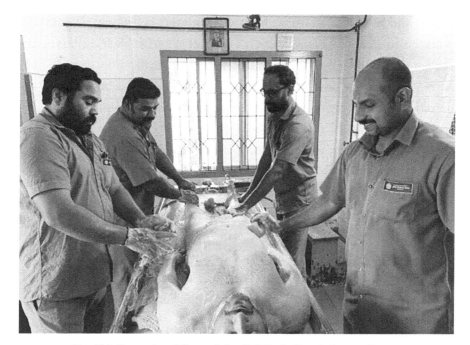

Fig. 17.1. Example of One of the Full-Body Panchakarma Detox
Medicated Oil Massage Protocols (*Pizhichil*)

can be harmful byproducts, as if the body and mind were two very different compartments. Luckily, a growing number of medical specialists and psychologists are coming to understand this concept. Ayurveda doesn't segregate body byproducts and mind byproducts, since both affect the organ systems health of the person, and ayurveda treats the whole person.

Udvartana: Ayurvedic Weight Loss Massage

Udvartana is among the best ayurvedic treatments for weight reduction. It is a deep tissue massage technique involving the use of ayurvedic herbal powders or oils, followed by a steam treatment or bath. It is performed by applying appropriate pressure on the skin to break down the excess of fat, cellulite, and toxins (ama) under the skin, making it an effective treatment for weight loss, but also an effective remedy for a vast number of ailments.[15] The ayurvedic scholar Sushruta described *urdhavagati abhyanga* or udvartana and referred to elevation and upward strokes during massage, along with the use of herbal powders (*churnas*) or herbal paste. These protocols are also considered as part of the dinacharyas (daily healthier regimen).

Treatment Types

In this process, the body is coated with medicated herbal oils, and herbal powders are applied and rubbed on the body in an upward direction. There are two main modalities: First, in dry (ruksha), udvartana is performed only with dry powders. Since the massage is dry and rough, it mostly assists in reducing weight and kapha dosha. And second, oily (sneha) udvartana uses herbals and medicated oils as a paste.

Udvartana can be given to the full body or to particular body areas such as the abdomen, to reduce localized fat depositions or promote fat reduction (*sthanika*). Also, it tones the skin, improving elasticity and strength; provides stress relief; and supports relaxation. The treatment is tailored to the body type and an individual's needs. Its effects are amplified by a tailored diet; for example, a kapha diet based on astringent, bitter, and pungent foods supports a reduction of stored kapha.

Health Benefits

Udvartana is usually recommended for people suffering from obesity, or who are overweight, have excess cellulite or specific fat accumulation—such as in the abdomen, buttocks, thighs, or loose skin on the arms—or who have other pathologies. It is also recommended as a general rejuvenation treatment due to its improvement of peripheral blood flow circulation, exfoliation of the skin, and reduction of body stiffness.[16] It is not recommended for individuals with dry skin, skin with cuts or other injuries, eczema, or psoriasis, or for pregnant women, or children under the age of ten.

Compounds and Oils (Thailam)

Oils (thailam) can be taken orally or internally through the skin to eliminate body weight. They are chosen according to the body type and weight loss target, and include triphala, *kottamchukkadi*, *khanwantharam*, *karpasasthyadi*, and *lavana* oils.

There is also another cleansing technique called *garshana*, or dry brushing, which stimulates lymphatic mobility and is also a vigorous way to support the removal of cellular waste products (ama) from the body. It is different to udvartana and is customarily done using raw linen gloves, though many prefer to use a natural body brush. The scrubbing massage creates dryness in the body, helping to manage an excess of body kapha, stimulate lymph, and support weight loss. These protocols are suggested for people who manifest signs and symptoms of ama, such as exhaustion, laziness, physical or mental dullness, constipation, and an overtaxed immune system.

AYURVEDIC PLANTS, RESINS, AND SPICES FOR REBALANCING YOUR BODY WEIGHT

The purpose of fat is to produce energy; it is our fuel. Obese people often feel tired because the undigested fat is not fully processed, so they have the impression of running low on fuel, which sparks a desire to eat more—a metabolic and hormonal process that is better understood now. Where there is lack of energy, there is low motivation. One role of some ayurvedic herbs is to make energy out of sedentary fat, thus increasing a person's drive to engage in physical activities.[17] Below, I present some of the relevant herbs and compounds for increasing your drive and encouraging body weight rebalance. Overall, they have bitter, astringent, and pungent qualities.

Ayurvedic Herbs
chitrac (*Plumbago zeylanica*): The ayurvedic pharmacopoeia describes this powerful herb as bringing fire into your body, drying out kapha, warming up vata, and reviving agni. It stimulates the thyroid gland, promotes pancreas activity, and is a mild laxative. As well, it helps to reduce fat deposition (omentums) around internal organs by improving their local agni, assisting in metabolizing unprocessed raw fat by burning it away and releasing energy from the byproduct of fat to maintain the tone of muscular tissue.[18]

kutki (*Picrorrhiza kurroa*): This is considered a highly effective herb for treating obesity, marketed by well-known ayurvedic drug manufacturers. It pacifies pitta and kapha but may stimulate vata. It can brush away the excess of unwanted arterial fat tissue, supporting the removal of plaque from blood vessels, and it is good for fatty degenerative hepatic alterations, preventing cirrhotic changes (kapha conditions). As well, it is antipyretic—good for pitta troubles like chronic fever. It breaks down gallstones and is a natural source of antihistamine, so can be used to treat eczema, dermatitis, and itching. Kutki is a blood thinner (anticoagulant) and can be used as a preventive measure for heart conditions; it acts like Coumadin, in that it breaks down clots.[19]

neem (*Azadiracta indica*): The leaves, fruits, bark, and seed oil from this tree offer a wealth of benefits for the skin, nails, scalp, teeth, and gums. Neem balances pitta and kapha but can aggravate vata. It removes excess fat, reduces cholesterol, and is a kapha reducer that regulates body weight. In cases of hyperglycemia, it supports healthy blood sugar levels. Neem is also antipyretic and antiseptic—it prevents against cavities, gingivitis, and gum disease. It is used to treat skin conditions such as eczema, dermatitis, and psoriasis.[20]

vidanga (*Embelia ribes*): This is a vata- and kapha-pacifying and agni-stimulating herb. It acts as a diuretic, a blood purifier, and a mild purgative herb, and it also increases digestive function.[21]

guggulu (*Commiphora mukul*): This is the resin obtained from the mukul myrhh tree. It assists in balancing all doshas as a rejuvenating, cleansing herb. It lowers lipid profiles, improves the HDL/LDL cholesterol ratio, and has anti-inflammatory effects.[22, 23]

vacha (*Acorus calamus*): In Sanskrit, this plant's name means "speaking clearly." It is bitter in taste and is used in dried form. The heating qualities of this root pacify vata and kapha and increase pitta. It reduces body fat, and is also considered helpful for learning ability, intellect, memory, and power of speech.[24]

simhadanti or **dandelion** (*Taraxacum officinale*): Ayurveda describes this herb as having anti-obesity attributes: it stimulates digestion, is a mild hepatic laxative, a diuretic, a depurator, a stomach tonic, and is considered a blood purifier, balancing bile production in the gallbladder and bile flow from the liver.[25]

ashwaghanda or Indian ginseng (*Withania somnifera*): Also known as winter cherry, it is used as a rasayana (rejuvenator), cognitive enhancer (nootropic), and as a natural, powerful adaptogen for general well-being and specific conditions such as body weight management.[26]

Kitchen Remedies: Spices

Ayurveda also describes other components to support digestion, lower body fat, and bring down some of the risk factors of vascular diseases linked with obesity:

cumin (*Cuminum cyminum L.*): In a weight-reduction diet cumin showed improvement in physical and biochemical parameters in overweight and obese women, results that are similar to the anti-obesity drug Orlistat. Note, however, that side effects of this drug include "anal leakage" or oily stools—what drug companies call "fecal spotting"—and patients are advised to wear dark pants and carry extra clothes in case of fecal discharges.[27] Also, in terms of kitchen remedies, infusion of cumin combined with coriander (*Coriandrum sativum*) and fennel (*Foeniculum vulgare*) in equal parts can be taken during the day, either warm or at room temperature, to regulate agni in supporting your digestion, and act as a mild diuretic. Other well-known kitchen remedies are to drink hot water with raw honey, lemon water, and apple cider vinegar (as the fermentation by *Acetobacter* produces acetic acid) alone or combined with lemon in the early morning.[28]

turmeric (*Curcuma longa*): It has a warm, bitter taste and is frequently used to flavor or color curry powders and mustards. Turmeric's most active compound, curcumin, has many health benefits, being a potent anti-inflammatory, antiseptic, antibacterial, and antioxidant substance. It pacifies kapha and pitta issues without triggering pitta. It is good for diabetes, heart health, and the prevention of Alzheimer's, cancer,[29] depression, and arthritis[30]—all potential complications of obesity. Obesity leads to diverse body changes including inflammatory processes, and these can lead to oxidative stress—an increase in the production of reactive oxygen species (ROS)—which in turn can trigger mitochondrial changes, a complication known as mitochondrial dysfunction.[31]

Curcumin increases levels of the fat-burning enzyme, lipase, associated with reduction of fat cells, and increases fat metabolism as well as increasing gene expression linked to production of brown fat, and enhanced expression of proteins involved in fat oxidation.[32]

saffron (*Crocus sativus*): The strong antioxidant property of the bioactive compounds (crocin and crocetin) can modify some metabolic disorders through multiple mechanisms such as improved appetite, and decrease BMI in people with coronary artery disease, through the mechanism of appetite suppression, which can beneficially alter obesity pathophysiology.[33]

black seed (*Nigella sativa*): This has a significant impact on plasma lipid levels. Lower total cholesterol, LDL-C, and TG levels with increased HDL-C are associated with black seed powder only.[34]

garlic (*Allium sativum*): A highly versatile vegetable—not a spice—garlic is antibacterial, antifungal, antiviral, antioxidant, an effective blood thinner, and an immune system stimulant. It promotes heart health by lowering one's lipid profile.[35]

Compounds

Ayurvedic medicine offers a great number of compounds. Here, I'll give you some examples of the most classic and widely used ones:

triphala: Translated as "three fruits," it is composed of the dried fruits of amalaki fruit (*Emblica officinalis*), bibhitaki fruit (*Terminalia belerica*), and *haritaki* fruit (*Terminalia chebula*). It contains five of the six tastes, all but salty, and is a highly recommended ayurvedic formulation due to its ability to gently cleanse and detoxify the system while simultaneously replenishing and nourishing it. Triphala removes excess vata, pitta, and kapha from the body, bringing balance and improved functioning to the system. It supports the functions of the digestive, circulatory, respiratory, and genitourinary systems, reducing body weight and hence lowering BMI.[36] It is commonly taken as a daily evening supplement.[37]

trikatu: This literally means "three pungent," as it contains the dried powders (churnas) of ginger root (*Zingiber officinale*), black pepper fruit (*Piper nigrum*), and pippali fruit (*Piper longum*) in equal parts. Its potent heating quality is usually used to kindle agni and to efficiently burn kapha, fat, and toxins, thus aiding in weight management. It can be made at home, used for all varieties of cooking, and can be added to ready-made meals.[38]

triphala guggulu: This formulation clears toxins from all the channels and tissues of the body. It supports healthy cholesterol levels, lowers body weight, and supports the digestive and elimination systems—for example, with intestinal and hepatic problems, belly reduction, flatulence, constipation, and piles.[39, 40]

arogyavardhini: This is a very bitter-tasting herbal blend. It comprises thirteen herbs including *kajali, guducchi, chitrak, shilajit*, neem, copper ash, and others; it is also treated with cow's urine. Arogyavardhini is used in treating obesity, detoxing the liver, and balancing pitta. It regulates cholesterol, kidney cleansing, skin conditions, and the thyroid.[41]

shilajit: This has been used for centuries in ayurveda as a rejuvenator and antiaging compound (rasayana), and for increasing physical strength and promoting good health. Originally found in the mountainous regions of Asia, sometimes in Himalayan rocks, it is formed of humic substances by centuries of gradual decomposition and transformation of plant, animal, and microbial residues, including fulvic acid, which makes up 60 to 80 percent of the total compound, plus some oligoelements including selenium, iron, copper, silica, zinc, and others.

Its functions include the pacification of vata, stimulation of pitta, and reduction of kapha. Shilajit balances blood sugar, uric acid, cholesterol, and triglycerides; revitalizes the reproductive tissue, increasing spermatogenesis; and stimulates an underactive thyroid gland, normalizing its function.[42]

Ayurvedic plants have exhibited highly effective use over centuries when used in regimens for obesity treatment.[43] There are many more ayurvedic plants and compounds with anti-obesity actions, which we do not have space to cover here. However, in a number of cases, clinical studies and further research are required to explain, in modern pharmacological terms, their efficacy and the pharmacotherapeutic value to incorporating them alongside conventional treatments.

Q&A

Effects of Regular Exercise on the Body-Mind

I've covered several of the active ayurvedic approaches to body-mind imbalances, in particular the adjustment of diet and nutrition according to your individual prakruti, manas prakruti, and vikruti conditions of imbalance. In this section we cover, in a more practical way, areas aimed at engaging you in active procedures to benefit your physical body organ systems.

Exercise increases total energy expenditure, which can help us to stay in energy balance or even lose weight, if we do not eat more to compensate for the burned calories. Physical activity has many benefits on body-mind health and well-being that go well beyond weight loss, and that is why exercise is particularly important for overweight and obese people.[44] A recent systematic review and meta-analysis suggests that exercise can effectively improve quality of life in adults with excess weight and obesity but is not able to positively reduce depression-related outcomes. It also shows that psychological outcomes such as body image, perceived stress, and life satisfaction are poorly studied, and evidence suggests either conflicting findings or null effects of exercise, preventing solid conclusions from being drawn. However, evidence of positive exercise-induced changes in exercise-independent motivations and self-efficacy was found to be relatively consistent.[45] For these reasons, ayurvedic practices of yoga and breathing exercises (pranayamas), among other activities, are important to support not only the physical aspects of your plan but also the psychological ones.

Before I describe these practices, this section includes the most common and relevant questions I hear from clients about how to deal with being overweight and rebalancing their body-mind.

How Does Exercise Support My Digestion and Metabolism?

The positive effects of exercise on health have been proven time and time again. Exercise is helpful for achieving and maintaining weight loss. It can increase catabolism—the breakdown of molecules to release energy—helping you to maintain and increase lean body mass by burning more calories. During exercise the physical action amplifies blood flow to the muscles in the digestive system, assisting a quicker passage, or peristalsis, of food along the GIT. Research also shows that exercise plays an important role in microbiome balance and mind function.

Could I Be Overexercising?

If you are overweight or obese, you may be prone to workout injuries, depending on the extent of excess weight and the kind of physical activity you are doing. Do not be discouraged, and search for guidance on how to increase your physical activity levels, even if this doesn't result in losing weight, because physical activity brings other health benefits such as reduced risk of type 2 diabetes and cardiovascular disease. One of the easiest and most effective routes is through the practice of low-impact exercise. You can start by walking. Also, aqua exercises are helpful since your body weight will be partially supported by the water, especially in conditions of morbid obesity where walking may be difficult. Take into consideration that the same amount of exercise for an obese or overweight person is much harder than for those who do not have excess body weight. Also consider that intense exercise could have a transitory negative effect on the GIT, involving nausea, vomiting, cramping, heartburn, diarrhea, and gastrointestinal bleeding.

A well-rounded approach to address the body-mind paradigm of physical activity and exercise could be achieved by addressing a combination of ayurveda and yoga knowledge; but before moving into this aspect, first I would like to answer more of the questions currently asked by my clients when they try to take the horse by the reins.

Q&A
....
Obesity

Which Genetic Factors Could Be Causing Obesity?

There is scientific research that seeks to understand and explain the role of genes and lifestyle choices on our body weight. In the case of obesity, the issue is the degree to which our genetics affect or even regulate what size, shape, and weight our body will be. So far, we know that obesity is a condition involving several genes (polygenes), which are associated with neurobehavioral, metabolic, and endocrine causes; in rare cases, it is monogenetic—or has one single gene origin. In fact, risk factors associated with obesity may be found on nearly every chromosome, with epigenetic processes nevertheless accounting for additional factors of obesity. Chromosomal abnormalities are only observed in less than 10 percent of children with severe obesity. Monogenetic obesity is found in people with loss-of-function mutations in gene coding for the hormone leptin, the leptin receptor (LEPR), hormone pro-opiomelanocortin (POMC), and melanocortin 4 receptor (MC4R). In the case of polygenic risk factors for obesity, the usual mutations include the fat mass and obesity-associated gene (FTO) and the MC4R receptor.[46]

Might Environmental Factors Be Contributing to the Global Obesity Epidemic?

In recent years there has been considerable attention given to both external and human-internal damage done by industrial chemical use and waste, and plastic production and its disposal. Two types of substances, phthalates and bisphenols incorporated into plastic goods, are extensively shown to migrate into food and the environment.[47] They are known as endocrine-disrupting chemicals (EDCs), exogenous substances or mixtures that modify endocrine system functions and therefore directly impact our organism. The use of plastics has a massive influence on our daily life, from our everyday food and water intake to household appliances, technologies, and medical uses to name a few. Allied to their use is the environmental cost resulting from single-use plastics thrown away by users that contaminate our oceans, rivers, and landfills.

These plastics break down into very small particles called microplastics (MPs) and nanoplastics (NPs)—also known collective as micro(nano) plastics (MNPs). There is mounting research on and empirical evidence of the detrimental impact from the colossal volume of MNPs impacting all aspects of our environment and ecology. Recent animal studies have found that MNPs can have an impact at subcellular, or molecular levels. Remember, these very tiny particles are moving through our gut, lungs, skin and other bodily tissues. Now it has been shown that they disturb our glucose and fat metabolism, which suggests they could be involved in the progression of obesity. Chronic contact with NPs also induces local inflammatory and immune responses by macrophage infiltration in the gut, and increases the liver's fat accumulation, damaging our metabolism and disrupting the gut microbiome.[48]

By describing the unescapable risk of plastics on our health, the environment and our shared ecology, I am not ignoring the strong corporate forces applied to the promotion of processed foods, marketed widely and representing billions in profit, despite the growing perspective that they directly feed our obesity epidemic. I feel that we all have a personal responsibility to address these trends as individuals, communities, and policymakers through regulation and education. As a suggestion consider the study of Zimin et al.[49]

Can Socioeconomic Status (SES) Affect Body Weight?

The short answer is yes, and how it affects your body weight depends on where you live. A study using data from sixty-seven countries examined how economic development, socioeconomic status, and obesity were related. It found that prevalence of obesity rose with a country's economic development, but also that socioeconomic status as it related to obesity changed. In lower-income countries, people with higher SES were more prone to being obese. Conversely, in high-income countries, those with higher SES were less prone to being obese.[50]

Why the inversion? It may be that in lower-income countries, higher SES leads to consuming high-calorie food and less physical exertion. But in higher-income countries, people with higher SES may respond with healthy eating choices and regular exercise. The implication is that while economic development improves health, "problems of malnutrition are replaced by problems of overconsumption that differentially affect SES groups," noted the authors. But some emerging countries, such as India, are facing continued high levels of malnutrition along with a rise in obesity.[51]

Overall, these studies show that factors that increase the risk of being obese affect SES groups differently and may cause disparities in obesity between socioeconomic groups, which worsen health and shorten longevity for those who are most disadvantaged.[52]

Can I Cause Body Weight Imbalance by Disrespecting Natural Daily Cycles?

The scientific journal *Cell* recently reported that the time at which eating occurs during the day may impact success in losing weight. Specifically, the research found that eating meals late at night may desynchronize the internal body clock—what we refer to as our circadian cycle. The researchers noted that insulin is released from the pancreas following the consumption of food, to help stabilize blood glucose levels. If food is ingested outside of typical mealtimes, then the subsequent release of insulin also occurs outside of a typical schedule. As a result of this, our natural daily cycles can be disturbed, affecting both weight loss and weight gain.

Let me explain the biology behind this: Cortisol, the stress hormone, typically peaks at eight o'clock in the morning, allowing us to wake from sleep; it then falls to its lowest concentration at three o'clock in the morning. This rise also occurs in line with exposure to sunlight. By noon, cortisol levels begin to fall, while serotonin and adrenaline rise inversely, which elevates mood and energy, increases energy levels, and in particular, stimulates feelings of hunger and encourages the person to eat. During the rest of the day, cortisol levels continue to decline, and serotonin is synthesized into the hormone melatonin, promoting feelings of sleepiness. Occurring alongside this is a decrease in blood sugar levels, which drop to their lowest point at approximately three o'clock in the morning. Physiological balance will be disturbed if you have habits such as eating snacks late at

night or eating meals outside normal times, which will affect your digestion and trigger stress.[53] This is one more corroboration of the ayurvedic
principle regarding the importance of eating at the right time, the type of
food intake, and the quantities consumed—all these factors can help you
avoid body-mind imbalances.

Vegetarianism and Losing Body Weight

There are many variants of vegetarian diets (vegan, ovolactovegetarian, pes-
catarian, and others). A classic vegetarian diet excluding all animal flesh can
significantly help weight reduction strategies, since its ingredients are based
on low-calorie foods; that is, vegetables, whole grains, and fruits.[54]

How Successful Are Weight-Loss Drugs for Obesity?

Let's be clear, weight-loss drugs do not work for everyone, and they will
not melt off the pounds overnight. Several studies show that when they
are successful, they result in an average weight loss of about 5 percent over
a period of six to twelve months.

There are also disturbing reports about weight-loss drugs.
Dexfenfluramine and Fenfluramine were taken off the market after they
were linked to heart valve damage. Sibutramine was removed after it was
linked to heart attack and stroke in people at highest risk for these conditions. Today's system in the United States and other countries considers it
appropriate if a drug helps you lose 5 percent of your weight within a few
months without side effects. However, remember that those drugs are not
a substitute for lifestyle changes, and they work best when used as part of
a broader medical weight-loss program. I think that if truly necessary, they
could be used as one component of a plan that includes a healthy diet,
regular exercise, adequate sleep, and stress reduction.[55] They are being marketed as a quick-fix weight loss solution, but with side effects.

Could My Weight Gain Be Caused by
Pharmaceutical Drugs?

Weight gain depends on several factors. These include specific drugs, your
age, your sleep patterns, and other medical conditions you may be experi-

encing. Some current medical drugs are linked to weight gain at all ages. If you are already overweight, you can gain even more weight, creating a real problem. Example of drugs that could instigate weight gain are: steroids, hormones used as birth control pills or corticosteroids, antipsychotics, antidepressants, some drugs for diabetes, and antihypertensive drugs. Discuss with your doctor the potential side effects of any new drug that could increase your body weight, and request another drug that's free of these side effects.

Ayurvedic medication's great advantage is the quite negligible side effects, since these are natural products. However, make sure that the practitioner prescribing the products is officially qualified, understands your condition, is careful about dose prescriptions and potential antagonism of natural products, and recommends medication that is certified organic. On that note, in this chapter you will find some ayurvedic herbs, compounds, or formulations intended to handle your overweight or obese condition. Ayurveda says about diet and medicine: "When diet is wrong, medicine is of no use. When diet is correct, medicine is of no need." For these reasons, and since we cannot scrub our body internally, we need to learn some skills to help cleanse our tissues, organs, and mind.

Why, Despite Efforts to Bring Down My Body Weight, Does It Remain Stable at a Certain Level?

Yes, we often blame overeating, insufficient exercise, and other causes, but the fact is that there are also many chemicals playing a role in expanding our waistlines. It is well known that there are fifty different chemicals, or more, that literally make us fatter: they are called obesogens and are present in our daily life. Some clear examples include bisphenol A (an endocrine disruptor), organophosphate flame retardants, and some phthalates. For example, some phthalates can change the way our body processes a meal and turns it into fat. These components can push your body either to make new fat cells or encourage cells to store more fat. Be aware that obesogens permeate our regular environment and are present in processed foods, food packaging, pesticides, cosmetics, personal care products, and even in our dust and water.

Is It True That There Is a Connection Between the Organelle Mitochondria and Obesity?

This is a complex subject. It starts from the understanding that DNA inside mitochondria organelle (mtDNA) in humans is inherited exclusively from the mother. Then, the more mitochondria you have, the more ATP and energy (agni) you will be able to produce. So if your body can make more of the enzymes that break down fat, the process of fat-burning will be more efficient, allowing you to lose weight. The most recent studies show that obesity causes mitochondrial fragmentation and dysfunction in white adipocytes. The process is associated with mitochondrial dynamics of fission/fusion related to some proteins (GTPases) that affect the pathophysiology of obesity, apparently offering new tactics for the treatment of obesity. The involved mechanisms are linked to connections between organelles, neuronal activity, adipose tissue thermogenesis, and other factors. If you would like to read more, I recommend you look at the studies by Wenmin Xia and by Jinling Wang.[56, 57]

Are GMO Foods Related to Obesity?

Genetically modified organisms, or GMOs, are plants, animals, or microbes whose genome has been artificially modified at the molecular level. In the United States, many crops are genetically modified, and more than 95 percent of meat and dairy produce in the US is from animals that are feed GMO crops.[58] The industrial production of GMO food enzymes (FEs) could be an example of what could affect our digestion and metabolism, causing body imbalances. For thousands of years, cheese was made of four ingredients: milk, starter culture, salt, and animal rennet, this last one involving a set of enzymes produced in the stomachs of ruminant mammals such as cows, lambs, or goats. In the process of making cheese, the natural enzyme chymosin from rennet is a key component (90 percent) in coagulating milk and separating solid curd from liquid whey. Other enzymes are pepsin and lipase. However, younger cheeses like mozzarella, ricotta, and other curd-based cheeses, such as cottage cheese, cream cheese, and provolone, are often made without rennet. For example, cheeses considered vegetarian, such as ricotta and paneer, use acids like lemon juice instead of rennet. Moreover, other plants or vegetable rennet, microbial-based substitutes, and GMOs are now also used for the preparation of vegetarian cheeses.

The industrial production of GMO food enzymes by the food industry has been increasing. An estimated 90 percent of North American cheese is made with a GMO rennet version called fermentation-produced chymosin (FPC), made by Pfizer (and exempt from GMO labeling, so consumers have no way to know in full what they are eating).[59] There are safety concerns regarding toxicity, or digestive issues, or potentially acting as an allergen (resulting in, for example, stomach upset or discomfort, runny nose, or increased in mucus production) with potential disruption of the gut microbiome.[60] Perhaps it is not only a question of how the cheese was made, but also the toxicity and indigestibility of FPC.

How Successful Is Bariatric Surgery (BS) in Treating Obesity?

Bariatric surgery is considered effective, but it is important to ponder long-term weight loss, side effects, and the risk of death from surgery. Common side effects include internal bleeding, infections, and blood clots. If the surgery involves redesigning the digestive system, potential intestinal leakage could be involved. Patients can present with significant nutritional deficiencies and complications, may fail to lose weight, or might reclaim their weight after a period of time.[61] Other study shows that 20 to 30 percent of individuals who have undergone BS have to face premature weight stabilization or can even regain weight if the dietary and lifestyle habits that led to obesity remain unchanged.[62] What should also be considered is the psychological impact of BS on patients as a result of changes in social settings such as body image and depression despite the significant weight loss and improvement in comorbidities.

How Successful Are Psychotherapy and Counselling for Obesity?

The more effective forms of counselling and psychotherapy for the treatment of obesity are the ones focusing on helping people to modify their behavior. Just to give a recent example, a study proved the effectiveness of supportive psychotherapy, in the form of psychodynamic psychotherapy, for the treatment of obesity in young women. The most significant effects in terms of long-term weight, BMI, WHR, and body fat reduction were observed for a combined approach integrating diet, dietetic follow-up, physical activity, and adjunctive psychotherapy; the latter, combined with diet and exercise, but without dietary consultation, also produced noticeable results.[63]

We grow only when we learn to observe our habits and behavior without the interference of our emotions and preconceptions. For that reason, I would like to conclude by briefly mentioning the yogic concept of *anitya bhavana*. It is about accepting the impermanence of everything in our life. Why should you be attached to something when nothing is permanent and everything is changing? This ayurvedic concept of awareness teaches us to reflect, cultivate mental detachment, and enjoy our body-mind efforts so we can change gracefully and find beauty in every phase of our life.

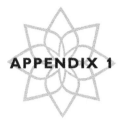

SELF-EVALUATIONS

WHAT IS YOUR PRAKRUTI?

Essentially, ayurveda defines your bodily well-being as the balance of three inborn constituents or typologies (doshas).

This prakruti evaluation, consisting of fifty-five categories, provides you with a clear indication of your primordial prakruti once completed. In answering the category choices, you will be exploring your psychosomatic and biological constitution, perhaps for the first time, as a focused evaluation of your physical and mental character. Your prakruti is the combination of the three doshas that form your personal constitution at the time of conception, which create the inborn tendencies that influence how you experience life.

The evaluation profile will reveal your personal distribution of the three doshas. If one of the doshas is too high, ayurvedic protocols guide you in rebalancing or fortifying the other two constituents by means of diet, lifestyle, and exercises such as yoga, meditation, and relaxation, in order to attain a better bodily and mental balance and create harmony between the three constituents.

Note: In the prakruti evaluation, you should give answers for each of the categories based on your typical state of physical and mental health. For example, if your immune system is normally good but you are experiencing a weakness in it because of a cold or flu, then your typical immune evaluation would be "good."

PRAKRUTI EVALUATION

V (Vata)	P (Pitta)	K (Kapha)
1. Physique		
☐ thin, bony	☐ average	☐ big, sturdy
2. Height		
☐ very tall or very small	☐ medium height	☐ small to medium
3. Propensity to Gain or Lose Weight		
☐ difficult to gain	☐ easy to gain or lose	☐ overweight, difficult to lose
4. Skin Luster		
☐ dull, dusky	☐ shiny	☐ lighter than average
5. Skin Texture		
☐ dry/rough/cold, visible veins	☐ warm/oily	☐ lubricated, coarse
6. Body Temperature		
☐ cold hands and feet	☐ warm	☐ cold or average
7. Hair Quality		
☐ dry, thin, brittle	☐ oily, balding, graying	☐ strong, glossy
8. Amount of Hair		
☐ average	☐ thin to early balding	☐ full, thick
9. Forehead		
☐ small	☐ moderate, furrows	☐ large
10. Eyes: Appearance		
☐ small, darting	☐ penetrating, light sensitive	☐ large, attractive, relaxed
11. Eyes: Lubrication		
☐ generally dry	☐ normal lubrication	☐ well lubricated, moist

PRAKRUTI EVALUATION (*cont.*)

V (Vata)	P (Pitta)	K (Kapha)
12. Teeth		
☐ irregular, small	☐ regular	☐ full, well-formed
13. Gums		
☐ thin gums	☐ sensitive/bleed easily	☐ strong gums
14. Tongue		
☐ rough	☐ soft, pink	☐ thick
15. Saliva Production		
☐ dry mouth	☐ average	☐ frequent
16. Face		
☐ small, dry	☐ delicate, glowing, acute	☐ large, pleasant, soft profile
17. Nose Moisture		
☐ often dry	☐ unremarkable	☐ frequently moist
18. Thorax		
☐ narrow	☐ moderately developed	☐ wide, well-developed
19. Bones		
☐ thin	☐ average	☐ strong
20. Joints		
☐ cracking	☐ loose	☐ strong
21. Nails		
☐ dry, rough, brittle	☐ soft, pink, flexible	☐ thick, wide, soft
22. Sleep		
☐ light, with interruptions	☐ not excessive but deep	☐ deep, excessive

PRAKRUTI EVALUATION (*cont.*)

V (Vata)	P (Pitta)	K (Kapha)
23. Dislikes		
☐ cold, dry conditions	☐ hot places, substances	☐ cold/oily substances, humidity
24. Appetite		
☐ variable/nervous	☐ strong, must eat on time	☐ moderate but constant
25. Food Temperature Preference		
☐ warm, oily, moist	☐ cool or cold	☐ warm and dry
26. Eating Speed		
☐ quick, often small meals	☐ moderately fast	☐ slowly, big quantities
27. Thirst		
☐ changeable	☐ usually thirsty	☐ moderate
28. Feces: Form and Tendency		
☐ hard/dry, small, constipation	☐ soft, loose, diarrhea	☐ bulky, sluggish
29. Urine Frequency		
☐ infrequent	☐ abundant, yellow	☐ moderate, clear
30. Sweating		
☐ reduced, not much smell	☐ often, strong smell	☐ moderate
31. Learning		
☐ fast, tendency to forget	☐ acute, clear	☐ slow but constant
32. Memory		
☐ best in short term	☐ well overall	☐ very good long-term
33. Understanding		
☐ spontaneous	☐ average	☐ takes a while

PRAKRUTI EVALUATION (*cont.*)

V (Vata)	P (Pitta)	K (Kapha)
34. Reaction to Stressful Situations		
☐ fear and anxiety	☐ frustration, irritability, anger	☐ manage stress well
35. Resistance to Discomfort		
☐ poor	☐ average	☐ good
36. Immune System		
☐ variable	☐ normal	☐ good
37. Ailments		
☐ nervous and mental	☐ inflammatory, infections	☐ systemic and respiratory
38. Frequent Illnesses		
☐ neuralgic, joint pain	☐ skin and blood-related	☐ mucus/joint inflammation
39. Sex Drive		
☐ variable, sexual fantasies	☐ high sexual impulse	☐ regular sexual impulse
40. Motivational Disposition		
☐ variable (ideas/mood)	☐ intense, externalized	☐ stable, reliable, slow to change
41. Climate Predilection		
☐ hot, sunny, humid	☐ cold, ventilated	☐ most climates except humid
42. Activity		
☐ restless	☐ moderate, constant	☐ slow mover
43. Exercise Inclination		
☐ strong: runs, bikes, hikes	☐ very much (with intensity)	☐ very little, but appreciative
44. Walking		
☐ quickly	☐ moderate to fast, determined	☐ slowly, steady, thoughtful

PRAKRUTI EVALUATION (*cont.*)

V (Vata)	P (Pitta)	K (Kapha)
45. Work/Job Activity		
☐ very quick, lots of initiative	☐ moderate speed, constant	☐ slowly and methodically
46. Temperament		
☐ nervous, changeable	☐ motivated, intense	☐ relaxed
47. Sensitive to		
☐ loud noises, chaotic scenes	☐ brightness, glaring lights	☐ strong lights, odors
48. Positive Emotions		
☐ adaptability	☐ courage, daring	☐ affection, warmth
49. Negative Emotions		
☐ fear	☐ intolerance	☐ attachment
50. Beliefs		
☐ variable, erratic	☐ strong, determined	☐ constant, slow to change
51. Speech/Conversation		
☐ fast, not very clear	☐ strong, clear, penetrating	☐ slow, prolonged
52. Tendency to Spend Money		
☐ unnecessary/superfluous	☐ on luxuries	☐ prefer to economize/save
53. Reaction to Difficulties/Problems		
☐ anxiety, indecision, worry	☐ anger, irritability, frustration	☐ calm, steady/stable attitude
54. Others Describe Me As		
☐ spacy/indecisive	☐ intolerant, annoying, intensive	☐ stubborn, sluggish
55. Others Wish I Would Be More		
☐ grounded	☐ tolerant, less judgmental	☐ more involved, enthusiastic

Total the scores from each column to find your corresponding doshas (vata, pitta, kapha):

Highest Score _____

2nd Highest Score _____

Lowest Score _____

Your Prakruti Profile _____
    (in descending order: K-P-V, K-V-P, and so on)

WHAT IS YOUR VIKRUTI?

Note: In the vikruti evaluation, you should give answers for each of the categories based on your current medium- or short-term experience with respect to your physical and mental health. For example, if your weight has dropped recently, not as part of a planned reduction but due to other factors, then your "Weight" response would be "underweight, undernourished."

VIKRUTI EVALUATION

V (Vata)	P (Pitta)	K (Kapha)
1. Body Appearance		
☐ slim, lean, bony	☐ average, highly energetic	☐ big, lethargic
2. Weight		
☐ underweight, undernourished	☐ stable	☐ plump, overweight
3. Joint Manifestation		
☐ cracking, popping, stiffness	☐ tender, sensitive	☐ swollen, puffy
4. Joint Sensation		
☐ body aches, dryness	☐ hot/warm, inflammation	☐ water retention (ankles)

VIKRUTI EVALUATION (*cont.*)

V (Vata)	P (Pitta)	K (Kapha)
5. Spine Tendency		
☐ sideways curvature tendency	☐ arching	☐ hunching
6. Bone Issues		
☐ sore	☐ sensitive, painful	☐ heaviness
7. Muscles		
☐ shivers, twitches, spasms	☐ tender, inflammation	☐ swollen
8. Skin		
☐ rough, dry, scaly	☐ tender, inflamed, rashes	☐ oily, smooth, clammy
9. Lymph Nodes		
☐ thin	☐ sensitive, inflamed	☐ expanding, congested
10. Veins		
☐ drained, protruding, weaker	☐ bruise easily, less visible	☐ filled, wide, lifeless
11. Eyes: Vision		
☐ dried, agitated, blinking	☐ redness, light hypersensitivity	☐ inflamed, viscous, secretions
12. Ears: Sound		
☐ resounding, ringing	☐ pain, distress, infections	☐ blocked, secretion
13. Nose		
☐ dehydrated, crusty	☐ inflamed, swollen	☐ blocked
14. Sinuses		
☐ dry	☐ irritated	☐ congested
15. Mouth		
☐ dry, gum disease	☐ inflamed/sensitive/puffy gums	☐ extreme salivation

VIKRUTI EVALUATION (*cont.*)

V (Vata)	P (Pitta)	K (Kapha)
16. Lips		
☐ dry, cracked	☐ dehydrated, irritated	☐ dull, unctuous
17. Lungs		
☐ dry	☐ warm and sharp feeling	☐ excess mucous, breathless
18. Taste		
☐ lacking taste	☐ bitter, sour, metal	☐ sour stomach, nausea
19. Teeth		
☐ cavities, weak enamel	☐ creamy/yellow, faded enamel	☐ strong teeth and enamel
20. Gums		
☐ pale, receding	☐ irritated	☐ enlarged
21. Tongue		
☐ dry, fissured, murky coating	☐ reddish, irritated, yellowish	☐ whitish, thick coating
22. Hair		
☐ dry, weak, brittle	☐ oily, grayish, baldness	☐ unctuous
23. Nails		
☐ dry, brittle, broken, bitten	☐ soft, sharp, irritated	☐ whitish, hard, oily
24. Food Intake		
☐ erratic/compulsive tendency	☐ excessive tendency	☐ emotional eating
25. Digestion		
☐ irregular, ballooning	☐ fast, heartburn, ulcers, reflux	☐ gradual, sustained, indigestion

VIKRUTI EVALUATION (*cont.*)

V (Vata)	P (Pitta)	K (Kapha)
26. Food Absorption		
☐ need warming substances	☐ reduced	☐ slow, steady
27. Food Assimilation		
☐ reduced, body debility	☐ reduced (putrefaction)	☐ accumulation (obesity)
28. Elimination		
☐ dry, constipated, irregular	☐ loose, burning, yellow urine	☐ large, oily/mucous feces
29. Liver and Spleen		
☐ noticeably enlarged	☐ noticeably tender	☐ enlarged and fatty
30. Thirst		
☐ fluctuating	☐ heavy, active (feverish)	☐ low
31. Breathing		
☐ anxious, worried	☐ assertive, tightness	☐ slower, from stomach, apnea
32. Voice		
☐ dry, hesitating, fiery	☐ sharp, powerful	☐ deep, gravelly
33. Speech		
☐ harsh, rushed, imprecise	☐ piercing, strong, deliberate	☐ slow, colorless, dull
34. Allergic Reactions		
☐ dry, wheeziness, gasping	☐ rashes, flushes, urticaria	☐ congestion, nasal secretion
35. Sleep/Napping		
☐ insomnia, disrupted sleep	☐ slow to sleep, not enough	☐ excessive, tiredness

VIKRUTI EVALUATION (*cont.*)

V (Vata)	P (Pitta)	K (Kapha)
36. Dreams		
☐ frequent, vivid, scary	☐ intense, deep, brutal	☐ idealistic, tender, romantic
37. Sex Drive		
☐ low and hurried	☐ high and self-serving	☐ low but sensual, attachment
38. Feelings		
☐ worry, distress, frantic	☐ impatience, rage, hate, envy	☐ attachment, despair, sadness
39. Motivation Level		
☐ restless, quickly exhausted	☐ intense, drained by thinking	☐ low, tiredness due to weight
40. Movement		
☐ faster, agitated, stiff	☐ fast and insistent	☐ slow, lethargic, heavy
41. Memory		
☐ good recent, poor long-term	☐ adequate, distinguishing	☐ slow, good long-term
42. Understanding		
☐ faster but deficient responses	☐ quicker correct responses	☐ slower precise responses

Total the scores in each column with the corresponding doshas:

Highest Score _____

2nd Highest Score _____

Lowest Score _____

Your Vikruti Profile: _____

(in descending order: K-P-V, K-P-V, and so on)

WHAT IS YOUR MANAS PRAKRUTI?

The manas prakruti evaluation is an invitation to start making helpful changes based on how ayurveda uses its understanding of the governing principles of sattva, rajas, and tamas.

Let us briefly consider the three dispositions of the mind in ayurvedic terms: A truly sattvic nature is deep in contentment and truth—in other words, desire-free. A rajas state of mind is active and needs stimulation, usually through the senses, in order to be satisfied. A tamasic type is more vulnerable due to their lethargic tendency and likelihood of being under the influence of inertia.

Ayurveda encourages us to become aware of our state of mind by observing our imbalances. In this particular case, it addresses individuals with depressive tendencies, and supports them in improving from a tamas to a rajas state or from a rajas to a sattva state. For most of us, answers to this evaluation will fit in the middle, or the rajasic area, which is the most common state in our active and outgoing culture today: we all carry psychological issues from the past, and deal with situations and problems daily. The goal of studying these three mental types is to offer a greater sense of self-awareness of your state of depression or anxiety, by opening your eyes to the protective patterns of behavior that perhaps were stages of your coping strategies. According to ayurveda, it is these protective patterns that negatively affect your body—for example in your gut, in relation to digestive fire and its helpful bacteria; or your mind, where stress and anxiety are created—resulting in an impact that generates imbalances, which in the long term could manifest as increased depression or other ill health.

In practical terms, remember that the gunas are always changing and, as such, this evaluation is not intended to provide a static profile. For that reason, I suggest doing the evaluation at least twice—the first time based on a long period of your life, and the second time answering the questions on how you have been feeling in the last month or so. Then calculate your profile in both cases. This will help you understand if recent life changes and/or challenges are affecting your usual state, and how much out of balance you could be. In that way, and according to your degree of active participation with this book's suggested activities, you can be a witness to your own gradual changes and rebalancing.

Note: In the manas prakruti evaluation, you should give answers for each of the categories based on your current medium- or short-term experience with respect to your physical and mental health.

MANAS EVALUATION

S (Sattva)	R (Rajas)	T (Tamas)
1. Mental Lucidity		
☐ good, prolonged	☐ moderate	☐ poor
2. Mental Harmony		
☐ peaceful	☐ reasonable	☐ rare
3. Satisfaction		
☐ usually	☐ partly	☐ occasionally
4. Conduct		
☐ compassionate, loving	☐ assertive, controlling	☐ destructive
5. Work		
☐ selfless	☐ self-centered tendency	☐ lazy
6. Communication		
☐ good	☐ variable	☐ difficult
7. Speech		
☐ clear, peaceful, soft	☐ fast, agitated	☐ slow, dull
8. Concentration		
☐ good	☐ wavering	☐ poor
9. Willpower		
☐ good	☐ fluctuating	☐ weak

MANAS EVALUATION (*cont.*)

S (Sattva)	R (Rajas)	T (Tamas)
10. Creativity		
☐ high	☐ moderate	☐ low
11. Knowledge		
☐ deep	☐ reasonable	☐ poor
12. Memory		
☐ good	☐ variable	☐ poor
13. Self-Awareness		
☐ complete	☐ uncertain	☐ weak
14. Sense of Service		
☐ whole	☐ variable	☐ rarely
15. Emotions		
☐ authentic	☐ contradictory	☐ suppressed
16. Anger		
☐ rarely	☐ occasionally	☐ frequently
17. Hate		
☐ rarely	☐ occasionally	☐ frequently
18. Violence		
☐ never	☐ occasionally	☐ frequently
19. Grief		
☐ uncommon	☐ occasionally	☐ frequently
20. Fear		
☐ hardly	☐ sometimes	☐ frequently

MANAS EVALUATION (*cont.*)

S (Sattva)	R (Rajas)	T (Tamas)
21. Pride		
☐ little	☐ some	☐ much
22. Desires		
☐ rarely, brief	☐ moderate, frequent	☐ long-standing
23. Attachment		
☐ rarely, brief	☐ moderate, frequent	☐ long-standing
24. Greed		
☐ rarely, brief	☐ moderate, frequent	☐ long-standing
25. Uncertainty		
☐ rarely, brief	☐ moderate, frequent	☐ long-standing
26. Feeling Down		
☐ rarely, brief	☐ moderate, frequent	☐ long-standing
27. Contentment		
☐ regularly	☐ occasionally	☐ rarely
28. Forgiveness		
☐ easily	☐ with effort	☐ begrudgingly
29. Consideration		
☐ mainly to others	☐ self and friends	☐ slight, self-considering
30. Honesty		
☐ constantly	☐ quite often	☐ infrequently
31. Commitment		
☐ total	☐ limited	☐ poor

MANAS EVALUATION (*cont.*)

S (Sattva)	R (Rajas)	T (Tamas)
32. Truthfulness		
☐ always	☐ most of the time	☐ rarely
33. Enjoyment		
☐ regular	☐ moderate	☐ occasional
34. Love		
☐ unconditional, giver	☐ selfish, taker	☐ needy, obsessed
35. Peace of Mind		
☐ generally	☐ relatively	☐ rarely
36. Spiritual Power		
☐ humankind	☐ self-interest	☐ unengaging
37. Mindfulness		
☐ daily	☐ occasionally	☐ rarely/never
38. Movement		
☐ with awareness	☐ fast, active	☐ sluggish, heavy, dull
39. Orderliness		
☐ always	☐ makes effort	☐ generally lazy
40. Exercise		
☐ gentle, daily	☐ competitive	☐ rarely
41. Sexual Activity		
☐ infrequent, soulful	☐ variable, pleasurable	☐ excessive, lusty
42. Sleep		
☐ sound, satisfying	☐ interrupted, unsatisfying	☐ excessive, heavy

MANAS EVALUATION (*cont.*)

S (Sattva)	R (Rajas)	T (Tamas)
43. Diet		
☐ light, wholesome	☐ mainly wholesome	☐ unwholesome
44. Digestion		
☐ good	☐ variable	☐ slow
45. Elimination		
☐ regular	☐ mainly regular	☐ irregular, heavy
46. Drugs/Alcohol		
☐ rarely	☐ sometimes, socially	☐ frequently
47. Money Focus		
☐ rarely	☐ some	☐ strong

Total the scores in each column to find your corresponding guna (sattva, rajas, tamas):

Highest Score _____

2nd Highest Score _____

Lowest Score _____

Your Manas Prakruti Profile: _____
    (in descending order S-R-T, T-R-S, and so on)

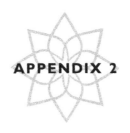

FOOD RECOMMENDATIONS
FOR THE THREE DOSHAS

KAPHA: FOOD RECOMMENDATIONS

Integrate new foods gradually, and progressively reduce unsuitable food items over a period of two or three weeks, one at a time. Avoid quick changes, especially with foods that have been part of your regular diet for a long time. Consult your physician if you suffer from food allergies or intolerances to any of the recommended food items. (See pages 232–33 for kapha-vata and vata-kapha and pages 233–35 for kapha-pitta and pitta-kapha food recommendations.)

Vegetables (in season)	artichokes, asparagus, beet greens, beets, bitter melons, broccoli, brussels sprouts, cabbages, carrots, cauliflower, celery, coriander leaves, corn, eggplant, fennel, German turnips (*kohlrabi*), green beans, green chilies, horseradish, Jerusalem artichokes, kale, leafy greens, leeks, lettuce, mixed-bean sprouts, mushrooms, mustard greens, lady's fingers (okra), onions, parsley, peas, peppers (sweet, hot), potatoes (white), radishes, spinach, squash, tomatoes, turnip greens, turnips, watercress, wheatgrass sprouts
Fruits	apples, apricots, berries, cherries, cranberries, figs, grapes, lemons, limes, peaches, pears, persimmons, pomegranates, prunes, raisins, strawberries
Grains	barley, buckwheat, cereal (cold, dry, or puffed), corn, couscous, crackers, durum flour, millet, muesli, oat bran, oats (dry), rice (wild), rice (basmati), rye, sago, sprouted wheat, tapioca, wheat bran

KAPHA: FOOD RECOMMENDATIONS (*cont.*)

Legumes	black beans, black-eyed peas, chickpeas, lentils (red or brown), lima beans, mung beans (green gram), peas (dried), pinto beans, adzuki beans (red mung beans), soy milk, split peas, sprouts, tofu (hot), pigeon peas (*tur dhal*)
Dairy Products	buttermilk, cottage cheese (from skimmed goat milk), goat's cheese (fresh, unsalted), goat's milk (skimmed)
Animal Products	chicken (white), eggs, fish (freshwater), rabbit, shrimps, turkey (white), venison
Condiments	black pepper, chili pepper, chutney (mango), coriander leaves, garlic, horseradish, lemon, mustard (without vinegar), seaweed
Nuts/Seeds	Avoid nuts and seeds except flaxseed, popcorn (without salt or butter), pumpkin seeds, and sunflower seeds
Oils	almond, corn, sunflower, ghee, mustard. Sesame for external use
Beverages	aloe vera juice, apple cider, apple juice, apricot juice, berry juice, black tea (spiced), carrot juice, cherry juice, cranberry juice, grape juice, mango juice, peach nectar, pear juice, pineapple juice, pomegranate juice, prune juice, soy milk (warm and spiced), vegetable juices and broths
Herbs	alfalfa, angelica, beleric (bibhitaki), barley, basil, bergamot, blackberries, burdock, chamomile, chicory, comfrey, dandelion, fenugreek, ginger, ginseng, hibiscus, hyssop, Indian asparagus (*shatavari*), jasmine, juniper berries, lavender, liquorice, lemon balm, lemongrass, long pepper (*pippali*), mukul myrrh tree (guggul), mustard, nettle, passion flower, pennyroyal, peppermint, raspberry, red clover, sage, sarsaparilla, sassafras, spearmint, strawberries, thyme, yarrow, slippery elm, valerian, wintergreen
Spices	allspice, anise, asafoetida (*hing*), bay leaf, bishop's seed (*ajwain*), black pepper, caraway, cardamom, cayenne, cinnamon, cloves, cumin, coriander, curry leaves, dill, fennel, fenugreek, garlic, ginger, mace, marjoram, mint, mustard seeds, nutmeg, orange peel, oregano, paprika, parsley, peppermint, poppy seeds, rosemary, saffron, salt, spearmint, star anise, tarragon, thyme, turmeric, vanilla
Food Supplements	aloe vera juice, bee pollen, brewer's yeast, minerals (calcium, copper, iron, magnesium, zinc), essential fatty acids, royal jelly
Sweeteners	honey (raw and not processed)

KAPHA: FOODS TO AVOID

Reduce intake or gradually start to avoid these foods.

Vegetables	cucumbers, olives (black and green), parsnips, potatoes (sweet), pumpkin, squash, tomatoes (raw), zucchini (*courgette*)
Fruits	avocados, bananas, coconut, dates, figs (fresh), grapefruits, kiwis, mangoes, melons, oranges, papayas, pineapples, plums, rhubarb, tamarinds, watermelons
Grains	bread (with yeast), oats (cooked), pancakes, pasta, rice (brown and white), rice cakes, wheat in general
Legumes	black lentils (*urad dhal*), kidney beans, soybeans, soy products, tofu (cold)
Dairy Products	butter, cheese (soft and hard), cow's milk, ice cream, sour cream, yogurt (plain, frozen, or with fruit)
Animal Products	beef, chicken (dark), duck, fish (sea), lamb, pork, salmon, sardines, seafood, tuna, turkey (dark)
Condiments	chocolate, chutney (sweet), kelp, ketchup, lime, lime pickle, mango pickle, mayonnaise, salt, soy sauce, vinegar
Nuts/Seeds	almonds, Brazil nuts, cashews, coconut, filberts, hazelnuts, peanuts, pecans, pine nuts, pistachios, sesame seeds, tahini, walnuts
Oils	coconut, flaxseed, olive, safflower, sesame, walnut
Beverages	alcohol, (strong, beer, sweet wines), almond milk, caffeinated beverages, carbonated drinks, cherry juice, chocolate milk, cold dairy drinks, grapefruit juice, iced tea, lemonade, orange juice, papaya juice, rice milk, soy milk, tomato juice
Herbs	rosehip
Spices	practically all under the salt presentation
Sweeteners	barley malt, fructose, jaggery, maple syrup, molasses, rice syrup, white sugar

PITTA: FOOD RECOMMENDATIONS

Integrate new foods gradually, and progressively reduce the unsuitable food items over a period of two or three weeks, one at a time. Avoid quick changes, especially with foods that have been part of your regular diet for a long time.

Vegetables (mostly sweet and bitter)	artichoke, avocados, beets (cooked), bitter melons, broccoli (steamed), brussels sprouts, cabbage, carrots, cauliflower (steamed), celery, cilantro, coriander, cucumbers, fennel, green beans, Indian asparagus (shatavari), Jerusalem artichoke, kale, leafy greens, leeks (cooked), lettuce, mushrooms, lady's fingers (okra), olives (black), onions (cooked), parsley, parsnips, peas, peppers (sweet), potatoes (sweet), prickly pear (leaves), pumpkin, radishes (cooked), sprouts, watercress, zucchini (courgette)
Fruits (mostly sweet)	apples, apricots, berries, cherries, coconut, dates, figs, grapes (red), limes, mangoes, melons, oranges, papayas, pears, pineapple, plums, pomegranates, prunes, raisins, tangerines, watermelons
Grains	barley, cereal (dry), couscous, durum flour, oat bran, oats (cooked), pastas, rice, rice cakes or crackers, sago, sprouted wheat bread, tapioca, wheat, noodles
Legumes	black beans, black-eyed peas, chickpeas, kidney beans, lentils (red and brown), green gram (mung beans), peas (dried), pinto beans, red mung beans (adzuki beans) soybeans, split peas, tofu and soy products
Dairy Products	butter (unsalted), cheese (soft, not mature, unsalted), cottage cheese, cow's milk, ghee, goat's cheese (soft, unsalted), goat's milk, ice cream, yoghurt
Animal Products	chicken, eggs (white only), fish (freshwater), rabbit, shrimps, turkey (white), venison
Condiments	black pepper, chutney (mango), coriander leaves, lime, lime pickle, mango pickle
Nuts/Seeds	(in moderation) almonds, coconut, flaxseed, popcorn (unsalted), pumpkin seeds, sunflower seeds

PITTA: FOOD RECOMMENDATIONS (*cont.*)

Oils	(in moderation) sunflower, safflower, ghee, olive, flaxseed, coconut, corn oil
Beverages	almond milk, aloe vera juice, apple cider, apricot juice, black tea, cherry juice, cool dairy drinks, grain coffee, grape juice, mango juice, orange juice, peach nectar, pear juice, pomegranate juice, prune juice, rice milk, soy milk, vegetable broths
Herbs	alfalfa, barley, blackberry, borage, burdock, chamomile, cardamom, coriander (cilantro), chicory, comfrey, dandelion, echinacea, goldenseal, False daisy (*bhringaraj*), fennel, ginger (fresh), Indian pennywort (*gotu kola*), hibiscus, hops, Indian gooseberry (amalaki), Indian madder (manjistha), jasmine, lavender, lemon balm, lemongrass, liquorice, neem, nettle, passion flower, peppermint, puncture vine (*gokshura*), raspberries, red clover, sandalwood, sarsaparilla, spearmint, strawberries, violet, wintergreen, yarrow
Spices	basil (fresh), black pepper, caraway, cardamom, cinnamon, coriander, cumin, curry leaves, dill, fennel, ginger (fresh), mint, parsley, saffron, spearmint, tarragon, turmeric, vanilla, wintergreen
Food Supplements	aloe vera juice, barley green, brewer's yeast, minerals (calcium, magnesium, zinc), spirulina, blue-green algae, vitamins D and E
Sweeteners	barley malt, maple syrup, rice syrup, sugarcane

PITTA: FOODS TO AVOID

Reduce intake or gradually start to avoid these foods, especially dry foods.

Vegetables	beet greens, beets (raw), burdock root, corn (fresh), daikon radishes, eggplant, garlic, green chilies, horseradish, German turnip (kohlrabi), leeks (raw), mustard greens, olives (green), onions (raw), peppers (hot), prickly pears (fruit), radishes (raw), spinach, tomatoes, turnip greens, turnips
Fruits (sour or green)	apples, apricots, bananas, berries, cherries, cranberries, grapefruits, grapes, kiwis, lemons, mangoes, oranges, peaches, persimmons, pineapples, plums, rhubarb, strawberries, tamarinds
Grains	bread (with yeast), buckwheat, corn, millet, muesli, oats (dry), rice (brown), rye

PITTA: FOODS TO AVOID (*cont.*)

Legumes	black lentil (*urad dhal*), pigeon pea (*tur dhal*), soy sauce
Dairy Products	butter (salted), buttermilk, cheese (ripe), sour cream, yogurt (plain or frozen with fruits)
Animal Products	beef, duck, egg yolk, sea fish, lamb, pork, salmon, sardines, tuna (low mercury)
Condiments	chili pepper, chocolate, horseradish, kelp, ketchup, mustard, lemon, pickle (mango, lime), mayonnaise, salt (in excess), seaweed, vinegar
Nuts/Seeds	Brazil nuts, cashews, hazelnuts, peanuts, pecans, pine nuts, pistachios, walnuts, sesame seeds, tahini
Oils	almond, corn, safflower, sesame
Beverages	alcohol (strong and wine), apple cider, berry juice (sour), caffeinated beverages, carbonated drinks, carrot juice, cherry juice (sour), chocolate milk, coffee, cranberry juice, grapefruit juice, iced tea, icy cold drinks, lemonade, papaya juice, pineapple juice, tomato juice
Herbs	Basil, bishop's seed (ajwain), cinnamon, clove, eucalyptus, fenugreek, ginger (dry), ginseng, hawthorn, hyssop, juniper berries, pennyroyal, rosehip, sage, sassafras
Spices	Allspice, anise, asafoetida (hing), basil (dry), bay leaf, bishop's seed (ajwain), cayenne, cloves, fenugreek, garlic, ginger (dry), mace, marjoram, mustard seeds, nutmeg, oregano, paprika, pippali, poppy seeds, rosemary, sage, star anise, thyme
Sweeteners	Fructose, honey, white sugar, molasses

VATA: FOOD RECOMMENDATIONS

Integrate new foods gradually, and progressively reduce the unsuitable food items over a period of two or three weeks, one at a time. Avoid quick changes, especially with foods that have been part of your regular diet for a long time.

VATA: FOOD RECOMMENDATIONS (*cont.*)

Vegetables	asparagus, avocados, beets, cabbage (cooked), carrots, cauliflower, cucumbers, radishes, fennel, green beans, leafy greens, leeks, okra (lady's fingers), parsnips, peas (cooked), sweet potatoes, pumpkin, spinach, sprouts, squash, turnip greens, zucchini (courgette)
Fruits (most sweet fruit)	apples (red), apricots, bananas (ripe), berries, cherries, coconut, dates (fresh), figs (fresh), grapefruit, grapes, kiwis, lemons, limes, mangoes, melons, oranges, papayas, peaches, pineapples, plums, prunes (soaked), raisins (soaked), rhubarb, strawberries
Grains	noodles, pasta, rice (brown, wild, white), oats (cooked), whole wheat cereals
Legumes	mung beans (green grams), red lentils, red mung beans (adzuki beans), pigeon pea (tur dhal), black lentils (urad dhal), tofu and soy products
Dairy Products	butter, buttermilk, cheese (soft), cottage cheese, cow's milk, diluted yogurt (*lassie*) ghee, goat's cheese, goat's milk
Animal Products	chicken, duck, eggs, fish (salmon, sardines, tuna), seafood, shrimp, turkey
Condiments	black pepper, chutney sauce (mango), lemon, lime, lime pickle, mango pickle, mustard, salt, soy sauce, tahini, tamari, vinegar
Nuts/ Seeds (in moderation)	almonds, brazil nuts, cashews, coconut, hazelnuts, macadamia nuts, pine nuts, pistachios, pumpkin seeds, sesame seeds, sunflower seeds, walnuts
Oils	most oils but in particular sesame, ghee, and olive in moderation
Beverages	juices including apricot, carrot, grape, grapefruit, mango, orange, papaya, peach nectar, pineapple; alcohol (white wine, beer); almond milk, aloe vera juice, apple cider, warm soy milk, broths, and vegetable juices
Herbs	bishop's weed (ajwain), *bala*, black myrobalan (haritaki), catnip (catmint), chamomile, chicory, clove, comfrey, elderflower, eucalyptus, fennel, fenugreek, ginger, ginseng, hawthorn, Indian asparagus (shatavari), Indian ginseng (*ashwagandha*), Indian pennywort (gotu kola), juniper berry, lavender, lemongrass, licorice, mukul myrrh tree (guggul), oat straw, orange blossom oil (neroli), orange peel, pennyroyal, peppermint, rosehip, saffron, sage, sarsaparilla, spearmint, valerian, wintergreen

VATA: FOOD RECOMMENDATIONS (*cont.*)

Spices (all good)	allspice, almond extract, anise, asafetida (hing), basil, bay leaf, bishop's seed (ajwain), black pepper, cardamom, cinnamon, cloves, coriander, cumin, dill, fennel, fenugreek, garlic, ginger, Indian long pepper (pippali), marjoram, mint, mustard seeds, nutmeg, orange peel, oregano, paprika, parsley, peppermint, poppy seeds, rosemary, saffron, salt, spearmint, tarragon, thyme, turmeric, vanilla, aromatic wintergreen
Food Supplements	aloe vera juice, bee pollen, essential fatty acids, minerals (calcium, copper, iron, magnesium, zinc), royal jelly, spirulina (if required)
Sweeteners	honey, unrefined sugar (jaggery), molasses, barley malt, rice syrup

VATA: FOODS TO AVOID

Reduce intake or gradually start to avoid these foods, especially dry foods.

Vegetables	artichoke, bitter melon, broccoli, brussels sprouts, burdock root, cabbage (raw), cauliflower (raw), celery, corn (fresh), dandelion greens, eggplant, German turnip (kohlrabi), horseradish, kale, mushrooms, olives (green), onions (raw), peppers (sweet and hot), potatoes (white), radishes (raw), tomatoes (raw), turnips, wheatgrass sprouts
Fruits	apples (raw), cranberries, dates (dry), figs (dry), pears, persimmons, pomegranates, prunes (dry), raisins (dry); most dried fruits
Grains	barley, bread (with yeast), buckwheat, cereal (cold, dry, or puffed), corn, couscous, millet, muesli, oat bran, oats (dry), rice cakes or crackers, rye, sago, tapioca, wheat bran; most dry, light grains
Legumes	black beans, black-eyed peas, chickpeas (garbanzo), kidney beans, lentils (brown; yellow), lima beans, peas (dried), pinto beans, red mung beans (adzuki), soybeans, white beans
Dairy Products	powdered milk, yogurt (plain, cold, frozen, or with fruit)
Animal Products	lamb, pork, rabbit, venison
Condiments	horseradish
Nuts/Seeds	suitable in moderation

VATA: FOODS TO AVOID (*cont.*)

Oils	flaxseed
Beverages (avoid cold)	alcohol (strong), apple juice, black tea, caffeinated or carbonated drinks, chocolate milk, coffee, cold dairy drinks, cranberry juice, iced tea, ice-cold drinks, pear juice, pomegranate juice, soy milk (cold), tomato juice
Herbs	basil, blackberries, borage, burdock, cornsilk, dandelion, ginseng, hibiscus, hops, nettle, red clover, yarrow
Spices	caraway (Persian cumin)
Sweeteners	industrial fructose and white sugar

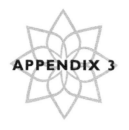

APPENDIX 3

SELF-MASSAGE OF
THE LYMPHATIC SYSTEM

PROTOCOL FOR THE MANUAL
ACTIVATION OF THE LYMPH FLOW
AND FUNCTION*

Our bodies face a continuous challenge with keeping the lymphatic filter clean. This is not an easy job considering the quality of the food we ingest, the polluted air we breathe, and the toxicity of chemical products we use in our houses, such as kitchen cleaners, laundry room soaps, and hygiene and medicinal products. It is surprising that our bodies keep draining waste and toxins daily to compensate for the creation of and exposure to all those factors that bring more stress to our lives. Other conditions that could affect your lymphatic system function, and by extension your overall body balance, are structural blockages caused by previous scars or adhesions in the fascia tissue preventing the lymphatic flow. The question is: How can we get that drainage system working properly? How can we stimulate our parasympathetic system? Well, the following self-massage protocol could make a significant difference for you, and I strongly suggest doing it daily after waking up and keeping to the order described below.

---

*As usual, in case of contraindications, please talk with your physician or physical therapist before beginning this massage.

297

General Mechanics of the Process

There are three main superficial regions on each side of the body where lymph nodes tend to cluster. These places are the cervical nodes in the neck area, the axillary nodes in the armpit, and the inguinal nodes in the groin. In order to achieve drainage, our bodies develop a system that has two thoracic lymph ducts, left and right, at the level of the collarbone area. The left-side thoracic duct, at the base of the neck, drains a much larger portion of the body than does the lymphatic duct on the right side.

A bit of anatomy: it is well known that lymph mostly drains from the collarbone area, above and below it. One of these trunks, the right lymphatic duct, drains the upper right portion of the body, returning lymph to the bloodstream via the right subclavian vein. The other trunk, the left thoracic duct, drains the rest of the body into the left subclavian vein. The lymph trunks drain into the lymph ducts, which in turn return lymph to the blood by emptying into the respective subclavian veins. The lymph flows into lymph nodes through afferent collecting lymphatic vessels and exits through efferent collecting lymphatic vessels. The lymph not only flows through the lymph nodes, but some of it is reabsorbed into the blood circulation at the lymph nodes. The majority of the lymph (75 percent) goes to the left side of the collarbone area and the rest goes to the right side; so the left is the main drain, but we always need to address both sides, starting at the left-side level of the neck.

It is now known that if lymphatic vessels in the brain or in other areas become congested, the result could compromise your immune system, which could leave viruses and bacteria in the brain and body, increasing the risks of infection, inflammation, autoimmunity, and even mental disturbances. Studies show that the brain drains our toxins at nighttime when we are sleeping—or rather, it's supposed to, if our body is in a state of balance. However, if blockages arise from brain toxicity at night when the lymph does not move, you'll feel sluggish or slow when trying to get started in the morning. On the other hand, we all find ways to face the world even while accompanied by an unconscious tension in our resting baseline state, which contracts our muscles and fascia and affects lymphatic flow. By starting the day with a lymph drainage self-massage of our fascia, mobilizing the muscles of the face, head, and other parts of the body, we are also stimulating the vagus nerve. This will induce a profound relaxation response, making your muscles of expressivity a bit more at ease and at your command. For the above reason, and as prevention practice, you'll benefit by taking the below steps every morning when you wake up, because most of the lymph could be stagnant if there is an overloaded lymphatic system causing tightness and stiffness in the body and in the joints. Particularly, when you feel a lot of congestion or stuffiness in your head, or some extra pressure in your head, it could be caused by the lymphatic system. Promoting drainage of extra lymphatic fluid in the head through the lymphatic drainage massage can bring that fluid down by pumping it out of the head.

Essentially, you are going to stimulate uptake of fluid into the lymphatics by practicing a gentle, manual technique using light pressure and rhythmic pumping, stretching the skin either by rubbing, twisting, or gently stroking; after that, you'll use a short series of gentle taps to provide a light vibration. You will be addressing seven areas: collarbone, head/neck, shoulders/pectorals, abdomen, inguinal/groin, full sternum, and complete body stimulation. Use gentle pressure on delicate areas such as your head, collarbone/neck, and groin. For all areas, I recommend you do a combination of rubbing back and forth, around ten to fifteen seconds. Then do some tapping, around ten times, creating vibration while avoiding excessive force.

Drink at least one glass of water beforehand, and do not practice massage if you have any underlying issues, feel sick, or are generally not doing well. Get comfortable, either sitting on a chair or standing up. This is the protocol, step by step, "from scalp to feet":

🌿 Self-Massage of the Lymphatic System

Collarbone: Slide your right hand to the left side of your clavicula/collarbone and rub above and below the soft tissue with your whole hand, toward the heart. That action of pressure opens up the near lymph nodes, draining fluid back into the body and freeing up any potential blockage. Then end with light tapping in the area with the whole hand.

Next, go to the right side of the collarbone area with the left hand and repeat the same process. This can be done directly on the skin or over clothes.

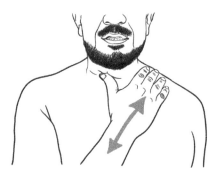

Fig. A.1. Collarbone

Next, start draining the fluid from your head toward your neck and around the ears and the back of the neck as follows.

Head/Scalp: Be very light; it is not a deep massage. You are going to work on the lymphatic fluids that are close to the surface of the skin. Use a pressure level that's as if you were moving a coin across the top of a table. For the scalp, gently massage your head with the tip of your fingers, then gently tap all over.

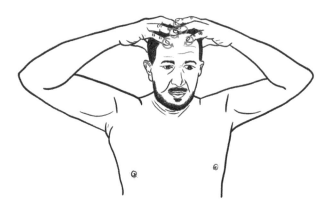

Fig. A.2. Head/Scalp

Behind the Ears: The next large node area to address in the upper body is from the back of the ears toward the neck, right above and behind the angle of the jaw, and behind the earlobe going down to the upper side of the collarbone area. These are known as cervical lymph nodes. Place the flat part of four fingers behind the ears, and the thumb in front of the ear, and start

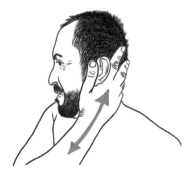

Fig. A.3. Behind the Ears

pulling straight down with the surface of your fingers and palm along that angle where the big sternocleidomastoid muscle leads toward the collarbone. Start from the left side first.

You may feel the drainage start to move, or feel a pressure change in your ears so that you may have to clear your throat. This head lymphatic drainage massage will give you some relief in cases of allergies, sinus congestion, or headaches from congestion in the head. Sometimes it can help with dizziness or vertigo, and with some of the symptoms that go along with having a cold and having a lot of fluid in your head.

Pectoral/Auxiliary: Go to the left side of your shoulder joint area, the region of the auxiliary nodes. Take your open hand and put it over the region where your shoulder joins your pecs, and rub it all the way over; then, with your whole open hand, tap the same area. Repeat the same protocol on your right side.

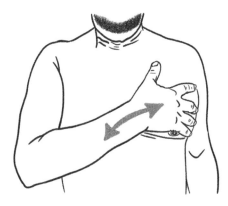

Fig. A.4. Pectoral/Auxiliary

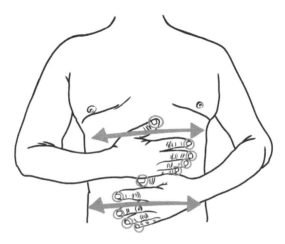

Fig. A.5. Abdominal/Gut

Abdominal/Gut: Place one open hand on your belly button and the other open hand above it, preferably standing up for more comfort. Rub the area with your two hands, either in circular movements, back and forth, or up and down; and then end the process with tapping the same area in order to transfer a vibration all the way through your gut.

Inguinal/Groin: Gently rub across the inguinal crest toward the pubic area on both sides, using both hands to stimulate the inguinal nodes. Then be very cautious where you are tapping.

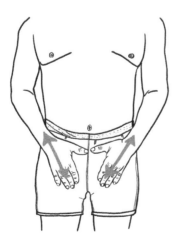

Fig. A.6. Inguinal/Groin

Back of the Knees: For this part, it is preferable to be standing or bending the hips and knee area. You can also try sitting down. When ready, rub above and below behind the back of the knees. This is an area where the popliteal lymphatic nodes get often stuck. Then, tap the backs of your knees.

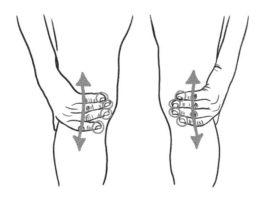

Fig. A.7. Back of the Knees

Sternum: Gently tap the sternum area with your fists to drain the lymph upward.

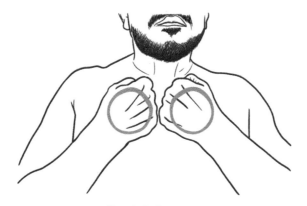

Fig. A.8. Sternum

Full Body Activation: Finally, for a general stimulation of the lymphatic flow, stand up on the toes or balls of your feet, and move up and down gently with your heels leaving the ground, using the calf muscles as the rebounder, for around ten to fifteen seconds.

GLOSSARY OF SANSKRIT TERMS

abhyanga: body massage

abhyantara: internal

agni: fire; digestion; transformation of food into energy

ahara: food

ahimsa: nonviolence

ama: undigested food; undigested nutrients; unmetabolized waste

amla: sour

apana: the most active of the five vata subdivisions; governs elimination functions

apathya: unhealthy or unwholesome diet

arogya: health

arsa: blood

asana: physical posture in hatha yoga practice

asti: bones

ati sthula: morbid obesity; hyper-obese

aushadha: medicines, treatments

ayurveda: *ayur*, meaning "life," and *veda*, meaning "knowledge" or "science"

bahya: external

basti: enema

bhrajaka: skin

bodhaka: tongue/mouth

brumana: restorative; repletion

bhutagni: agni from five elements

buddhi: intellect

chakra: "wheel" or "disk"; seven chakras considered to be conductors of bodily energy

deha: body

dhatus: the seven basic types of bodily tissues

dhatwagni: agni from the seven organ systems

dinacharya: daily duties

dosha: psychophysiological functional principle of the body

drava: liquid

dravyaguna: pharmacology

dushya: disturbance; that which is vitiated

garshana: dry massage technique that stimulates skin and lymphatic system, improving circulation

guna: attribute or quality

guru: heavy

hetu: disease causative factors

indriya: sense organs

jataragni: agni manifesting in the stomach and duodenum; the agni "chief"

kala: time; natural rhythms

kapha: one of the three doshas

kasaya: astringent

katu: sharp; pungent

kaya: physiology; metabolism

karshana: depletion

khavaigunya: defective tissular or organ spaces

kleda: liquefaction; excess body fluids; associated with kapha dosha waste products

kledaka: moistens food in the stomach

koshas: five body sheets

koshta: alimentary canal

krimi: all microorganisms

krimirogas: diseases caused by pathogenic microorganisms

laghu: light

lakshana: symptoms

lavana: salty

loka: universe

madhura: sweet

majja: bone marrow

mala: impurity; waste product

manas: mind; can be individual or universal

medas: adipose tissue; fat

medoroga: obesity

mutra: urine

nasya: medication taken through the nose

nidana: pathology; causative factors

ojas: a vital, subtle essence that promotes and sustains physical vitality, mental clarity, and overall health; subtle immunity

pachaka: stomach/small bowel

paka: stage of digestion

pakwashaya: gut

panchakarma: the five methods of eliminating excess doshas or ama

panchamahabhutas: the five basic elements

pathya: nourishing food intake

pitta: one of the three doshas

prabhava: exceptional dynamic efficacy or property of a substance

prakruti: biological constitution of an individual

prameha: diabetes

prana: vital force for life existence; primarily taken in through the breath

pranayama: Indian breathing techniques to get control of the life energy/force

purisha: feces

purusha: consciousness

purvarupa: prodromes

rajas: one of the three qualities of consciousness; principle of kinetic energy

rakta: blood

rasa: nutrient fluid; plasma

rasayana: rejuvenation therapy; science of longevity

ritucharya: seasonal duties

roga: disease

rupa: symptoms

sahaja: congenital microbiome

samana: separates nutrients and waste; removes waste

Samhita: classic ayurvedic text

sarira: body; anatomy

sattva: one of the three qualities of consciousness; principle of equilibrium; essence

shukra: reproductive tissue

sloka: poetic form used in Sanskrit (verses)

snehana: oleation therapy

snigdha: unctuous

srotas: channel

sthana: position; rank; place; sections

sthoulya: obesity; thick; solid; strong; big; bulky

sthula: gross

sutra: rule or aphorism in Sanskrit literature

surya namaskar: sun salutation series of body postures

sveda: sweat

svedana: sudation therapy

swasa: asthma

tamas: one of the three qualities of consciousness; principle of inertia

tejas: essence of fire (agni) and pitta dosha leading all body fires; subtle vitality

thailam: oil

tikta: bitter

triguna: universal qualities that pervade everything

trividha pariksha: one short modality of ayurvedic diagnosis

udana: carries the air out; induces speech; effort

udvartana: ayurvedic deep tissue massage treatment for weight reduction

ushna: hot

vasa: fat present in muscles

vata: one of the three doshas

vayu: air

veda: knowledge; science; when capitalized, refers to the Vedas, ancient scriptures in India

vikruti: state of disturbed and distressed physiology of the physical body and mind

vipaka: final post-digestive effect of food

virya: energy; power or potency of a substance, such as a food or medicinal herb

vrddhi: aggravation

RESOURCES

CLASSICAL AYURVEDIC
MEDICAL TEXTBOOKS TO READ

If you are interested in studying in more detail the panoply of ayurveda and ayurvedic medicine, the following is a reference to classical textbooks of ayurveda that contain important expositions of ill health and disease. Here are some from the Samhitas:

- ▼ Body tissues increasing factors (Ca. Su. 23/3–6)
- ▼ Origins of the lipid tissue imbalance (medo roga) (Ma. Ni. 31/1–2)
- ▼ Origins of obesity (sthoulya) (Su. Sū. 15/32)
- ▼ Factor vitiating adipose and muscular tissue (medo/*mamsavaha srotas*) (Ca. Vi. 5/15–16)
- ▼ Origins of diabetes (prameha) (Ca. Ni. 4/5)
- ▼ Kapha's increasing factors (Ca. Chi. 6/4)

MODERN AYURVEDIC BOOKS

If you are a reader interested in exploring even deeper the causes of these imbalances, this list represents relevant books written by modern ayurvedic doctors, available in the English language:

Ambikadatta Shastri. *Rasa Ratna Samucchaya.* Varanasi: Chowkhamba Samskrit Series, 1978. Explains obesity in 18th chapter.

Babu, Madham Shetty Suresh. *Yoga Ratnakara*. 6th ed. Varanasi: Chowkhamba Sanskrit Series, 2005. Obesity is explained in a dedicated chapter, as well as formulations to treat sthoulya.

Chakrapanidatta, Acharya. *Chakradatta (Chikitsa Sara Sangraha)*. Varanasi: Choukhambha Orientalia, 1995. Explains treatment of obesity in 36th chapter.

Desai, Ranjit Roy. *Nidana Chikitsa Hastamalaka*. Nagapur: Baidyanath Ayurveda Bhavan, 1995. Written in more current times, the 2nd volume addresses obesity.

Kaviraj, A., and D. Shastri. *Bhaishajya Ratnavali*. Varanasi: Chowkhamba Sanskrit Series, 1991. The 39th chapter explains diverse treatments and medicinal preparations for obesity.

Krishnamurthy, K. H. *Bhela Samhita*. Varanasi: Chaukhambha Visvabharati, 2000. 11th chapter of Sutrasthana explains various aspects of obesity.

Mishra, Bhav S. *Bhavaprakasha Nighantu*. Varanasi: Chaukhambha Samskrita Samsthana, 1998. Explains the process of popular fumigation (*dhupa*) in 39th chapter of the treatment section, diverse kinds of external pastes (*lepas*), and the massage protocol with dry powders applied in the opposite direction of hair roots (*udvarthana*) as treatment to lose fat tissue.

Saxena, N. *Vangasena Samhita or Cikitsasara Samgraha of Vangasena*. 1st ed. Varanasi: Chowkhamba Sanskrit Series Office, 2004. In this classical textbook, the treatment for obesity is explained in the 16th chapter.

Sharangdhara Samhita. Early written ayurvedic text in the form of an herb manual describing diverse preparations and their action on various organs and diseases (see the Ayushveda website).

Shodhal, Vaidyavarya Shri. *Gadanigraha*. Varanasi: Chowkhamba Sanskrit Series, 1969. In 31st chapter, obesity and its treatments are described.

Srikantha Murthy, K. R. *Astanga Samgraha of Vagbhata*. Varanasi: Chaukhambha Orientalia, 2002. A scholarly text describing the different aspects of obesity including the explanation that the imbalance is caused by overnourishing, found in Sutrasthana chapter "Dwividhopakramaniya."

Srikantha Murthy, K. R. *Sarngadhara-Samhita: A Treatise on Ayurveda*. Varanasi: Choukhambha Orientalia, 2001.

Tewari, P. V. *Kasyapa Samhita or Vrddhajivakiya Tantra*. Varanasi: Chaukhambha Visvabharati, 2002. Describes the protocols and process of bloodletting (*rakta mokshana*) as a treatment for obesity.

NOTES

PREFACE

1. Cardona-Sanclemente, "Obesity: Imminent Danger and Massive Terror—A Role of Ayurveda."
2. Cardona-Sanclemente, "Effects of Diet on Lipid Profile and Protein Levels in Different Kinds of Long-Term Vegetarian Diets and a Control Group."

I. THE BASIC PRINCIPLES OF AYURVEDA

1. World Health Organization, *WHO Global Report on Traditional and Complementary Medicine 2019*.
2. Cardona-Sanclemente, *Ayurveda for Depression*.
3. Dinerstein, "The War Against Obesity."
4. Cardona-Sanclemente, "Fresh Perspectives on Obesity."'
5. Cardona-Sanclemente, "How Ayurveda Sees Obesity," 25–29.
6. Catalán et al. "Time to Consider the 'Exposome Hypothesis' in the Development of the Obesity Pandemic," 1597.

2. THE AYURVEDIC MEDICAL TREATISES OF THE *CHARAKA SAMHITA* AND *SUSHRUTA SAMHITA*

1. World Health Organization, *Benchmarks for Training in Ayurveda*.
2. Frawley and Rajaram, *Hidden Horizons*.
3. Avari, *India*.
4. Wiseman and Ellis, *Fundamentals of Chinese Medicine*.

5. Sharma and Dash, eds., *Charaka Samhita of Agnivesa*, 341–42.

6. Sharma and Dash, eds., *Charaka Samhita of Agnivesa*, 341–42.

7. Suśruta, *An English Translation of the Sushruta Samhita*.

8. Valiathan, *The Legacy of Sushruta*.

9. Murthy, *Madhava Nidanam (Roga Viniscaya of Madhavakara)*.

10. Patañjali, *The Yoga Sutras of Patanjali*.

3. THREE UNIVERSAL BODY ENERGIES

1. World Health Organization, *Constitution of the World Health Organization*.

2. World Health Organization, "Traditional, Complementary and Integrative Medicine."

3. Bich, Pradeu, and Moreau, "Understanding Multicellularity.'"

4. Cardona-Sanclemente and Born, "Effect of Inhibition of Nitric Oxide Synthesis on the Uptake of LDL and Fibrinogen by Arterial Walls and Other Organs of the Rat," 1490–94.

5. Burov, Kletskii, Kurbatov, Lisovin, and Fedik, "Mechanisms of Nitric Oxide Generation in Living Systems," 1–16.

6. Ferreira and Nutt, "Regulating the Oxides of Nitrogen," 1–7.

7. Chauhan, Mishra, and Choudhary, "Importance of Agni and Its Role in Chikitsa."

8. Gundersen and Shen, "Total Body Water in Obesity," 77–83.

9. Wallis, "Your Body Has a Clever Way to Detect How Much Water You Should Drink Every Day."

10. Turányi et al., "Association between Lunar Phase and Sleep Characteristics," 1411–16.

11. Della Monica, Atzori, and Dijk, "Effects of Lunar Phase on Sleep in Men and Women in Surrey," 687–94.

12. Walker et al., "Circadian Rhythm Disruption and Mental Health."

13. Larson, *Classical Sāṃkhya*.

14. Malinar, "Narrating Sāṃkhya Philosophy: Bhīṣma, Janaka and Pañcaśikha at Mahābhārata 12.211–12," 609–49.

15. Mishra, ed., *Scientific Basis for Ayurvedic Therapies*, "Obesity (Medoroga) in Ayurveda," Chapter 9, 149–66.

16 Agrawal, Yadav, and Meena, "Physiological Aspects of Agni," 395–98.

17. Cardona-Sanclemente, "Sustainability and Ayurveda," 25–32.

4. BEING OVERWEIGHT AS IT RELATES TO THE GUT

1. Bray and Bouchard, eds., *Handbook of Obesity—Volume 2: Clinical Applications.*
2. Cardona-Sanclemente, "Sustainability and Ayurveda," 25–32.
3. Callahan, Leonard, and Powell, *Nutrition: Science and Everyday Application.*
4. Sultan et al., "Lipoprotein Lipase and Hepatic Lipase Activities in a Hypercholesterolaemic (RICO) Strain of Rat. Effect of Dietary Cholesterol," 349–53.
5. Cardona-Sanclemente, Sultan, and Griglio, "Characterization and Quantification of Apolipoprotein E in the Genetically Hypercholesterolemic Rat (RICO)," 15–22.
6. Cardona-Sanclemente, Pastier, Ayrault-Jarrier, and Lutton, "Apolipoprotein E in the Genetically Hypercholesterolemic Rat (RICO)."
7. Cardona-Sanclemente, Feresou, and Lutton, "Cholesterol Metabolism in the Genetically Hypercholesterolemic (RICO) Rat. II," 382–89.
8. Cardona-Sanclemente et al., "Cholesterol Metabolism in the Genetically Hypercholesterolemic Rat (RICO).," 205–12.
9. Cardona-Sanclemente et al., "Apolipoprotein E," 1988.
10. Pool, *Fat: Fighting the Obesity Epidemic.*
11. Ye et al., "Fat Cell Size," 35–60.
12. MacLean et al., "The Role for Adipose Tissue in Weight Regain after Weight Loss," 45–54.
13. Arner and Rydén, "Human White Adipose Tissue: A Highly Dynamic Metabolic Organ," 611–21.
14. Muscogiuri et al., "Obesity."
15. Cardona-Sanclemente, Harbrecht, Medina, Farmer, and Born, "Effect of Hydrocortisone on the Accumulation of LDL and Fibrinogen by Arterial Wall and Other Tissues of the Rat," 114.
16. Cardona-Sanclemente and Born, "Increase by Adrenaline or Angiotensin II of the Accumulation of Low-Density Lipoprotein and Fibrinogen by Aortic Walls in Unrestrained Conscious Rats," 1089–94.
17. Cardona-Sanclemente and Born, "Effect of Inhibition," 1490–94.
18. Eduardo Cardona-Sanclemente, Medina, and Born, "Effect of Increasing Doses of Angiotensin II into Normal and Hypertensive Rats on Low Density Lipoprotein and Fibrinogen Uptake by Aortic Walls," 3285–88.
19. Swami et al., "Hangry in the Field."
20. Nielsen, Nielsen, and Holm, "The Impact of Familial Predisposition to

Obesity and Cardiovascular Disease on Childhood Obesity," 319–28.

21. Hinney, Körner, and Fischer-Posovszky, "The Promise of New Anti-obesity Therapies Arising from Knowledge of Genetic Obesity Traits," 623–37.

22. Bray, "Obesity."

23. Namjou et al., "Evaluation of the MC4R Gene across eMERGE Network Identifies Many Unreported Obesity-Associated Variants," 155–69.

24. Pigeyre et al., "Recent Progress in Genetics, Epigenetics and Metagenomics Unveils the Pathophysiology of Human Obesity," 943–986.

25. McLaren, "Socioeconomic Status and Obesity," 29–48.

26. Lee, Cardel, and Donahoo, "Social and Environmental Factors Influencing Obesity."

27. Macpherson-Sánchez, "Integrating Fundamental Concepts of Obesity and Eating Disorders: Implications for the Obesity Epidemic."

28. Savas et al., "Systematic Evaluation of Corticosteroid Use in Obese and Non-obese Individuals," 615–21.

29. Bradshaw and Mairs, "Obesity and Serious Mental Ill Health."

30. Medina, Cardona-Sanclemente, and Born, "Effect of Deoxycorticosterone Acetate on Blood Pressure in Relation to Accumulation of Low-Density Lipoprotein and Fibrinogen by Aorta and Other Tissues of Normotensive Wistar Rats," 531–36.

31. Liu et al., "Quotient of Waist Circumference and BMI: A Valuable Indicator for the High-Risk Phenotype of Obesity."

32. Elffers et al., "Body Fat Distribution, in Particular Visceral Fat, Is Associated with Cardiometabolic Risk Factors in Obese Women."

33. Kim et al., "Effects of Abdominal Visceral Fat Compared with Those of Subcutaneous Fat on the Association between PM10 and Hypertension in Korean Men."

34. Chait and den Hartigh, "Adipose Tissue Distribution, Inflammation and Its Metabolic Consequences, Including Diabetes and Cardiovascular Disease."

35. Lee and Gallagher, "Assessment Methods in Human Body Composition," 566–72.

36. Fryar, Carroll, Gu, Afful, Ogden, "Anthropometric Reference Data for Children and Adults," 1–44.

37. Fryar, "Anthropometric."

38. Chin, Kahathuduwa, and Binks, "Physical Activity and Obesity," 1226–44.

39. Kelley, Sbrocco, and Sbrocco, "Behavioral Modification for the Management of Obesity," 159–75.

40. Sombra and Anastasopoulou, "Pharmacologic Therapy for Obesity."

41. Wilding et al. "Once-Weekly Semaglutide in Adults with Overweight or Obesity," 989–1002.

42. Liu et al., "Lipase Inhibitors for Obesity."

43. Szmulewicz et al., "Mental Health Quality of Life after Bariatric Surgery: A Systematic Review and Meta-analysis of Randomized Clinical Trials."

44. Coulman et al., "Patient Experiences of Outcomes of Bariatric Surgery: A Systematic Review and Qualitative Synthesis," 547–59.

5. MEDA DHATU (OBESITY)

1. Valiathan, *Towards Ayurvedic Biology: A Decadal Vision Document*.

2. Ranade and Ranade, *Concept of Pathology in Ayurveda*.

3. Frawley, *Ayurveda and the Mind*.

4. Gupta, *Psychopathology in Indian Medicine*.

5. Pandya and Jani, "Achievements through Panchakarma in Clinical Management and Future Prospects" 62–65.

6. Thomas, "The Chemical Composition of Adipose Tissue of Man and Mice," 179–88.

7. Schuster, Fichtner, and Sasso, "Use of Fibonacci Numbers in Lipidomics–Enumerating Various Classes of Fatty Acids."

8. Pandey, *Obesity Therapy = Medoroga vijñanam*.

9. Rao, *Sareera Kriya Vignanam: Physiology in Ayurveda*.

10. Kotur and Kotur, *A Textbook of Ayurvedic Physiology*.

11. Saket and Kumar, "An Elixir Effect of Diet on *Sthoulya* (*Medoroga*) in Ayurveda," 2393–9591.

12. Mādhavakara, trans., *Madhava Nidana: Ayurvedic System of Pathology*.

13. Dwarakanath, *Concept of Agni in Ayurveda*.

14. Dash, *Concept of Agni in Ayurveda with Special Reference to Agnibala Pariksa*.

15. Itani, Keshwa, and Pathak, "Exploring the Impact of Ayurvedic Approaches on Obesity: A Scientific Research Perspective," 206–215.

16. Dwarakanath, *Digestion and Metabolism in Ayurveda*.

17. Singh, *The Holistic Principles of Ayurvedic Medicine*.

18. Dwivedi and Guru, *Introduction to Ayurveda*.

19. Singh, *Holistic Principles*.

20. Ninivaggi, *An Elementary Textbook of Ayurveda*.

21. Nityanand, Srivastava, and Asthana, "Clinical Trials with Gugulipid," 323–28.

22. Bhat and Rather, "Medicinal Benefits and Scientific Justification of Commiphora Mukul (Muqil)," 170–72.

23. Shikha Srivastava, *Current Traditional Medicine*, 75–83(9).

24. Vandana and Reddy, "Survey to Assess Quality of Life in Obesity in Relation to Ashtadoshas of Ati-Sthoulya and Prakriti," 3718–23.

6. PRAKRUTI

1. Sheldon, Stevens, and Tucker, *The Varieties of Human Physique.*

2. Gardner, *Multiple Intelligences: New Horizons.*

3. Liiv et al., "Anthropometry, Somatotypes, and Aerobic Power in Ballet, Contemporary Dance, and Dancesport," 207–11.

4. Sharma, "Ayurveda," 87–91.

5. Dash and Sharma, eds., *Charaka Samhita.*

6. Svoboda, *Prakrut.*

7. Kapadia and Dagar, "Understanding Self and Well-Being Based on Ayurveda," 157–97.

8. Travis and Wallace, "Dosha Brain-Types," 280–85.

9. Sharma et al., "Conceptual study of Vata Dosha w.s.r. to Nervous System," 134–40.

10. Mahalle et al., "Association of Constitutional Type," 150–57.

11. Sharma and Prajapati, "Predictive, Preventive and Personalized Medicine: Leads from Ayurvedic Concept of Prakriti (Human Constitution)," 441–50.

12. Sharma and Wallace, "Ayurveda and Epigenetics," 687.

13. Srivastava and Saxena, "Concepts of Prakriti (Human Constitution) and Its Association with Hematological Parameters, Body Mass Index (BMI), Blood Groups and Genotypes," 162–68.

14. Kang, Li, and Zhang, "Entropy-Based Model for Interpreting Life Systems in Traditional Chinese Medicine," 273–79.

15. Plunk and Richards, "Epigenetic Modifications Due to Environment, Ageing, Nutrition, and Endocrine Disrupting Chemicals and Their Effects on the Endocrine System."

16. Sonpipare and Pandey, "Deha-Prakruti and Its Importance in Daily Life," 293–301.

17. Krishnamurthy, trans., *Bhela Samhita, Sutrasthana.*

18. Palmer, Ferrige, and Moncada, "Nitric Oxide Release Accounts for the Biological Activity of Endothelium-Derived Relaxing Factor," 524–6.

19. Michel and Balligand, "Nitric Oxide Signalling in Cardiovascular Health and Disease," 292–316.
20. Slika and Patra, "Traditional Uses, Therapeutic Effects and Recent Advances of Curcumin," 1072–82.
21. McCraty, *Science of the Heart*.
22. Barrett et al., *Ganong's Review of Medical Physiology*.

7. VIKRUTI

1. Martone, "Early Life Experience."
2. Capparelli and Iannelli, "Role of Epigenetics in Type-2 Diabetes and Obesity," 977.
3. King and Skinner, "Epigenetic Transgenerational Inheritance of Obesity Susceptibility," 478–94.
4. McEwen, "Construction of a Review About Epigenetics for Biology Teachers and Other Non-experts," 997–1026.
5. Gupta et al., "Organs-on-a-Chip in Precision Medicine," 233–49.
6. Cardona-Sanclemente, "How Ayurveda Sees Rheumatoid Arthritis," 24–28.
7. Cardona-Sanclemente, "Ayurveda and the Treatment of Asthma."
8. Murthy, *Ashtanga Hridayam*, 1:156.
9. Aggarwal, "An Overview of Ayurvedic Management of Sthaulya W. S. R., Obesity."
10. Nagaraj, Yashesh, and Sarika, "Critical Review on the Concept of Prakruthi," 17–20.

8. MANAS PRAKRUTI

1. Cardona-Sanclemente, *Ayurveda for Depression*.
2. Lad, *Ayurveda*.
3. Frawley, *Ayurveda and the Mind*.
4. Silvertooth, "Special Relativity," 590.
5. Albrecht et al., "The Muon Puzzle in Cosmic-Ray Induced Air Showers and Its Connection to the Large Hadron Collider."
6. Aftab, Joshi, and Gehlot, "Manas Prakriti," 31–37.

9. YOUR GUT AND BODY REGULATIONS

1. Trappe, "Frank and Mycorrhizae," 277–81.
2. Simard et al., "Net Transfer of Carbon between Ectomycorrhizal Tree Species in the Field," 579–582.

3. Grant, "Do Trees Talk to Each Other?"

4. Gest, "The Discovery of Microorganisms by Robert Hooke and Antoni van Leeuwenhoek, Fellows of The Royal Society," 58187–201

5. Lecoq, "Découverte du premier virus, le virus de la mosaïque du tabac: 1892 ou 1898?" 929–33.

6. Turnbaugh et al., "The Human Microbiome Project," 804–10.

7. Hassani, Durán, and Hacquard, "Microbial Interactions within the Plant Holobiont," *Microbiome* 6 (2018): Article 58.

8. Carpenter, "That Gut Feeling," 50.

9. Sarkar et al., "Psychobiotics and the Manipulation of Bacteria-Gut-Brain Signals," 763–781.

10. Kwon et al., "Rhizolutin, a Novel 7/10/6-Tricyclic Dilactone, Dissociates Misfolded Protein Aggregates and Reduces Apoptosis/Inflammation Associated with Alzheimer's Disease," 22994–98.

11. Jain, *Acharya Umasvami's Tattvarthsutra*.

12. Sharma, trans., "Vimanasthanum, Chapter 3," *Charaka Samhita*.

13. Tengse et al., "A Survey on Etiopathological Correlation of Krimi (Intestinal Helminths) and Pandu (Anemia)," 165–170.

14. Bhanumathy et al., "Breaking Barriers."

15. Siddiqui and Patni, "A Review on Ayurvedic Concept of Krimi & Its Management," 19–23.

16. Shastri, ed., *Sushruta Samhita Uttaratantra; Krimirogapratishedha Adhyaya*.

17. Shastri, *Sushruta Samhita*.

18. Kar, *Parasitology in Ayurveda*.

19. Hu, Yu, He et al., "Integrative Metagenomic Analysis Reveals Distinct Gut Microbial Signatures Related to Obesity."

20. Barrow, Bell, and Bell, "Transforming Personalized Nutrition Practice," 1046–51.

21. Barrea et al., "Nutrigenetics," 1–13.

22. Gupta, Osadchiy, and Mayer, "Brain–Gut–Microbiome Interactions in Obesity and Food Addiction," 655–72.

23. Pulipati et al., "The Indian Gut Microbiota," 133–40.

24. Woldemariam et al., "Celiac Disease and Immunogenic Wheat Gluten Peptides and the Association of Gliadin Peptides with HLA DQ2 and HLA DQ8," 1553–76.

25. Oliveira et al., "A Perspective Review on Diet Quality, Excess Adiposity, and Chronic Psychosocial Stress and Implications for Early-Onset Colorectal Cancer," 1069–1079.

26. Matute and Iyavoo, "Exploring the Gut Microbiota."

10. THE MICROBIOME

1. Stinson, Boyce, Payne, Keelan, "The Not-so-Sterile Womb," 1124.
2. Bhanumathy et al., "Breaking Barriers."
3. Wilson et al., "Diet and the Human Gut Microbiome: An International Review," 723–40.
4. Qin et al., "A Human Gut Microbial Gene Catalogue Established by Metagenomic Sequencing," 59–65.
5. Hehemann et al., "Transfer of Carbohydrate-Active Enzymes from Marine Bacteria to Japanese Gut Microbiota," 908–12.
6. Li et al., "Amadis."
7. Diwan and Harke, "Bank on Microbiome to Keep the Body Healthy," 791.
8. Costea et al., "Enterotypes in the Landscape of Gut Microbial Community Composition," 8–16.
9. Gomaa, "Human Gut Microbiota/Microbiome in Health and Diseases," 2019–40.
10. Henning et al., Health Benefit of Vegetable/Fruit Juice-Based Diet."
11. Mirzaei et al., "Dual Role of Microbiota-Derived Short-Chain Fatty Acids on Host and Pathogen."
12. Blaser, "Gut Check."
13. Mohajeri et al., "The Role of the Microbiome for Human Health: From Basic Science to Clinical Applications," 1–14.
14. Fan and Pedersen, "Gut Microbiota in Human Metabolic Health and Disease," 55–71.
15. Barber et al., "Dietary Influences on the Microbiota–Gut–Brain Axis."
16. Walter, Martínez, and Rose, "Holobiont Nutrition," 340–46.
17. Martínez et al., "Gut Microbiome Composition Is Linked to Whole Grain-Induced Immunological Improvements," 269–80.
18. van den Munckhof et al., "Role of Gut Microbiota in Chronic Low-Grade Inflammation as Potential Driver for Atherosclerotic Cardiovascular Disease," 1719–34.
19. Jackson and Theiss, "Gut Bacteria Signaling to Mitochondria in Intestinal Inflammation and Cancer," 285–304.
20. Daniel et al., "Dietary Fat and Low Fiber in Purified Diets Differently Impact the Gut-Liver Axis to Promote Obesity-Linked Metabolic Impairments," G1014–33.
21. Hijová, "Synbiotic Supplements in the Prevention of Obesity and Obesity-Related Diseases," 313.

22. da Silva et al., "The Impact of Probiotics, Prebiotics, and Synbiotics on the Biochemical, Clinical, and Immunological Markers, as Well as on the Gut Microbiota of Obese Hosts," 337–55.

23. Illiano, Brambilla, and Parolini, "The Mutual Interplay of Gut Microbiota, Diet and Human Disease," 833–55.

24. Moles and Otaegui, "The Impact of Diet on Microbiota Evolution and Human Health: Is Diet an Adequate Tool for Microbiota Modulation?"

25. Abernathy-Close et al., "Intestinal Inflammation and Altered Gut Microbiota Associated with Inflammatory Bowel Disease Render Mice Susceptible to Clostridioides Difficile Colonization and Infection."

26. Cheng and Ning, "Stereotypes about Enterotype," 4–12.

27. Luo et al., "Influences of Food Contaminants and Additives on Gut Microbiota as Well as Protective Effects of Dietary Bioactive Compounds," 180–92.

28. Partridge et al., "Food Additives," 329–49.

29. Breton et al., "Dietary Inflammatory Potential and Food Patterns in Relation to Gut Microbiome among Children with Crohn's Disease," S39–40.

30. Cao et al., "Impact of Food Additives on the Composition and Function of Gut Microbiota: A Review," 295–310.

31. Zinöcker and Lindseth, "The Western Diet-Microbiome-Host Interaction and Its Role in Metabolic Disease," 365.

32. Senghor et al., "Gut Microbiota Diversity According to Dietary Habits and Geographical Provenance," 1–9.

33. Souza, Rocha, and Cotrim, "Diet and Intestinal Bacterial Overgrowth: Is There Evidence?" 4713–16.

34. Sani et al., "The Role of Gut Microbiota in the High-Risk Construct of Severe Mental Disorders."

35. Stinson, "The Not-so-Sterile Womb," 1124.

36. Dinan and Cryan, "Gut Microbiota: A Missing Link in Psychiatry," 111–12.

37. Born et al., "Factors Influencing the Transendothelial Accumulation of Atherogenic Plasma Proteins in Artery Walls," 9–18.

38. Młynarska et al., "The Role of the Microbiome-Brain-Gut Axis in the Pathogenesis of Depressive Disorder."

39. Frankiensztajn, Elliott, and Koren, "The Microbiota and the Hypothalamus-Pituitary-Adrenocortical (HPA) Axis, Implications for Anxiety and Stress Disorders," 76–82. Studies show that taking the time to meditate and relax can help ease symptoms of gut disorders.

40. Smith and Wissel, "Microbes and the Mind," 397–418.

41. Kuo et al., "Genomic and Clinical Effects Associated with a Relaxation Response Mind-Body Intervention in Patients with Irritable Bowel Syndrome and Inflammatory Bowel Disease."

42. Liu, "The Microbiome as a Novel Paradigm in Studying Stress and Mental Health," 655–67.

43. Welch, *Balance Your Hormones, Balance Your Life.*

44. Jirtle and Tyson, eds., *Environmental Epigenomics in Health and Disease: Epigenetics and Disease Origins.*

45. Lazar et al., "Aspects of Gut Microbiota and Immune System Interactions in Infectious Diseases, Immunopathology, and Cancer," 1830.

46. Wekerle, "The Gut-Brain Connection," ii68–75.

47. Obrenovich, "Leaky Gut, Leaky Brain?" 107.

48. Bostick, Schonhoff, and Mazmanian, "Gut Microbiome-Mediated Regulation of Neuroinflammation."

49. *Environmental Chemicals, the Human Microbiome, and Health Risk: A Research Strategy.*

50. Liu et al., "Machine Learning-Based Investigation of the Relationship between Gut Microbiome and Obesity Status."

51. Kardan et al., "Novel Therapeutic Strategy for Obesity through the Gut Microbiota-Brain Axis: A Review Article," 215–227.

52. Benakis et al., "The Microbiome-Gut-Brain Axis in Acute and Chronic Brain Diseases," 1–9.

53. Zhang et al., "Dietary Fiber-Derived Short-Chain Fatty Acids."

54. Liu et al., "High-Fiber Diet Mitigates Maternal Obesity-Induced Cognitive and Social Dysfunction in the Offspring via Gut-Brain Axis," 923–38.e6.

55. Hong et al., "Dietary Strategies May Influence Human Nerves and Emotions by Regulating Intestinal Microbiota," 3311–21.

56. Lee et al., "Emotional Well-Being and Gut Microbiome Profiles by Enterotype."

57. Aatsinki et al., "Infant Fecal Microbiota Composition and Attention to Emotional Faces."

II. THE ADIPOSE TISSUE

1. Wozniak et al., "Adipose Tissue: The New Endocrine Organ? A Review Article," 1847–56.

2. Khedikar et al., "Correlative Study of Visceral Fats with Medodhara Kala (Membrane)," 435–42.

3. Camastra and Ferrannini, "Role of Anatomical Location, Cellular Phenotype and Perfusion of Adipose Tissue in Intermediary Metabolism," 43–50.

4. Yang and Stanford, "Batokines," 1–9.

5. Dragoo et al., "The Essential Roles of Human Adipose Tissue."

6. Rosenbaum and Leibel, "20 Years of Leptin: Role of Leptin in Energy Homeostasis in Humans," T83–96.

7. Kawai, Autieri, and Scalia, "Adipose Tissue Inflammation and Metabolic Dysfunction in Obesity," C375–91.

8. Hagberg and Spalding, "White Adipocyte Dysfunction and Obesity-Associated Pathologies in Humans," 270–289.

12. THE FASCIA

1. Bordoni et al., "Fascial Nomenclature."

2. Bordoni, Lintonbon, and Morabito, "Meaning of the Solid and Liquid Fascia to Reconsider the Model of Biotensegrity."

3. Tozzi, "Does Fascia Hold Memories?" 259–65.

4. Warraich, "It's Time to Rethink the Origins of Pain."

5. Batvada and Sharma, "Elaborative Study of Pittadhara Kala," 452–56.

6. Carobbio et al., "Unraveling the Developmental Roadmap toward Human Brown Adipose Tissue," 641–55.

7. Carobbio, Pellegrinelli, and Vidal-Puig, "Adipose Tissue Function and Expandability as Determinants of Lipotoxicity and the Metabolic Syndrome," 161–96.

8. Zhang et al., "Cytological and Functional Characteristics of Fascia Adipocytes in Rats: A Unique Population of Adipocytes."

9. Su et al., "Fascia Origin of Adipose Cells," 1407–19.

10. Virtue and Vidal-Puig, "Adipose Tissue Expandability, Lipotoxicity and the Metabolic Syndrome—An Allostatic Perspective," 338–49.

13. THE LYMPHATICS

1. Moore and Bertram, "Lymphatic System Flows," 459–82.

2. J. Dixon, "Lymphatic Lipid Transport: Sewer or Subway?" 480–87.

3. Benros et al., "Autoimmune Diseases and Severe Infections as Risk Factors for Mood Disorders: A Nationwide Study," 812–20.

4. Liu, Ho, and Mak, "Interleukin (IL)-6, Tumour Necrosis Factor Alpha (TNF-α) and Soluble Interleukin-2 Receptors (sIL-2R) Are Elevated in Patients with Major Depressive Disorder," 230–39.

5. Bali, Dahiya, and Bali, "Delivery of Phytoconstituents via Brain Lymphatics," 16683–87.

6. Nores et al., "Obesity but Not High-Fat Diet Impairs Lymphatic Function."

7. Jiang et al., "The Lymphatic System in Obesity, Insulin Resistance, and Cardiovascular Diseases," 1402.

8. Vidal-Puig, "Adipose Tissue Expandability, Lipotoxicity and the Metabolic Syndrome," PL9.

9. Goossens, "The Metabolic Phenotype in Obesity," 207–15.

10. Babu and Sivaram, "Understanding Vyana Vayu," 122–26.

14. THE VAGUS NERVE

1. Darwin, *The Expressions of Emotions in Man and Animals.*

2. Johnson and Wilson, "A Review of Vagus Nerve Stimulation as a Therapeutic Intervention," 203–13.

3. Sigrid, et al., "Vagus Nerve as Modulator of the Brain–Gut Axis in Psychiatric and Inflammatory Disorders," 44.

4. Bonaz, Sinniger, and Pellissier, "The Vagus Nerve in the Neuro-Immune Axis: Implications in the Pathology of the Gastrointestinal Tract," 1452.

5. McCraty, *Science of the Heart.*

6. Mörkl et al., "Cardiac Vagal Activity Is Associated with Gut Microbiome Patterns in Women—An Exploratory Pilot Study," 1–9.

7. Young et al., "Vagus Nerve Stimulation as Adjunctive Therapy in Patients with Difficult-to-Treat Depression (RESTORE-LIFE)."

8. Pal and Nanda, "Vagus Nerve," 1–2.

9. Mondal, "Proposed Physiological Mechanisms of Pranayama," 100877.

10. Varambally and Gangadhar, "Yoga and Traditional Healing Methods in Mental Health."

11. Badran and Austelle, "The Future Is Noninvasive: A Brief Review of the Evolution and Clinical Utility of Vagus Nerve Stimulation," 3–7.

12. Srihagulang et al., "Potential Roles of Vagus Nerve Stimulation on Traumatic Brain Injury."

13. Masi, Valdés-Ferrer, and Steinberg, "The Vagus Neurometabolic Interface and Clinical Disease," 1101–11.

14. Gouveia et al., "A Systematic Review on Neuromodulation Therapies for Reducing Body Weight in Patients with Obesity."

15. BEYOND SIMPLY EATING LESS

1. Sharma and Dash, trans., *Charaka Samhita*.

2. Spence, "The Tongue Map and the Spatial Modulation of Taste Perception," 598–610.

3. Chaudhari and Roper, "The Cell Biology of Taste," 285–96.

4. Fischer, Ciotu, and Szallasi, "The Mysteries of Capsaicin-Sensitive Afferents."

5. Reed et al., "NIH Workshop Report: Sensory Nutrition and Disease," 232–45.

6. Törnwall et al., "Why Do Some Like It Hot? Genetic and Environmental Contributions to the Pleasantness of Oral Pungency," 381–89.

7. Boesveldt and de Graaf, "The Differential Role of Smell and Taste for Eating Behavior," 307–19.

8. Ustun et al., "Flavor Sensing in Utero and Emerging Discriminative Behaviors in the Human Fetus," 1651–63.

9. Berthoud, "Metabolic and Hedonic Drives in the Neural Control of Appetite," 888–96.

10. Spence et al., "Eating with Our Eyes: From Visual Hunger to Digital Satiation," 53–63.

11. Hegde et al., "Traditional Indian Way of Eating," 20–23.

12. Mayeli et al., "Neural Indicators of Human Gut Feelings."

13. Pereira and van der Bilt, "The Influence of Oral Processing, Food Perception and Social Aspects on Food Consumption," 630–48.

14. Bastiaanssen et al., "Making Sense of . . . the Microbiome in Psychiatry," 37–52.

15. Ochoa-Reparaz, Ramelow, and Kasper, "A Gut Feeling."

16. Holzer, "Gut Signals and Gut Feelings: Science at the Interface of Data and Beliefs."

17. World Health Organization, "Healthy Diet."

18. Ludwig et al., "Dietary Fiber, Weight Gain, and Cardiovascular Disease Risk Factors in Young Adults," 1539–46.

19. He et al., "Effects of Dietary Fiber on Human Health," 1–10.

20. da Poian and Castanho, *Integrative Human Biochemistry*.

21. Lad, *Textbook of Ayurveda*, 245–50.

22. Cardona-Sanclemente and Born, "Adrenaline Increases the Uptake of Low-Density Ipoprotein in Carotid Arteries," 215–18.

23. Agrawal, Yadav, and Meena, "Physiological Aspects of Agni," 395–98.

24. Shastri and Chaturvedi, eds., *Charaka Samhita,* 461.

25. Cardona-Sanclemente, "Effects of Diet."

26. Cardona-Sanclemente, "Decrease of Plasma Cholesterol Levels Induced by Vegetarian Diets in a Normal Adult Population."

27. Gugusheff , Ong, and Muhlhausler, "A Maternal 'Junk-Food' Diet Reduces Sensitivity to the Opioid Antagonist Naloxone in Offspring Postweaning," 1275–84.

28. Offer et al., "The Association Between Childhood Trauma and Overweight and Obesity in Young Adults," 3257–66.

16. AYURVEDA AND DIET

1. Harland, Buttriss, and Gibson, "Achieving Eatwell Plate Recommendations," 324–43.

2. de Ridder et al., "Healthy Diet," 907–41.

3. Wansink and Adrey Wansink, "MyPlate, Half-Plate, and No Plate: How Visual Plate-Related Dietary Benchmarks Influence What Food People Serve."

4. Davis et al., "Definition of the Mediterranean Diet: A Literature Review," 9139–53.

5. Medina et al., "Obesity, Mediterranean Diet, and Public Health," 3715.

6. Estruch and Ros, "The Role of the Mediterranean Diet on Weight Loss and Obesity-Related Diseases," 315–27.

7. Lassale et al., "Correction: Healthy Dietary Indices and Risk of Depressive Outcomes," 3657.

8. Xia et al., "Dietary Intakes of Eggs and Cholesterol in Relation to All-Cause and Heart Disease Mortality."

9. Pett et al., "Ancel Keys and the Seven Countries Study," 603–12.

11. Gibney, "Dietary Guidelines," 245–54.

12. Valk, Hammill, and Grip, "Saturated Fat," 2312–21.

13. Waehler, "Fatty Acids."

14. Stamp, "Average Person Will Try 126 Fad Diets in Their Lifetime, Poll Claims."

15. Alcorta et al., "Foods for Plant-Based Diets: Challenges and Innovations," 293.

16. Baker, "Wellness Gurus, Internet Celebrities and Influencers," 75–113.

17. Cardona-Sanclemente and Born, "Increase by Adrenaline," 1089–94.

18. Moon et al., "Lead, Mercury, and Cadmium Exposures Are Associated with Obesity but Not With Diabetes Mellitus."

19. Crespo et al., "Television Watching, Energy Intake and Obesity in US Children," 360–65.

20. Kolovos et al., "Association of Sleep, Screen Time and Physical Activity with Overweight and Obesity in Mexico," 169–79.

21. Zhang et al., "Screen Time and Health Issues in Chinese School-Aged Children and Adolescents: A Systematic Review and Meta-Analysis."

22. Cardona-Sanclemente and Born, "Adrenaline Increases the Uptake," 215–18.

23. Asmita, "The Concept of Pradnyapradh with Respect to the Factors That Cause Life-Style Disorders."

24. Sastri, *Tridosha Theory*.

25. Wittmann et al., "Circadian Rhythms and Depression," 308–18.

26. Angerer et al., "Night Work and the Risk of Depression," 404–11.

27. Ma et al., "A Longitudinal Study of Sleep, Weight Status, and Weight-Related Behaviors: Childhood Obesity Study in China Mega-cities," 971–79.

28. de Wit, Ten Have, Cuijpers, Graaf. "Body Mass Index and Risk of Onset of Mood and Anxiety Disorders in the General Population."

29. Yeung and Tadi, *Physiology, Obesity Neurohormonal Appetite and Satiety Control*.

30. Peterson, Denniston, and Chopra, "Therapeutic Uses of Triphala in Ayurvedic Medicine," 607–14.

31. Baliga et al., "Scientific Validation of the Ethnomedicinal Properties of the Ayurvedic Drug Triphala: A Review," 946–54.

32. Prasad and Srivastava, "Oxidative Stress and Cancer," 72.

33. Li et al., "Association of Ultraprocessed Food Consumption with Risk of Dementia," e1056–66.

34. Nunes et al., "Neuropsychiatric Inventory in Community-Dwelling Older Adults with Mild Cognitive Impairment and Dementia," 669–78.

35. Piché, Tchernof, and Després, "Obesity Phenotypes, Diabetes, and Cardiovascular Diseases."

36. Poti, Braga, and Qin, "Ultra-Processed Food Intake and Obesity," 420–31.

37. Couzin-Frankel, "A Lighter Burden," 480–83.

38. Loos and Yeo, "The Genetics of Obesity: From Discovery to Biology."

39. de Souza Pinhel et al., "The Truth About the Influence of Endocrine Disruptors on Obesity," 217–29.

17. THE FUTURE OF AYURVEDIC MODALITIES IN THE AGE OF EPIDEMIC IMBALANCES

1. Boyce, Yao, Xing, "Osteoclasts Have Multiple Roles in Bone in Addition to Bone Resorption," 171–80.

2. Dos Santos et al., "Gut-Microbiome-Brain Axis: The Crosstalk between the Vagus Nerve, Alpha-Synuclein and the Brain in Parkinson's Disease," 2611–14.

3. Anheyer et al., "Yoga in Women with Abdominal Obesity."

4. Hainsworth et al., "A Pilot Study of Iyengar Yoga for Pediatric Obesity," 92.

5. Hainsworth et al., "Pilot Study," 92.

6. Sengupta, "Health Impacts of Yoga and Pranayama: A State-of-the-Art Review," 444–58.

7. Smita et al., "Effect of Pranayama on Body Mass Index in Young Medical Students," 24–27.

8. Sawarkar and Patange, "Role of Yoga for the Prevention & Management of COVID-19," 1720–24.

9. Cardona-Sanclemente, "Coronavirus–An Unwelcome New Visitor or an Old Foe?"

10. Conklin et al., "Insight Meditation and Telomere Biology," 233–45.

11. Merrow, Spoelstra, and Roenneberg, "The Circadian Cycle," 930–35.

12. Sun et al., "Alteration of Faecal Microbiota Balance Related to Long-Term Deep Meditation."

13. Bhishagratna, "The Medicinal Use of Sneha (Oleaginous Substances)."

14. Lohith, *A Text Book of Panchakarma*.

15. Sharma and Sharma, "A Clinical Study to Assess the Impact of Lekhan Basti, Udvarthana, and Navak Guggulu in the Management of Obesity vis-à-vis Sthaulya."

16. Vinayaka and Suchitra, "Effect of Udvarthana on Obesity," A148.

17. Vasudeva, Yadav, and Sharma, "Natural Products," 473–80.

18. Shukla et al., "Phytochemistry and Pharmacological Studies of *Plumbago Zeylanica* L.: A Medicinal Plant Review."

19. Khandekar et al., "Role of Katuka (Picrorhiza Kurroa Royle Ex Benth.) In Obesity W. S. R. to Ayurvedic and Modern Aspect," 31–35.

20. Yarmohammadi et al., "The Protective Effect of *Azadirachta Indica* (Neem) Against Metabolic Syndrome," 280–92.

21. Kundu et al., "A Review on Therapeutic Use of Vidanga (*Embelia Ribes*) for Pathological Consequences Associated with Obesity as per Ayurvedic Classics," 38–40.

22. Kaiser Permanente (website), accessed 2020.

23. Radheshyam et al., "A Review On: Herbal, Pharmacognostical and Pharmacological Studies on Guggulu," 139–44.

24. Kapoor et al., "Role of Natural Products in the Treatment of Obesity," 451–80.

25. Aabideen et al., "Anti-Obesity Attributes."

26. Choudhary, Bhattacharyya, and Joshi, "Body Weight Management in Adults under Chronic Stress through Treatment with Ashwagandha Root Extract," 96–106.

27. Zare et al., "Effect of Cumin Powder on Body Composition and Lipid Profile in Overweight and Obese Women," 297–30.

28. DerSarkissian, "Normal Blood Sugar Levels for Adults with Diabetes."

29. Slika and Patra, "Traditional Uses," 1072–82.

30. Akaberi, Sahebkar, and Emami, "Turmeric and Curcumin."

31. de Mello et al., "Mitochondrial Dysfunction in Obesity," 26–32.

32. Prasad and Aggarwal, "Turmeric, the Golden Spice."

33. Abedimanesh et al., "Saffron and Crocin Improved Appetite, Dietary Intakes and Body Composition in Patients with Coronary Artery Disease," 200–208.

34. Sahebkar et al., "Nigella Sativa (Black Seed) Effects on Plasma Lipid Concentrations in Humans," 37–50.

35. Ahmed and Wang, "Black Garlic and Its Bioactive Compounds on Human Health Diseases."

36. Phimarn, Sungthong, and Itabe, "Effects of Triphala on Lipid and Glucose Profiles and Anthropometric Parameters."

37. Phetkate et al., "Study of the Safety of Oral Triphala Aqueous Extract on Healthy Volunteers," 35–40.

38. Kaushik, Jain, and Khan, "Trikatu: Transforming Food into Medicines."

39. Bhatt and Khader, "Obesity."

40. Phimarn, Sungthong, and Itabe, "Effects of Triphala," 1–9.

41. Suba, "Reverse Pharmacology."

42. Mishra et al., "Shilajit (Mumie)," 104–20.

43. Korabu and Kulkarni, "A Review of Pre-clinical Studies on Obesity Markers Using Ayurvedic Medicinal Plants," 960–69.

44. Niemiro, Rewane, and Algotar, "Exercise and Fitness Effect on Obesity."

45. Carraça et al., "Effect of Exercise Training on Psychological Outcomes in Adults with Overweight or Obesity."

46. Müller et al., "Anti-obesity Drug Discovery," 201–23.

47. Lobstein and Brownell, "Endocrine-Disrupting Chemicals and Obesity Risk."

48. Yee et al., "Impact of Microplastic and Nanoplastics on Human Health," 496.

49. Yu et al., "Drinking Boiled Tap Water Reduces Human Intake of Nanoplastics and Microplastics," 273–279.

50. Pampel, Denney, and Krueger, "Obesity, SES, and Economic Development."

51. Ravishankar, "Is India Shouldering a Double Burden of Malnutrition?" 313–28.

52. Gómez et al., "Socioeconomic Status Impact on Diet Quality and Body Mass Index in Eight Latin American Countries."

53. Crosby et al., "Insulin/IGF-1 Drives PERIOD Synthesis to Entrain Circadian Rhythms with Feeding Time," 896–909.

54. R. Y. Huang et al., "Vegetarian Diets and Weight Reduction," 109–116.

55. The President and Fellows of Harvard College, "Are Weight-Loss Drugs Worth Trying?"

56. Xia et al., "Obesity Causes Mitochondrial Fragmentation and Dysfunction in White Adipocytes due to Rala Activation."

57. Wang et al., "Effects of Mitochondrial Dynamics in the Pathophysiology of Obesity," 107.

58. Food and Drug Administration, "GMO Crops, Animal Food, and Beyond."

59. Lerner, Benzvi, and Vojdani, "The Potential Harmful Effects of Genetically Engineered Microorganisms (GEMs) on the Intestinal Microbiome and Public Health," 238.

60. Ledford, "Why Are So Many Young People Getting Cancer?" 258–260.

61. Elnahas, Jackson, and Hong, "Management of Failed Laparoscopic Roux-en-Y Gastric Bypass," 36–40.

62. Paul, van der Heiden, and Hoek, "Cognitive Behavioral Therapy and Predictors of Weight Loss in Bariatric Surgery Patients," 474–79.

63. Juchacz et al., "The Effectiveness of Supportive Psychotherapy in Weight Loss in a Group of Young Overweight and Obese Women," 532.

BIBLIOGRAPHY

Aabideen, Zain, Muhammad Waseem Mumtaz, Muhammad Tayyab Akhtar, Hamid Mukhtar, Syed Ali Raza, Tooba Touqeer, and Nazamid Saari. "Anti-Obesity Attributes; UHPLC-QTOF-MS/MS-Based Metabolite Profiling and Molecular Docking Insights of Taraxacum Officinale." *Molecules* 25, no. 21 (2020): Article 4935.

Aatsinki, Anna-Katariina, Eeva-Leena Kataja, Eveliina Munukka, Leo Lahti, Anniina Keskitalo, Riikka Korja, Saara Nolvi, Tuomo Häikiö, Saija Tarro, Hasse Karlsson, and Linnea Karlsson. "Infant Fecal Microbiota Composition and Attention to Emotional Faces." *Emotion*, advance online publication.

Abedimanesh, Nasim, S. Zahra Bathaie, Saeed Abedimanesh, Behrooz Motlagh, Ahmad Separham, and Alireza Ostadrahimi. "Saffron and Crocin Improved Appetite, Dietary Intakes and Body Composition in Patients with Coronary Artery Disease." *Journal of Cardiovascular and Thoracic Research* 9, no. 4 (2017): 200–208.

Abernathy-Close, Lisa, Madeline R. Barron, James M. George, Michael G. Dieterle, Kimberly C. Vendrov, Ingrid L. Bergin, and Vincent B. Young. "Intestinal Inflammation and Altered Gut Microbiota Associated with Inflammatory Bowel Disease Render Mice Susceptible to Clostridioides Difficile Colonization and Infection." *mBio* 12, no. 3 (June 2021): e02733–20.

Aftab, Anam, Shobhna Joshi, and Sangeeta Gehlot. "Manas Prakriti: An Influential Aspect to Upsurge the Mental Health." *International Journal of Ayurveda & Medical Sciences* 3, no. 4 (June 2021): 31–37.

Aggarwal, Monica. "An Overview of Ayurvedic Management of Sthaulya W. S. R Obesity." *International Journal of Ayurveda and Pharma Research* 7, no. 2 (February 2019).

Agrawal, Akash Kumar, C. R. Yadav, and M. S. Meena. "Physiological Aspects of Agni." *Ayu* 31, no. 3 (July 2010): 395–98.

Ahmed, Tanvir, and Chin-Kun Wang. "Black Garlic and Its Bioactive Compounds on Human Health Diseases: A Review." *Molecules* 26, no. 16 (2021): Article 5028.

Akaberi, Maryam, Amirhossein Sahebkar, and Seyed Ahmad Emami. "Turmeric and Curcumin: From Traditional to Modern Medicine." In *Studies on Biomarkers and New Targets in Aging Research in Iran*, edited by Paul C. Guest. N.p.: Springer, 2021.

Albrecht, Johannes, Lorenzo Cazon, Hans Dembinski, Anatoli Fedynitch, Karl-Heinz Kampert, Tanguy Pierog, Wolfgang Rhode et al. "The Muon Puzzle in Cosmic-Ray Induced Air Showers and Its Connection to the Large Hadron Collider." *Astrophysics and Space Science* 367 (March 2022): Article 27.

Alcorta, Alexandra, Adrià Porta, Amparo Tárrega, María Dolores Alvarez, and M. Pilar Vaquero. "Foods for Plant-Based Diets: Challenges and Innovations." *Foods* 10, no. 2 (2021): 293.

Ambicadutt, Shastri. *Sushruta Samhita*. Varanasi, India: Chaukhamba Sanskrit Sansthan, 2005.

Angerer, Peter, Renate Schmook, Irina Elfantel, and Jian Li. "Night Work and the Risk of Depression." *Deutsches Ärzteblatt International* 114, no. 24 (July 2017): 404–11.

Anheyer, Dennis, Anna K. Koch, Meral S. Thoms, Gustav Dobos, and Holger Cramer. "Yoga in Women with Abdominal Obesity–Do Lifestyle Factors Mediate the Effect? Secondary Analysis of a RCT." *Complementary Therapies in Medicine* 60 (August 2021): Article 102741.

Arner, Peter, and Mikael Rydén. "Human White Adipose Tissue: A Highly Dynamic Metabolic Organ." *Journal of Internal Medicine* 291, no. 5 (May 2022): 611–21.

Avari, Burjor. *India: The Ancient Past*. London: Routledge, 2007.

Babu, Abhirami, and Anjali Sivaram. "Understanding Vyana Vayu: Bridging Ayurveda and Modern Physiology." *International Journal of Ayurveda and Pharma Research* 12, no. 2 (February 2024), 122–26.

Badran, Bashar W., and Christopher W. Austelle. "The Future Is Noninvasive: A Brief Review of the Evolution and Clinical Utility of Vagus Nerve Stimulation." *Focus* 20, no. 1 (Winter 2022): 3–7.

Baker, Stephanie Alice. "Wellness Gurus, Internet Celebrities and Influencers." In *Wellness Culture (Society Now)*, 75–113. Leeds, UK: Emerald Group, 2022.

Bali, Sharadendu, Randhir Dahiya, and Ranjana Bali. "Delivery of Phytoconstituents via Brain Lymphatics: An Unexplored Ocean of Opportunities in Treatment of Brain Disorders." *Turkish Journal of Physiotherapy and Rehabilitation* 32, no. 3 (September 2022): 16683–87.

Baliga, Manjeshwar Shrinath, Sharake Meera, Benson Mathai, Manoj Ponadka Rai, Vikas Pawar, and Princy Louis Palatty. "Scientific Validation of the Ethnomedicinal Properties of the Ayurvedic Drug Triphala: A Review." *Chinese Journal of Integrative Medicine* 18, no. 12 (December 2012): 946–54.

Barber, Thomas M., Georgios Valsamakis, George Mastorakos, Petra Hanson, Ioannis Kyrou, Harpal S. Randeva, and Martin O. Weickert. "Dietary Influences on the Microbiota–Gut–Brain Axis." *International Journal of Molecular Sciences* 22, no. 7 (2021): Article 3502.

Barrea, Luigi, Giuseppe Annunziata, Laura Bordoni, Giovanna Muscogiuri, Annamaria Colao, and Silvia Savastano. "Nutrigenetics—Personalized Nutrition in Obesity and Cardiovascular Diseases." *International Journal of Obesity Supplements* 10 (2020): 1–13.

Barrett, Kim, Susan Barman, Jason Yuan, and Heddwen Brooks. *Ganong's Review of Medical Physiology.* 26th ed. New York: McGraw-Hill Education, 2019.

Barrow, Michelle, Linda Bell, and Celia Bell. "Transforming Personalized Nutrition Practice." *Nutrition Reviews* 78, no. 12 (December 2020): 1046–51.

Bastiaanssen, Thomaz F. S., Caitlin S. M. Cowan, Marcus J. Claesson, Timothy G. Dinan, and John F. Cryan. "Making Sense of … the Microbiome in Psychiatry." *International Journal of Neuropsychopharmacology* 22, no. 1 (January 2019): 37–52.

Batvada, Ashwini J., and Gopal B. Sharma. "Elaborative Study of Pittadhara Kala." *World Journal of Pharmaceutical Research* 8, no. 4 (2019): 452–56.

Benakis, Corinne, Camille Martin-Gallausiaux, Jean-Pierre Trezzi, Philip Melton, Arthur Liesz, and Paul Wilmes. "The Microbiome-Gut-Brain Axis in Acute and Chronic Brain Diseases." *Current Opinion in Neurobiology* 61 (April 2020): 1–9.

Benros, Michael E., Berit L. Waltoft, Merete Nordentoft, Søren D. Ostergaard, William W. Eaton, Jesper Krogh, and Preben B. Mortensen. "Autoimmune Diseases and Severe Infections as Risk Factors for Mood Disorders: A Nationwide Study." *JAMA Psychiatry* 70, no. 8 (August 2013): 812–20.

Berthoud, Hans-Rudolf. "Metabolic and Hedonic Drives in the Neural Control of Appetite: Who Is the Boss?" *Current Opinion in Neurobiology* 21, no. 6 (December 2011): 888–96.

Bhanumathy, Parvathy, Hemavathi Shivapura Krishnarajabhatt, and Parvathy Unnikrishnan. "Breaking Barriers: Maternal Gut-Brain-Axis Modulation as a Catalyst for Fetal Gut Microbiome Reshaping: A Comprehensive Review." *AIP Conference Proceedings 3171*, no. 060003 (2024).

Bhat, Shabir Ahmad, and Shameem Ahmad Rather. "Medicinal Benefits and Scientific Justification of Commiphora Mukul (Muqil): A Review." *Journal of Drug Delivery & Therapeutics* 11, no. 1-S (January–February 2021): 170–72.

Bhatt, Kusum Lata, and Abdul Khader. "Obesity: An Ayurveda Prospective." *Journal of Ayurveda and Integrated Medical Sciences* 5, no. 4 (July–August 2020): 328–31.

Bhishagratna, Kaviraj Kunja Lal. "The Medicinal Use of Sneha (Oleaginous Substances)," in *Sushruta Samhita*, Volume 4: Cikitsasthana. [India?]: 1911.

Bich, Leonardo, Thomas Pradeu, and Jean-François Moreau. "Understanding Multicellularity: The Functional Organization of the Intercellular Space." *Frontiers in Physiology* 10 (September 2019): Article 1170.

Blaser, Martin. "Gut Check: Exploring Your Microbiome." Interview for Coursera / University of Colorado, Boulder.

Boesveldt, Sanne, and Kees de Graaf. "The Differential Role of Smell and Taste for Eating Behavior." *Perception* 46, no. 3–4 (2017): 307–19.

Bonaz, Bruno, Valérie Sinniger, and Sonia Pellissier. "The Vagus Nerve in the Neuro-Immune Axis: Implications in the Pathology of the Gastrointestinal Tract." *Frontiers in Immunology* 8 (2017): 1452.

Bordoni, Bruno, David Lintonbon, and Bruno Morabito. "Meaning of the Solid and Liquid Fascia to Reconsider the Model of Biotensegrity." *Cureus* 10, no. 7 (July 2018): Article e2922.

Bordoni, Bruno, Stevan Walkowski, Bruno Morabito, and Matthew A. Varacallo. "Fascial Nomenclature: An Update." *Cureus* 11, no. 9 (September 2019): Article e5718.

Born, G. V. R. et al. "Factors Influencing the Tranendothelial Accumulation of Atherogenic Plasma Proteins in Artery Walls." *Clinical Hemorheology and Microcirculation* 37, no. 1–2 (2007): 9–18.

Bostick, John W., Aubrey M. Schonhoff, and Sarkis K. Mazmanian. "Gut Microbiome-Mediated Regulation of Neuroinflammation." *Current Opinion in Immunology* 76 (June 2022): Article 102177.

Boyce, B. F., Z. Yao, and L. Xing. "Osteoclasts Have Multiple Roles in Bone in Addition to Bone Resorption." Critical Reviews in Eukaryotic Gene Expression, 19(3) (2009): 171–80.

Bradshaw, Tim, and Hilary Mairs. "Obesity and Serious Mental Ill Health: A Critical Review of the Literature." *Healthcare* 2, no. 2 (2014): 166–82.

Bray, George A. "Obesity: A 100 Year Perspective." *International Journal of Obesity* website, May 7, 2024.

Bray, George A., and Claude Bouchard, eds. *Handbook of Obesity—Clinical Applications*. 2nd ed. New York: Marcel Dekker, Inc., 2004.

———. *Handbook of Obesity—Volume 2: Clinical Applications*. 5th ed. Boca Raton, FL: CRC Press, 2024.

Breit, Sigrid, Aleksandra Kupferberg, Gerhard Rogler, and Gregor Hasler. "Vagus Nerve as Modulator of the Brain–Gut Axis in Psychiatric and Inflammatory Disorders." *Frontiers in Psychiatry* 9 (2018): 44.

Breton, Jessica, Vincent Tu, Ceylan Tanes, Ryan Quinn, Maire Conrad, Kelly Kachelries, Kyle Bittinger, Robert Baldassano, Charlene Compher, and Lindsey Albenberg. "Dietary Inflammatory Potential and Food Patterns in Relation to Gut Microbiome among Children with Crohn's Disease: A Comparative Study with Healthy Controls." *Inflammatory Bowel Diseases* 27, Issue Supplement_1 (January 2021): S39–40.

Burov, Oleg N., Mikhail E. Kletskii, Sergey V. Kurbatov, Anton V. Lisovin, and Nikita S. Fedik. "Mechanisms of Nitric Oxide Generation in Living Systems." *Nitric Oxide* 118 (January 2022): 1–16.

Callahan, Alice, Heather Leonard, and Tamberly Powell. *Nutrition: Science and Everyday Application*. Open Oregon Educational Resources, 2020.

Camastra, Stefania, and Ele Ferrannini. "Role of Anatomical Location, Cellular Phenotype and Perfusion of Adipose Tissue in Intermediary Metabolism: A Narrative Review." *Reviews in Endocrine and Metabolic Disorders* 23 (2022): 43–50.

Cao, Yu, Hongli Liu, Ningbo Qin, Xiaomeng Ren, Beiwei Zhu, and Xiaodong Xia. "Impact of Food Additives on the Composition and Function of Gut Microbiota: A Review." *Trends in Food Science & Technology* 99 (May 2020): 295–310.

Capparelli, Rosanna, and Domenico Iannelli. "Role of Epigenetics in Type-2 Diabetes and Obesity." *Biomedicines* 9, no. 8 (August 2021): 977.

Cardona-Sanclemente, L. Eduardo. "Ayurveda and the Treatment of Asthma." *Prana-Pukka Magazine*, Winter/Spring 2010.

———. *Ayurveda for Depression: An Integrative Approach to Restoring Balance and Reclaiming Your Health*. Berkeley, CA: North Atlantic Books, 2020.

———. "Coronavirus–An Unwelcome New Visitor or an Old Foe?" *North Atlantic Books* website, May 6, 2020.

———. "Decrease of Plasma Cholesterol Levels Induced by Vegetarian Diets in a Normal Adult Population." Presentation, Svastha International Ayurveda Conference, London, 2007.

———. "Effect of Hydrocortisone on the Accumulation of LDL and Fibrinogen by Arterial Wall and Other Tissues of the Rat." In *Proceedings of the Physiological Society* 100 (1998): 174.

———. "Effects of Diet on Lipid Profile and Protein Levels in Different Kinds of Long-Term Vegetarian Diets and a Control Group." Master's thesis, Valle University, Colombia, 1979.

———. "Fresh Perspectives on Obesity–A Correlation of Ayurvedic Science and Modern Medicine." Master's thesis, London: Middlesex University, 2009.

———. "How Ayurveda Sees Obesity." *Ayurveda Journal of Health* 9, no. 4 (Summer 2011): 25–29.

———. "How Ayurveda Sees Rheumatoid Arthritis." *Ayurveda Journal of Health* 10, no. 4 (Summer 2012): 24–28.

———. "Obesity: Imminent Danger and Massive Terror–A Role of Ayurveda." Lecture, NAMA Conference, San Mateo, CA, April 15–18, 2010.

———. "Sustainability and Ayurveda." *Ayurveda Journal of Health* 15, no. 1 (Winter 2017): 25–32.

Cardona-Sanclemente, L. Eduardo, D. Pastier, M. Ayrault-Jarrier, and C. Lutton. "Apolipoprotein E in the Genetically Hypercholesterolemic Rat (RICO)." *Bulletin de la societe de chimie biologique* 53, no. 27 (1988).

Cardona-Sanclemente, L. Eduardo, F. Sultan, and S. Griglio. "Characterization and Quantification of Apolipoprotein E in the Genetically Hypercholesterolemic Rat (RICO)." *Journal of Physiology and Biochemistry* 52, no. 1 (March 1996): 15–22.

Cardona-Sanclemente, L. Eduardo, C. Verneau, D. Mathe, and C. Lutton. "Cholesterol Metabolism in the Genetically Hypercholesterolemic Rat (RICO). I. Measurement of Turnover Processes." *Biochimica Biophysica Acta* 919, no. 3 (June 1987): 205–12.

Cardona-Sanclemente, L. Eduardo, and G. V. R. Born. "Adrenaline Increases the Uptake of Low-Density Lipoprotein in Carotid Arteries." *Atherosclerosis* 96 (1992): 215–18.

———. "Effect of Inhibition of Nitric Oxide Synthesis on the Uptake of LDL and Fibrinogen by Arterial Walls and Other Organs of the Rat." *British Journal of Pharmacology* 114, no. 7 (April 1995): 1490–94.

———. "Increase by Adrenaline or Angiotensin II of the Accumulation of Low-Density Lipoprotein and Fibrinogen by Aortic Walls in Unrestrained Conscious Rats." *British Journal of Pharmacology* 117, no. 6 (March 1996): 1089–94.

Cardona-Sanclemente, L. Eduardo, J. Feresou, and C. Lutton. "Cholesterol Metabolism in the Genetically Hypercholesterolemic (RICO) Rat. II. A Study of Plasma Lipoproteins and Effect of Dietary Cholesterol." *Biochimica et Biophysica Acta (BBA)* 960, no. 3 (June 1988): 382–89.

Cardona-Sanclemente, L. Eduardo, R. Medina, and G. V. R Born. "Effect of Increasing Doses of Angiotensin II into Normal and Hypertensive Rats on Low Density Lipoprotein and Fibrinogen Uptake by Aortic Walls." In *Proceedings of the National Academy of Sciences of the United States of America* 91 (1994): 3285–88.

Carobbio, Stefania, Anne-Claire Guenantin, Myriam Bahri, Sonia Rodriguez-Fdez, Floris Honig, Ioannis Kamzolas, Isabella Samuelson et al. "Unraveling the Developmental Roadmap toward Human Brown Adipose Tissue." *Stem Cell Reports* 16, no. 3 (March 2021): 641–55.

Carobbio, Stefania, Vanessa Pellegrinelli, and Antonio Vidal-Puig. "Adipose Tissue Function and Expandability as Determinants of Lipotoxicity and the Metabolic Syndrome." In *Obesity and Lipotoxicity*, edited by Engin A. and Engin A., 161–96. N.p.: Springer, 2017.

Carpenter, Siri. "That Gut Feeling." *Monitor on Psychology* 43, no. 8 (September 2012): 50.

Carraça, Eliana V., Jorge Encantado, Francesca Battista, Kristine Beaulieu, John E. Blundell, Luca Busetto, Marleen van Baak et al. "Effect of Exercise Training on Psychological Outcomes in Adults with Overweight or Obesity: A Systematic Review and Meta-Analysis." *Obesity Reviews* 22, no. S4 (July 2021): Article e13261.

Catalán, Victoria, Iciar Avilés-Olmos, Amaia Rodríguez, Sara Becerril, José Antonio Fernández-Formoso, Dimitrios Kiortsis, Piero Portincasa, Javier Gómez-Ambrosi, and Gema Frühbeck. "Time to Consider the 'Exposome Hypothesis' in the Development of the Obesity Pandemic." *Nutrients* 14, no. 8 (April 2022): 1597.

Chait, Alan, and Laura J. den Hartigh. "Adipose Tissue Distribution, Inflammation and Its Metabolic Consequences, Including Diabetes and Cardiovascular Disease." *Frontiers in Cardiovascular Medicine* 7, no. 22 (February 25, 2020).

Chaudhari, Nirupa, and Stephen D. Roper. "The Cell Biology of Taste." *The Journal of Cell Biology* 190, no. 3 (August 2010): 285–96.

Chauhan, Bindu, Anjana Mishra, and Vijay Choudhary. "Importance of Agni and Its Role in Chikitsa." *Journal of Ayurveda and Integrated Medical Sciences* 7, no. 3 (April 2022): 167–71.

Cheng, Mingyue, and Kang Ning. "Stereotypes about Enterotype: The Old and New Ideas." *Genomics, Proteomics & Bioinformatics* 17, no. 1 (February 2019): 4–12.

Chin, S. H., C. N. Kahathuduwa, and M. Binks. "Physical Activity and Obesity: What We Know and What We Need to Know." *Obesity Reviews* 17, no. 12 (December 2016): 1226–44.

Choudhary, Dnyanraj, Sauvik Bhattacharyya, and Kedar Joshi. "Body Weight Management in Adults under Chronic Stress through Treatment with Ashwagandha Root Extract." *Journal of Evidence-Based Complementary & Alternative Medicine* 22, no. 1 (2017): 96–106.

Claudino Dos Santos, J. C. et al. "Gut-Microbiome-Brain Axis: The Crosstalk between the Vagus Nerve, Alpha-Synuclein and the Brain in Parkinson's Disease." *Neural Regeneration Research*, 18(12) (December 2023): 2611–2614.

Conklin, Quinn A., Brandon G. King, Anthony P. Zanesco, Jue Lin, Anahita B. Hamidi, Jennifer J. Pokorny, María Jesús Álvarez-López, et al. "Insight Meditation and Telomere Biology: The Effects of Intensive Retreat and the Moderating Role of Personality." *Brain, Behavior, and Immunity* 70 (May 2018): 233–45.

Costea, Paul I., Falk Hildebrand, Manimozhiyan Arumugam, Fredrik Bäckhed, Martin J. Blaser, Frederic D. Bushman, Willem M. de Vos et al. "Enterotypes in the Landscape of Gut Microbial Community Composition." *Nature Microbiology* 3 (2018): 8–16.

Coulman, Karen D., Fiona MacKichan, Jane M. Blazeby, and Amanda Owen-Smith. "Patient Experiences of Outcomes of Bariatric Surgery: A Systematic Review and Qualitative Synthesis." *Obesity Reviews* 18, no. 5 (May 2017): 547–59.

Couzin-Frankel, Jennifer. "A Lighter Burden." *Science* 373, no. 6554 (July 2021): 480–83.

Crespo, C. J., E. Smit, R. P. Troiano, S. J. Bartlett, C. A. Macera, and R. E. Andersen. "Television Watching, Energy Intake and Obesity in US Children: Results from the Third National Health and Nutrition Examination Survey, 1988–1994." *Archives of Pediatrics and Adolescent Medicine* 155, no. 3 (March 2001): 360–365.

Crosby, Priya, Ryan Hamnett, Marrit Putker, Nathaniel P. Hoyle, Martin Reed, Carolyn J. Karam, Elizabeth S. Maywood et al. "Insulin/IGF-1 Drives PERIOD Synthesis to Entrain Circadian Rhythms with Feeding Time." *Cell* 177, no. 4 (May 2019): 896–909.

Daniel, Noëmie, Laís Rossi Perazza, Thibault V. Varin, Jocelyn Trottier, Bruno Marcotte, Philippe St-Pierre, Olivier Barbier, Benoit Chassaing, and André Marette. "Dietary Fat and Low Fiber in Purified Diets Differently Impact the Gut-Liver Axis to Promote Obesity-Linked Metabolic Impairments." *American Journal of Physiology* 320, no. 6 (June 2021): G1014-33.

da Poian, Andrea T., and Miguel Castanho. *Integrative Human Biochemistry*. New York: Springer, 2015.

Darwin, Charles. *The Expressions of Emotions in Man and Animals*. London: John Murray, 1872.

Dash, Bhagwan. *Concept of Agni in Ayurveda with Special Reference to Agnibala Pariksa*. Varanasi, India: Chaukhamba Amarabharati Prakashan, 1993.

Dash, Bhagwan, and R. K. Sharma, eds. *Charaka Samhita*. Varanasi, India: Chowkhamba Sanskrit Series Office, 2009.

Dash, Bhagwan, and R. K. Sharma, eds. *Charaka Samhita*. Varanasi, India: Chaukhambha Orientalia, 1995.

da Silva, Tatiane Ferreira, Sabrina Neves Casarotti, Gislane Lelis Vilela de Oliveira, and Ana Lúcia Barretto Penna. "The Impact of Probiotics, Prebiotics, and Synbiotics on the Biochemical, Clinical, and Immunological Markers, as Well as on the Gut Microbiota of Obese Hosts." *Critical Reviews in Food Science and Nutrition* 61, no. 2 (2021): 337–55.

Davis, Courtney, Janet Bryan, Jonathan Hodgson, and Karen Murphy. "Definition of the Mediterranean Diet: A Literature Review." *Nutrients* 7, no. 11 (November 2015): 9139–53.

Della Monica, Ciro, Giuseppe Atzori, and Derk-Jan Dijk. "Effects of Lunar Phase on Sleep in Men and Women in Surrey." *Journal of Sleep Research* 24, no. 6 (December 2015): 687–94.

de Ridder, Denise, Floor Kroese, Catharine Evers, Marieke Adriaanse, and Marleen Gillebaart. "Healthy Diet: Health Impact, Prevalence, Correlates, and Interventions." *Psychology and Health* 32, no. 8 (August 2017): 907–41.

DerSarkissian, Carol. "Normal Blood Sugar Levels for Adults with Diabetes." WebMD. January 15, 2022.

de Souza Pinhel, Marcela Augusta, Ligia Moriguchi Watanabe, Natália Yumi Noronha, Rafael Fernandes-Ferreira et al. "The Truth About the Influence of Endocrine Disruptors on Obesity: What Can Be Done?" *Obesity: Clinical, Surgical and Practical Guide*. Shamim I. Ahmad, ed. Springer. 217–29.

de Wit, Leonore, Margreet Ten Have, Pim Cuijpers, Ron de Graaf. "Body Mass Index and Risk of Onset of Mood and Anxiety Disorders in the General

Population: Results from the NEMESIS-2." *BMC Psychiatry* (August 2022).

Dinan, Timothy G., and John F. Cryan. "Gut Microbiota: A Missing Link in Psychiatry." *World Psychiatry* 19, no. 1 (February 2020): 111–12.

Dinerstein, Chuck. "The War Against Obesity." American Council on Science and Health website. January 29, 2021.

Diwan, Arvind Dattatrey, and Sanjay Harke. "Bank on Microbiome to Keep the Body Healthy." *Journal of Nutrition & Food Sciences* 11 (February 2021): 791.

Dixon, J. Brandon. "Lymphatic Lipid Transport: Sewer or Subway?" *Trends in Endocrinology and Metabolism* 21, no. 8 (August 2010): 480–87.

Dragoo, Jason L., Shane A. Shapiro, Hannah Bradsell, and Rachel M. Frank. "The Essential Roles of Human Adipose Tissue: Metabolic, Thermoregulatory, Cellular, and Paracrine Effects." *Journal of Cartilage & Joint Preservation* 1, no. 3 (September 2021): Article 100023.

Dwarakanath, C. *Concept of Agni in Ayurveda.* Calcutta: Baidyanath, 2002.

Dwarakanath, C. *Digestion and Metabolism in Ayurveda.* Varanasi, India: Krishnadas Academy, 1997.

Dwivedi, L. D., and L. V. Guru. *Introduction to Ayurveda.* Varanasi, India: Krishnadas Academy, 1988.

Elffers, Theodora W., Renée de Mutsert, Hildo J. Lamb, Albert de Roos, Ko Willems van Dijk, Frits R. Rosendaal, J. Wouter Jukema, and Stella Trompet. "Body Fat Distribution, in Particular Visceral Fat, Is Associated with Cardiometabolic Risk Factors in Obese Women." *PLoS One* 12, no. 9 (September 2017): Article e0185403.

Elnahas, Ahmad Ibrahim, Timothy D. Jackson, and Dennis Hong. "Management of Failed Laparoscopic Roux-en-Y Gastric Bypass." *Bariatric Surgical Practice and Patient Care* 9, no. 1 (March 2014): 36–40.

Estruch, Ramon, and Emilio Ros. "The Role of the Mediterranean Diet on Weight Loss and Obesity-Related Diseases." *Reviews in Endocrine and Metabolic Disorders* 21 (2020): 315–27.

Fan, Yong, and Oluf Pedersen. "Gut Microbiota in Human Metabolic Health and Disease." *Nature Reviews Microbiology* 19 (2021): 55–71.

Ferreira, Plinio M., and David Nutt. "Regulating the Oxides of Nitrogen–Popping the Myths." *Drug Science, Policy and Law* 8 (April 2022): 1–7.

Fischer, Michael J. M., Cosmin I. Ciotu, and Arpad Szallasi. "The Mysteries of Capsaicin-Sensitive Afferents." *Frontiers in Physiology* 11 (2020): Article 554195.

Food and Drug Administration, "GMO Crops, Animal Food, and Beyond," FDA website.

Frankiensztajn, Linoy Mia, Evan Elliott, and Omry Koren. "The Microbiota and the Hypothalamus-Pituitary-Adrenocortical (HPA) Axis, Implications for Anxiety and Stress Disorders." *Current Opinion in Neurobiology* 62 (2020): 76–82.

Frawley, David. *Ayurveda and the Mind: The Healing of Consciousness.* Twin Lakes, WI: Lotus Press, 1996. Delhi: Motilal Banarsidass Publishers, 2004.

Frawley, David, and Navaratna S. Rajaram. *Hidden Horizons: Unearthing 10,000 Years of Indian Culture.* Amdvad, India: Swaminarayan Aksharpith, 2007.

Fryar, Cheryl D., Margaret D. Carroll, Qiuping Gu, Joseph Afful, Cynthia L. Ogden. "Anthropometric Reference Data for Children and Adults: United States, 2015–2018." *Vital & Health Statistics. Series 3, Analytical and Epidemiological Studies.* (January 2021) 11 (36): 1–44.

García Nores, G. D. A. Cuzzone, N. J. Albano, G. E. Hespe, R. P. Kataru, J. S. Torrisi, J. C. Gardenier, I. L. Savetsky, S. Z. Aschen, M. D. Nitti, and B. J. Mehrara. "Obesity but Not High-Fat Diet Impairs Lymphatic Function." *International Journal of Obesity* 40 (2016): 1582–90.

Gardner, Howard. *Multiple Intelligences: New Horizons.* New York: Basic Books, 2010.

Gest, H. "The Discovery of Microorganisms by Robert Hooke and Antoni van Leeuwenhoek, Fellows of The Royal Society." *Notes and Records: The Royal Society Journal of the History of Science* 58, no. 2 (May 2004): 187–201.

Gibney, M. J. "Dietary Guidelines: A Critical Appraisal." *Journal of Human Nutrition and Dietetics* 3, no. 4 (1990): 245–54.

Gomaa, Eman Zakaria. "Human Gut Microbiota/Microbiome in Health and Diseases: A Review." *Antonie van Leeuwenhoek* 113 (December 2020): 2019–40.

Gómez, Georgina, Irina Kovalskys, Ana Carolina B. Leme et al. "Socioeconomic Status Impact on Diet Quality and Body Mass Index in Eight Latin American Countries: ELANS Study Results." *Nutrients* 13, no. 7 (2021): Article 2404.

Goossens, Gijs H. "The Metabolic Phenotype in Obesity: Fat Mass, Body Fat Distribution, and Adipose Tissue Function." *Obesity Facts* 10, no. 3 (2017): 207–15.

Gouveia, Flavia Venetucci, Esther Silk, Benjamin Davidson, Christopher B. Pople, Agessandro Abrahao, Jill Hamilton, George M. Ibrahim et al. "A Systematic Review on Neuromodulation Therapies for Reducing Body Weight in Patients with Obesity." *Obesity Reviews* 22, no. 10 (October 2021): Article e13309.

Grant, Richard. "Do Trees Talk to Each Other?" *Smithsonian Magazine*, March 2018.

Grotto, David, and Elisa Zied. "The Standard American Diet and Its Relationship to the Health Status of Americans." *Nutrition in Clinical Practice* 25, no. 6 (December 2010): 603–12.

Gugusheff, Jessica R., Zhi Yi Ong, and Beverly S. Muhlhausler. "A Maternal 'Junk-Food' Diet Reduces Sensitivity to the Opioid Antagonist Naloxone in Offspring Postweaning." *FASEB Journal* 27, no. 3 (March 2013): 1275–84.

Gundersen, Kare, and Grace Shen. "Total Body Water in Obesity." *The American Journal of Clinical Nutrition* 19, no. 2 (August 1966): 77–83.

Gupta, Arpana, Vadim Osadchiy, and Emeran A. Mayer. "Brain–Gut–Microbiome Interactions in Obesity and Food Addiction." *Nature Reviews Gastroenterology & Hepatology* 17 (2020): 655–72.

Gupta, Kaviraj Russick Lal, trans. *Madhava Nidana: Ayurvedic System of Pathology.* Delhi: Sri Satguru, 1987.

Gupta, Satya Pal. *Psychopathology in Indian Medicine.* Delhi: Chaukhamba Sanskrit Pratishtan, 2000.

Gupta, Vikas, Ravinder Sharma, Renu Bansal, Gunpreet Kaur et al. "Chapter 12 - Organs-on-a-Chip in Precision Medicine," *Human Organs-on-a-Chip Technology*, Academic Press (2024): 233–49.

Haas de Mello, Aline, Ana Beatriz Costa, Jéssica Della Giustina Engel, and Gislaine Tezza Rezin. "Mitochondrial Dysfunction in Obesity." *Life Sciences* 192 (January 2018): 26–32.

Hagberg, Carolina E. and Kirsty L. Spalding, "White Adipocyte Dysfunction and Obesity-Associated Pathologies in Humans." *Nature Reviews Molecular Cell Biology* 25, (2024): 270–289.

Hainsworth, Keri R., Xue Cheng Liu, Pippa M. Simpson, Ann M. Swartz, Nina Linneman, Susan T. Tran, Gustavo R. Medrano, Bryant Mascarenhas, Liyun Zhang, and Steven J. Weisman. "A Pilot Study of Iyengar Yoga for Pediatric Obesity: Effects on Gait and Emotional Functioning." *Children* 5, no. 7 (2018): 92.

Harland, Janice I., J. Buttriss, and Sigrid Ann Gibson. "Achieving Eatwell Plate Recommendations: Is This a Route to Improving Both Sustainability and Healthy Eating?" *Nutrition Bulletin* 37, no. 4 (December 2012): 324–43.

Harvard College. "Are Weight-Loss Drugs Worth Trying?" *Harvard Health Publishing* website, May 22, 2018.

Hassani, M. Amine, Paloma Durán, and Stéphane Hacquard. "Microbial Interactions within the Plant Holobiont." *Microbiome* 6 (2018): Article 58.

He, Yang, Bixiang Wang, Liankui Wen, Fengzhong Wang, Hansong Yu, Dongxia Chen, Xin Su, and Chi Zhang. "Effects of Dietary Fiber on Human Health." *Food Science and Human Wellness* 11, no. 1 (January 2022): 1–10.

Hegde, Shweta, Leena P. Nair, Haritha Chandran, and Haroon Irshad. "Traditional Indian Way of Eating–An Overview." *Journal of Ethnic Foods* 5, no. 1 (March 2018): 20–23.

Hehemann, Jan-Hendrik, Gaëlle Correc, Tristan Barbeyron, William Helbert, Mirjam Czjzek, and Gurvan Michel. "Transfer of Carbohydrate-Active Enzymes from Marine Bacteria to Japanese Gut Microbiota." *Nature* 464, no. 7290 (2010): 908–12.

Henning, Susanne M., Jieping Yang, Paul Shao, Ru-Po Lee, Jianjun Huang, Austin Ly, Mark Hsu et al. "Health Benefit of Vegetable/Fruit Juice-Based Diet: Role of Microbiome." *Scientific Reports* 7 (2017): Article 2167.

Hijová, Emília. "Synbiotic Supplements in the Prevention of Obesity and Obesity-Related Diseases." *Metabolites* 12, no. 4 (2022): 313.

Hinney, Anke, Antje Körner, and Pamela Fischer-Posovszky. "The Promise of New Anti-obesity Therapies Arising from Knowledge of Genetic Obesity Traits." *Nature Reviews Endocrinology* 18 (2022): 623–37.

Holzer, Peter. "Gut Signals and Gut Feelings: Science at the Interface of Data and Beliefs." *Frontiers in Behavioral Neuroscience* 16 (2022): Article 929332.

Hong, Mengyu, Chi-Tang Ho, Xin Zhang, Ruilin Zhang, and Yanan Liu. "Dietary Strategies May Influence Human Nerves and Emotions by Regulating Intestinal Microbiota: An Interesting Hypothesis." *Food Science + Technology* 56, no. 7 (July 2021): 3311–21.

Hu, Xinliang, Chong Yu, Yuting He et al. "Integrative Metagenomic Analysis Reveals Distinct Gut Microbial Signatures Related to Obesity." *BMC Microbiology* 24, no. 119 (2024).

Huang, R. Y. et al. "Vegetarian Diets and Weight Reduction: a Meta-Analysis of Randomized Controlled Trials." *Journal of General Internal Medicine* 31 (2016), 109–116.

Illiano, Placido, Roberta Brambilla, and Cinzia Parolini. "The Mutual Interplay of Gut Microbiota, Diet and Human Disease." *The FEBS Journal* 287, no. 5 (March 2020): 833–55.

Itani, Naresh, Komal Keshwa, and Divya Pathak, "Exploring the Impact of Ayurvedic Approaches on Obesity: A Scientific Research Perspective." *Journal of Ayurveda and Integrated Medical Sciences* 8, no. 8 (August 2023): 206–15.

Jackson, Dakota N., and Arianne L. Theiss. "Gut Bacteria Signaling to

Mitochondria in Intestinal Inflammation and Cancer." *Gut Microbes* 11, no. 3 (2020): 285–304.

Jain, Vijay K. *Acharya Umasvami's Tattvarthsutra.* Uttarakhand, India: Vikalp Printers, 2011.

Jiang, Xinguo, Wen Tian, Mark R. Nicolls, and Stanley G. Rockson. "The Lymphatic System in Obesity, Insulin Resistance, and Cardiovascular Diseases." *Frontiers in Physiology* 10 (November 2019): 1402.

Jirtle, Randy L., and Frederick L. Tyson, eds. *Environmental Epigenomics in Health and Disease: Epigenetics and Disease Origins.* Heidelberg: Springer Berlin, 2013.

Johnson, R. L., and C. G. Wilson. "A Review of Vagus Nerve Stimulation as a Therapeutic Intervention." *Journal of Inflammation Research* 11 (May 2018): 203–13.

Juchacz, Krzysztof, Patrycja Kłos, Violetta Dziedziejko, and Rafał W. Wójciak. "The Effectiveness of Supportive Psychotherapy in Weight Loss in a Group of Young Overweight and Obese Women." *Nutrients* 13, no. 2 (2021): 532.

Kang, Guolian, Shao Li, and Ji-Feng Zhang. "Entropy-Based Model for Interpreting Life Systems in Traditional Chinese Medicine." *Evidence-Based Complementary and Alternative Medicine* 5, no. 3 (January 2008): 273–79.

Kapadia, Mala, and Chirag Dagar. "Understanding Self and Well-Being Based on Ayurveda: Implications for Indian Management." In *Indigenous Indian Management*, edited by Ashish Pandey, Pawan Budhwar, and Dharm P. S. Bhawuk, 157–97. [London?]: Palgrave Macmillan, 2022.

Kapoor, Kashish, Reecha Madaan, Suresh Kumar, Rajni Bala, and Raman P. Walia. "Role of Natural Products in the Treatment of Obesity: Nanotechnological Perspectives." *Current Drug Metabolism* 22, no. 6 (2021): 451–80.

Kar, A. C. *Parasitology in Ayurveda.* Varanasi: Chaukhambha Visvabharati, 2013.

Kardan, Romina, Jaber Hemmati, Mohsen Nazari, Amjad Ahmadi, Babak Asghari, Mehdi Azizi, Mansoor Khaledi et al. "Novel Therapeutic Strategy for Obesity through the Gut Microbiota-Brain Axis: A Review Article," *Caspian Journal of Internal Medicine* 15, no. 2 (Summer 2024): 215–227.

Kaushik, Rahul, Jainendra Jain, and Azhar Danish Khan. "Trikatu: Transforming Food into Medicines." In *Innovations in Food Technology*, edited by Pragya Mishra, Raghvendra Raman Mishra, and Charles Oluwaseun Adetunji. Singapore: Springer, 2020.

Kawai, Tatsuo, Michael V. Autieri, and Rosario Scalia. "Adipose Tissue Inflammation and Metabolic Dysfunction in Obesity." *American Journal of Physiology* 320, no. 3 (March 2021): C375–91.

Kelley, Claire P., Geena Sbrocco, and Tracy Sbrocco. "Behavioral Modification for the Management of Obesity." *Primary Care: Clinics in Office Practice* 43, no. 1 (March 2016): 159–75.

Khandekar, Surekha, Tabasum Pansare, Abhijeet Pachpor, and Sharad Kumar Maurya. "Role of Katuka (Picrorhiza Kurroa Royle Ex Benth.) in Obesity W.S.R to Ayurvedic and Modern Aspect: A Review." *International Journal of Herbal Medicine* 7, no. 6 (2019): 31–35.

Khedikar, Sachin, Gaurav Sawarkar, Priti Desai. "Correlative Study of Visceral Fats with Medodhara Kala (Membrane): A Review." *African Journal of Biological Sciences* 6, no. 10 (June 9, 2024): 435–42.

Kim, Hyun-Jin, Hyuktae Kwon, Su-Min Jeong, Seo Eun Hwang, and Jin-Ho Park. "Effects of Abdominal Visceral Fat Compared with Those of Subcutaneous Fat on the Association between PM10 and Hypertension in Korean Men: A Cross-Sectional Study." *Scientific Reports* 9 (April 2019): Article 5951.

King, Stephanie E., and Michael K. Skinner. "Epigenetic Transgenerational Inheritance of Obesity Susceptibility." *Trends in Endocrinology & Metabolism* 31, no. 7 (March 2020): 478–94.

Kolovos, Spyros, Aura Cecilia Jimenez-Moreno, Rafael Pinedo-Villanueva, Sophie Cassidy, and Gerardo A. Zavala. "Association of Sleep, Screen Time and Physical Activity with Overweight and Obesity in Mexico." *Eating and Weight Disorders* 26 (2021): 169–179.

Korabu, J. R., and A. M. Kulkarni. "A Review of Pre-clinical Studies on Obesity Markers Using Ayurvedic Medicinal Plants." *World Journal of Pharmaceutical Research* 10, no. 5 (2021): 960–69.

Kotur, S. B., and Shashikala Kotur. *A Textbook of Ayurvedic Physiology*. Varanasi, India: Chaukhambha Orientalia, 2007.

Krishnamurthy, K. H., trans. *Bhela Samhita, Sutrasthana*. Varanasi, India: Chaukhambha Vishwabharati, 2006.

Kundu, Suman, Hazera Khatun, Nisith Kumar Mandal, and Kazi M. M. Mohiuddin Ahmed. "A Review on Therapeutic Use of Vidanga (Embelia Ribes) for Pathological Consequences Associated with Obesity as per Ayurvedic Classics." *International Research Journal of Pharmacy* 10, no. 2 (February 2019): 38–40.

Kuo, Braden, Manoj Bhasin, Jolene Jacquart, Matthew A. Scult, Lauren Slipp, Eric Isaac Kagan Riklin, Veronique Lepoutre et al. "Genomic and Clinical Effects Associated with a Relaxation Response Mind-Body Intervention in Patients with Irritable Bowel Syndrome and Inflammatory Bowel Disease." *PLoS ONE* 12, no. 2 (2017): Article e0172872.

Kwon, Yun, Jisu Shin, Kwangho Nam, Joon Soo An, Seung-Hoon Yang, Seong-Heon Hong, Munhyung Bae et al. "Rhizolutin, a Novel 7/10/6-Tricyclic Dilactone, Dissociates Misfolded Protein Aggregates and Reduces Apoptosis/Inflammation Associated with Alzheimer's Disease." *Angewandte Chemie* 59, no. 51 (December 2020): 22994–98.

Lad, Vasant. *Ayurveda: The Science of Self-Healing.* Twin Lakes, WI: Lotus Press, 2009.

———. *Textbook of Ayurveda: Fundamental Principles.* Albuquerque, NM: Ayurveda Press, 2002.

Larson, Gerald James. *Classical Sāṃkhya: An Interpretation of Its History and Meaning.* Delhi, India: Motilal Banarsidass Publishers, 1969.

Lassale, Camille, G. David Batty, Amaria Baghdadli, Felice Jacka, Almudena Sánchez-Villegas, Mika Kivimäki, and Tasnime Akbaraly. "Healthy Dietary Indices and Risk of Depressive Outcomes: A Systematic Review and Meta-Analysis of Observational Studies." *Molecular Psychiatry* 26 (2021): 3657.

Lazar, Veronica, Lia-Mara Ditu, Gratiela Gradisteanu Pircalabioru, Irina Gheorghe, Carmen Curutiu, Alina Maria Holban, Ariana Picu, Laura Petcu, and Mariana Carmen Chifiriuc. "Aspects of Gut Microbiota and Immune System Interactions in Infectious Diseases, Immunopathology, and Cancer." *Frontiers in Immunology* 9 (August 2018): 1830.

Lecoq, Hervé. "Découverte du premier virus, le virus de la mosaïque du tabac: 1892 ou 1898?" *Comptes Rendus de l'Académie des Sciences - Series III - Sciences de la Vie* 324, no. 10 (October 2001): 929–33.

Ledford, H., "Why Are So Many Young People Getting Cancer?" *Nature* 627 (2024), 258-260.

Lee, Alexandra, Michelle Cardel, and William T. Donahoo. "Social and Environmental Factors Influencing Obesity." In *Endotext [Internet],* edited by Kenneth R. Feingold, Bradley Anawalt, Marc R. Blackman, Alison Boyce, George Chrousos, Emiliano Corpas, Wouter W. de Herder et al. South Dartmouth, MA: MDText (website).

Lee, Seon Yeong, and Dympna Gallagher. "Assessment Methods in Human Body Composition." *Current Opinion in Clinical Nutrition and Metabolic Care* 11, no. 5 (September 2008): 566–72.

Lee, Sung-Ha, Seok-Hwan Yoon, Yeonjae Jung, Namil Kim, Uigi Min, Jongsik Chun, and Incheol Choi. "Emotional Well-Being and Gut Microbiome Profiles by Enterotype." *Scientific Reports* 10 (2020): Article 20736.

Lerner, A., C. Benzvi, A. Vojdani. "The Potential Harmful Effects of Genetically

Engineered Microorganisms (GEMs) on the Intestinal Microbiome and Public Health." *Microorganisms* 12, no. 2 (2024): 238.

Li, Huiping, Shu Li, Hongxi Yang, Yuan Zhang, Shunming Zhang, Yue Ma, Yabing Hou et al. "Association of Ultraprocessed Food Consumption with Risk of Dementia: A Prospective Cohort Study." *Neurology* 99, no. 10 (September 2022): e1056–66.

Li, Long, Qingxu Jing, Sen Yan, Xuxu Liu, Yuanyuan Sun, Defu Zhu, Dawei Wang, Chenjun Hao, and Dongbo Xue. "Amadis: A Comprehensive Database for Association Between Microbiota and Disease." *Frontiers in Physiology* 12 (July 2021): Article 697059.

Liiv, Helena, Matthew A. Wyon, Toivo Jürimäe, Meeli Saar, Jarek Mäestu, and Jaak Jürimäe. "Anthropometry, Somatotypes, and Aerobic Power in Ballet, Contemporary Dance, and Dancesport." *Medical Problems of Performing Artists* 28, no. 4 (December 2013): 207–11.

Liu, Richard T. "The Microbiome as a Novel Paradigm in Studying Stress and Mental Health." *American Psychologist* 72, no. 7 (2017): 655–67.

Liu, Tian-Tian, Xiao-Tian Liu, Qing-Xi Chen, and Yan Shi. "Lipase Inhibitors for Obesity: A Review." *Biomedicine & Pharmacotherapy* 128 (August 2020): Article 110314.

Liu, Wanjun, Xiaojie Fang, Yong Zhou, Lihong Dou, and Tongyi Dou. "Machine Learning-Based Investigation of the Relationship between Gut Microbiome and Obesity Status." *Microbes and Infection* 24, no. 2 (March 2022): Article 104892.

Liu, Xiao-Cong, Yu Huang, Kenneth Lo, Yu-Qing Huang, Ji-Yan Chen, and Ying-Qing Feng. "Quotient of Waist Circumference and BMI: A Valuable Indicator for the High-Risk Phenotype of Obesity." *Frontiers in Endocrinology* 12 (May 2021): Article 697437.

Liu, Xiaoning, Xiang Li, Bing Xia, Xin Jin, Qianhui Zou, Zhenhua Zeng, Weiyang Zhao et al. "High-Fiber Diet Mitigates Maternal Obesity-Induced Cognitive and Social Dysfunction in the Offspring via Gut-Brain Axis." *Cell Metabolism* 33, no. 5 (May 2021): 923–38.e6.

Liu, Yang, Roger Chun-Man Ho, and Anselm Mak. "Interleukin (IL)-6, Tumour Necrosis Factor Alpha (TNF-α) and Soluble Interleukin-2 Receptors (sIL-2R) Are Elevated in Patients with Major Depressive Disorder: Meta-Analysis and Meta-Regression." *Journal of Affective Disorders* 139, no. 3 (August 2012): 230–39.

Lohith, B. A. *A Text Book of Panchakarma*. Varanasi, India: Chaukambha Orientalia, 2016.

Loos, Ruth J. F., and Giles S. H. Yeo. "The Genetics of Obesity: From Discovery to Biology." *Nature Reviews Genetics* 23 (2022).

Ludwig, David S., Mark A. Pereira, Candyce H. Kroenke, Joan E. Hilner, Linda Van Horn, Martha L. Slattery, and David R. Jacobs, Jr. "Dietary Fiber, Weight Gain, and Cardiovascular Disease Risk Factors in Young Adults." *JAMA* 282, no. 16 (October 1999): 1539–46.

Luo, Min, Dan-Dan Zhou, Ao Shang, Ren-You Gan, and Hua-Bin Li. "Influences of Food Contaminants and Additives on Gut Microbiota as Well as Protective Effects of Dietary Bioactive Compounds." *Trends in Food Science & Technology* 113 (July 2021): 180–92.

Ma, Lu, Yixin Ding, Dorothy T. Chiu, Yang Wu, Zhiyong Wang, Xin Wang, and Youfa Wang. "A Longitudinal Study of Sleep, Weight Status, and Weight-Related Behaviors: Childhood Obesity Study in China Mega-cities." *Pediatric Research* 90 (2021): 971–79.

MacLean, P. S., J. A. Higgins, E. D. Giles, V. D. Sherk, and M. R. Jackman. "The Role for Adipose Tissue in Weight Regain after Weight Loss." *Obesity Reviews* 16, no. S1 (January 2015): 45–54.

Macpherson-Sánchez, Ann E. "Integrating Fundamental Concepts of Obesity and Eating Disorders: Implications for the Obesity Epidemic." *American Journal of Public Health* 105, no. 4 (March 2015): e71–e85.

Mahalle, Namita P., Mohan V. Kulkarni, Narendra M. Pendse, and Sadanand S. Naik. "Association of Constitutional Type in Ayurveda with Cardiovascular Risk Factors, Inflammatory Markers and Insulin Resistance." *Journal of Ayurveda and Integrative Medicine* 3, no. 3 (July–September 2012): 150–57.

Malinar, Angelika. "Narrating Sāṃkhya Philosophy: Bhīṣma, Janaka and Pañcaśikha at Mahābhārata 12.211–12." *Journal of Indian Philosophy* 45 (2017): 609–49.

Martínez, Inés, James M. Lattimer, Kelcie L. Hubach, Jennifer A. Case, Junyi Yang, Casey G. Weber, Julie A. Louk et al., "Gut Microbiome Composition Is Linked to Whole Grain-Induced Immunological Improvements." *The ISME Journal* 7, no. 2 (February 2013): 269–80.

Martone, Robert. "Early Life Experience: It's in Your DNA." *Scientific American*, July 10, 2018.

Masi, Emily Battinelli, Sergio Iván Valdés-Ferrer, and Benjamin Ethan Steinberg. "The Vagus Neurometabolic Interface and Clinical Disease." *International Journal of Obesity* 42 (2018): 1101–11.

Matute, Sharlize Pedroza, and Sasitaran Iyavoo. "Exploring the Gut Microbiota:

Lifestyle Choices, Disease Associations, and Personal Genomics." *Frontiers in Nutrition* 10 (October 5, 2023).

Mayeli, Ahmad, Obada Al Zoubi, Evan J. White et al. "Neural Indicators of Human Gut Feelings." Preprint, submitted June 25, 2021.

McCraty, Rollin. *Science of the Heart: Exploring the Role of the Heart in Human Performance*, vol. 2. N.p.: HeartMath Institute, 2016.

McEwen, Birgitta. "Construction of a Review About Epigenetics for Biology Teachers and Other Non-experts." *Science & Education* 31 (September 2021): 997–1026.

McLaren, Lindsay. "Socioeconomic Status and Obesity." *Epidemiologic Reviews* 29, no. 1 (May 2007): 29–48.

Medina, Francesc Xavier, Josep M. Solé-Sedeno, Anna Bach-Faig, and Alicia Aguilar-Martínez. "Obesity, Mediterranean Diet, and Public Health: A Vision of Obesity in the Mediterranean Context from a Sociocultural Perspective." *International Journal of Environmental Research and Public Health* 18, no. 7 (2021): 3715.

Medina, R., L. Eduardo Cardona-Sanclemente, and G. V. R. Born. "Effect of Deoxycorticosterone Acetate on Blood Pressure in Relation to Accumulation of Low-Density Lipoprotein and Fibrinogen by Aorta and Other Tissues of Normotensive Wistar Rats." *Journal of Hypertension* 15, no. 5 (May 1997): 531–36.

Merrow, Martha, Kamiel Spoelstra, and Till Roenneberg. "The Circadian Cycle: Daily Rhythms from Behavior to Genes." *EMBO Reports* 6, no. 10 (October 2005): 930–35.

Michel, Lauriane Y. M., Charlotte Farah, and Jean-Luc Balligand. "Nitric Oxide Signalling in Cardiovascular Health and Disease." *Nature Reviews Cardiology* 15 (February 2018): 292–316.

Mishra, Lakshmi C., ed. *Scientific Basis for Ayurvedic Therapies*. 1st ed. New York: Routledge, 2003.

Mishra, Tanuja, Harcharan S. Dhaliwal, Karan Singh, and Nasib Singh. "Shilajit (Mumie): Current Status of Biochemical, Therapeutic and Clinical Advances." *Current Nutrition & Food Science* 15, no. 2 (2019): 104–20.

Mirzaei, Rasoul, Elahe Dehkhodaie, Behnaz Bouzari, Mandana Rahimi, Abolfazl Gholestani, Seyed Reza Hosseini-Fard, Hossein Keyvani, Ali Teimoori, and Sajad Karampoor. "Dual Role of Microbiota-Derived Short-Chain Fatty Acids on Host and Pathogen." *Biomedicine & Pharmacotherapy* 145 (January 2022): Article 112352.

Młynarska, Ewelina, Joanna Gadzinowska, Julita Tokarek, Joanna Forycka, Aleksandra Szuman, Beata Franczyk, and Jacek Rysz. "The Role of the

Microbiome-Brain-Gut Axis in the Pathogenesis of Depressive Disorder." *Nutrients* 14, no. 9 (2022): Article 1921.

Mohajeri, M. Hasan, Robert J. M. Brummer, Robert A. Rastall, Rinse K. Weersma, Hermie J. M. Harmsen, Marijke Faas, and Manfred Eggersdorfer. "The Role of the Microbiome for Human Health: From Basic Science to Clinical Applications." *European Journal of Nutrition* 57 (2018): 1–14.

Moles, Laura, and David Otaegui. "The Impact of Diet on Microbiota Evolution and Human Health: Is Diet an Adequate Tool for Microbiota Modulation?" *Nutrients* 12, no. 6 (2020): Article 1654.

Mondal, Samiran. Proposed Physiological Mechanisms of Pranayama: A Discussion." *Journal of Ayurveda and Integrative Medicine* 15, no. 1 (January/February) 2024) 100877.

Moore, James E., and Christopher D. Bertram. "Lymphatic System Flows." *Annual Review of Fluid Mechanics* 50 (2018): 459–82.

Moon, Min Kyong, Inae Lee, Aram Lee, Hyunwoong Park, Min Joo Kim, Sunmi Kim, Yoon Hee Cho et al. "Lead, Mercury, and Cadmium Exposures Are Associated with Obesity but Not with Diabetes Mellitus: Korean National Environmental Health Survey (KoNEHS) 2015–2017." *Environmental Research* 204, part A (March 2022): Article 111888.

Mörkl, Sabrina, Andreas Oberascher, Josef M. Tatschl, Sonja Lackner, Thomaz F. S. Bastiaanssen, Mary I. Butler, Maximilian Moser, Matthias Frühwirth, Harald Mangge, and John F. Cryan. "Cardiac Vagal Activity Is Associated with Gut Microbiome Patterns in Women—An Exploratory Pilot Study." *Dialogues in Clinical Neuroscience* 24, no. 1 (2022): 1–9.

Müller, Timo D., Matthias Blüher, Matthias H. Tschöp, and Richard D. DiMarchi. "Anti-obesity Drug Discovery: Advances and Challenges." *Nature Reviews Drug Discovery* 21 (2022): 201–23.

Murthy, Srikantha K. R. *Ashtanga Hridayam*. Varanasi, India: Chowkhamba Krishnadas Academy, 2010.

Murthy, K. R. Srikantha. *Madhava Nidanam (Roga Viniscaya of Madhavakara): A Treatise on Ayurveda*. Varanasi, India: Chaukhambha Orientalia, 2013.

Muscogiuri, G., L. Verde, C. Vetrani et al. "Obesity: A Gender-View." *Journal of Endocrinology Investigation* 47 (2024), 299–306.

Nagaraj, Kamath, Patel Yashesh, and Lal Sarika. "Critical Review on the Concept of Prakruthi." *Unique Journal of Ayurvedic and Herbal Medicines (UJAHM)* 7, no. 6 (2019): 17–20.

Namjou, Bahram, Ian B. Stanaway, Todd Lingren, Frank D. Mentch, Barbara

Benoit, Ozan Dikilitas, Xinnan Niu et al. "Evaluation of the MC4R Gene across eMERGE Network Identifies Many Unreported Obesity-Associated Variants." *International Journal of Obesity* 45 (January 2021): 155–69.

The National Academies of Sciences, Engineering, and Medicine. *Environmental Chemicals, the Human Microbiome, and Health Risk: A Research Strategy.* Washington, DC: National Academies Press, 2017.

Nielsen, Louise Aas, Tenna Ruest Haarmark Nielsen, and Jens-Christian Holm. "The Impact of Familial Predisposition to Obesity and Cardiovascular Disease on Childhood Obesity." *Obesity Facts* 8, no. 5 (October 2015): 319–28.

Niemiro, Grace M., Ayesan Rewane, and Amit M. Algotar. "Exercise and Fitness Effect On Obesity." In *StatPearls* website. Treasure Island, FL: StatPearls, 2024.

Ninivaggi, Frank John. *An Elementary Textbook of Ayurveda.* N.p.: Psychosocial Press, 2001.

Nityanand, S., J. S. Srivastava, and O. P. Asthana. "Clinical Trials with Gugulipid: A New Hypolipidaemic Agent." *The Journal of the Association of Physicians of India* 37, no. 5 (May 1989): 323–28.

Nunes, Paula Villela, Monise Caroline Schwarzer, Renata Elaine Paraizo Leite, Renata Eloah de Lucena Ferretti-Rebustini, Carlos Augusto Pasqualucci, Ricardo Nitrini, Roberta Diehl Rodriguez et al. "Neuropsychiatric Inventory in Community-Dwelling Older Adults with Mild Cognitive Impairment and Dementia." *Journal of Alzheimer's Disease* 68, no. 2 (2019): 669–78.

Obrenovich, Mark E. M. "Leaky Gut, Leaky Brain?" *Microorganisms* 6, no. 4 (2018): 107.

Ochoa-Reparaz, Javier, Christina C. Ramelow, and Lloyd H. Kasper. "A Gut Feeling: The Importance of the Intestinal Microbiota in Psychiatric Disorders." *Frontiers in Immunology* 11 (2020): Article 510113.

Offer, Samuel, Elise Alexander, Kelsie Barbara, Erik Hemmingsson, Stuart W. Flint, and Blake J. Lawrence. "The Association Between Childhood Trauma and Overweight and Obesity in Young Adults: The Mediating Role of Food Addiction." *Eating and Weight Disorders: Studies on Anorexia, Bulimia and Obesity* 27 (2022): 3257–66.

Oliveira, Manoela Lima, Alana Biggers, Vanessa M. Oddo, Betina Yanez, Emily Booms, Lisa Sharp, Keith Naylor et al. "A Perspective Review on Diet Quality, Excess Adiposity, and Chronic Psychosocial Stress and Implications for Early-Onset Colorectal Cancer," *Journal of Nutrition*, 154, no. 4, (2024): 1069–1079.

Pal, Gopal Krushna, and Nivedita Nanda. "Vagus Nerve: The Key Integrator of Anti-Inflammatory Reflex." *International Journal of Clinical and*

Experimental Physiology 7, no. 1 (May 2020): 1–2.

Palmer, R. M., A. G. Ferrige, and S. Moncada. "Nitric Oxide Release Accounts for the Biological Activity of Endothelium-Derived Relaxing Factor." *Nature* 327, no. 6122 (June 1987): 524–26.

Pampel, Fred C., Justin T. Denney, and Patrick M. Krueger. "Obesity, SES, and Economic Development: A Test of the Reversal Hypothesis." *Social Science and Medicine* 74, no. 7 (2012): 1073–81.

Pandey, Gyanendra. *Obesity Therapy = Medoroga vijñanam.* Varanasi, India: Chowkhamba Sanskrit Series Office, 2006.

Pandya, Kapil A., and Jalpa Jani. "Achievements through Panchakarma in Clinical Management and Future Prospects." *Journal of Ayurveda and Integrated Medical Sciences* 3, no. 2 (March–April 2018): 62–65.

Partridge, D., K. A. Lloyd, J. M. Rhodes, A. W. Walker, A. M. Johnstone, and B. J. Campbell. "Food Additives: Assessing the Impact of Exposure to Permitted Emulsifiers on Bowel and Metabolic Health: Introducing the FADiets Study." *Nutrition Bulletin* 44, no. 4 (November 2019): 329–49.

Patañjali. *The Yoga Sutras of Patanjali: The Book of the Spiritual Man: An Interpretation.* London: Watkins, 1975.

Patil, Asmita. "The Concept of Pradnyapradh with Respect to the Factors That Cause Life-Style Disorders." *International Ayurvedic Medical Journal* (2018).

Patil, Smita, Gaikwad Pandurang B., Suvarna T. Jadhav, Nilima Ramchandra Patil, and Vinayak B. Gaikwad. "Effect of Pranayama on Body Mass Index in Young Medical Students." *International Journal of Research & Review* 3, no. 2 (February 2016): 24–27.

Patwardhan, Bhushan, and Gerard Bodeker. "Ayurvedic Genomics: Establishing a Genetic Basis for Mind-Body Typologies." *Journal of Alternative and Complementary Medicine* 14, no. 5 (June 2008): 571–76.

Paul, Linda, Colin van der Heiden, and Hans W. Hoek. "Cognitive Behavioral Therapy and Predictors of Weight Loss in Bariatric Surgery Patients." *Current Opinion in Psychiatry* 30, no. 6 (November 2017): 474–79.

Pereira, L. J., and A. van der Bilt. "The Influence of Oral Processing, Food Perception and Social Aspects on Food Consumption: A Review." *Journal of Oral Rehabilitation* 43, no. 8 (August 2016): 630–48.

Peterson, Christine Tara, Kate Denniston, and Deepak Chopra. "Therapeutic Uses of Triphala in Ayurvedic Medicine." *Journal of Alternative and Complementary Medicine* 23, no. 8 (August 2017): 607–14.

Pett, K. D., J. Kahn, W. C. Willett, and D. L. Katz. "Ancel Keys and the Seven

Countries Study: An Evidence-Based Response to Revisionist Histories." White paper commissioned by the True Health Initiative, August 1, 2017.

Phetkate, Pratya, Tanawan Kummalue, Prasob-orn Rinthong, Somboon Kietinun, and Kusuma Sriyakul. "Study of the Safety of Oral Triphala Aqueous Extract on Healthy Volunteers." *Journal of Integrative Medicine* 18, no. 1 (January 2020): 35–40.

Phimarn, Wiraphol, Bunleu Sungthong, and Hiroyuki Itabe. "Effects of Triphala on Lipid and Glucose Profiles and Anthropometric Parameters." *Journal of Evidence-Based Integrative Medicine* 26 (2021).

Piché, Marie-Eve, André Tchernof, and Jean-Pierre Després. "Obesity Phenotypes, Diabetes, and Cardiovascular Diseases." *Circulation Research* 126, no. 11 (May 2020): 1477–1500.

Pigeyre, Marie, Fereshteh T. Yazdi, Yuvreet Kaur, and David Meyre. "Recent Progress in Genetics, Epigenetics and Metagenomics Unveils the Pathophysiology of Human Obesity." *Clinical Science* 130, no. 12 (June 2016): 943–986.

Plunk, Elizabeth C., and Sean M. Richards. "Epigenetic Modifications Due to Environment, Ageing, Nutrition, and Endocrine Disrupting Chemicals and Their Effects on the Endocrine System." *International Journal of Endocrinology* 2020, Article 9251980.

Pool, Robert. *Fat: Fighting the Obesity Epidemic.* New York: Oxford University Press, 2001.

Poti, Jennifer M., Bianca Braga, and Bo Qin. "Ultra-Processed Food Intake and Obesity: What Really Matters for Health–Processing or Nutrient Content?" *Current Obesity Reports* 6, no. 4 (December 2017): 420–31.

Prasad, Sahdeo, and Bharat B. Aggarwal. "Turmeric, the Golden Spice: From Traditional Medicine to Modern Medicine." In *Herbal Medicine: Biomolecular and Clinical Aspects*, 2nd edition, edited by I. F. F. Benzie and S. Wachtel-Galor. Boca Raton, FL: CRC Press/Taylor & Francis, 2011.

Prasad, S., and S. K. Srivastava. "Oxidative Stress and Cancer: Chemopreventive and Therapeutic Role of Triphala." *Antioxidants* 9, no. 1 (January 2020): 72.

Prasher, Bhavana, Sapna Negi, Shilpi Aggarwal, Amit K. Mandal, Tav P. Sethi, Shailaja R. Deshmukh, Sudha G. Purohit et al. "Whole Genome Expression and Biochemical Correlates of Extreme Constitutional Types Defined in Ayurveda." *Journal of Translational Medicine* 6 (September 2008): Article 48.

Pulipati, Priyanjali, Priyanka Sarkar, Aparna Jakkampudi, Vishal Kaila, Subhaleena Sarkar, Misbah Unnisa, D. Nageshwar Reddy, Mojibur Khan, and Rupjyoti Talukdar. "The Indian Gut Microbiota—Is it Unique?" *Indian Journal of Gastroenterology* 39 (May 2020): 133–40.

Qin, Junjie, Ruiqiang Li, Jeroen Raes, Manimozhiyan Arumugam, Kristoffer Solvsten Burgdorf, Chaysavanh Manichanh, Trine Nielsen et al. "A Human Gut Microbial Gene Catalogue Established by Metagenomic Sequencing." *Nature* 464 (2010): 59–65.

Ranade, Subhash, and Sunanda Ranade. *Concept of Pathology in Ayurveda*. Pune, India: Narendra Prakashan, 2003.

Rao, M. Ramasunder. *Sareera Kriya Vignanam: Physiology in Ayurveda*. Vijayawada, India: M. Mandhava, 2001.

Ravishankar, A. K. "Is India Shouldering a Double Burden of Malnutrition?" *Journal of Health Management* 14, no. 3 (2012): 313–28.

Reed, Danielle R., Amber L. Alhadeff, Gary K. Beauchamp, Nirupa Chaudhari, Valerie B. Duffy, Monica Dus, Alfredo Fontanini, et al. "NIH Workshop Report: Sensory Nutrition and Disease." *The American Journal of Clinical Nutrition* 113, no. 1 (January 2021): 232–45.

Rosenbaum, Michael, and Rudolph L. Leibel. "20 Years of Leptin: Role of Leptin in Energy Homeostasis in Humans." *Journal of Endocrinology* 223, no. 1 (October 2014): T83–96.

Sahebkar, Amirhossein, Guglielmo Beccuti, Luis E. Simental-Mendía, Valerio Nobili, and Simona Bo. "Nigella Sativa (Black Seed) Effects on Plasma Lipid Concentrations in Humans: A Systematic Review and Meta-Analysis of Randomized Placebo-Controlled Trials." *Pharmacological Research* 106 (April 2016): 37–50.

Saket, Dass, and Baghel Pramod Kumar. "An Elixir Effect of Diet on *Sthoulya* (*Medoroga*) in Ayurveda." *Ayushdhara* 7, no. 6: (2020).

Sani, Gabriele, Mirko Manchia, Alessio Simonetti, Delfina Janiri, Pasquale Paribello, Federica Pinna, and Bernardo Carpiniello. "The Role of Gut Microbiota in the High-Risk Construct of Severe Mental Disorders: A Mini Review." *Frontiers in Psychiatry* 11 (2020): Article 585769.

Sarkar, Amar, Soili M. Lehto, Siobhán Harty, Timothy G. Dinan, John F. Cryan, and Philip W. J. Burnet. "Psychobiotics and the Manipulation of Bacteria-Gut-Brain Signals." *Trends in Neurosciences* 39, no. 11 (November 2016): 763–781.

Savas, Mesut, Vincent L. Wester, Sabine M. Staufenbiel, Jan W. Koper, Erica L. T. van den Akker, Jenny A. Visser, Aart J. van der Lely, Brenda W. J. H. Penninx, and Elisabeth F. C. van Rossum. "Systematic Evaluation of Corticosteroid Use in Obese and Non-obese Individuals: A Multi-cohort Study." *International Journal of Medical Sciences* 14, no. 7 (2017): 615–21.

Sawarkar, Punam, and Anil Patange. "Role of Yoga for the Prevention &

Management of COVID-19: A Review." *International Journal of Research in Pharmaceutical Sciences* 11, no. SPL1 (December 2020): 1720–24.

Schuster, Stefan, Maximilian Fichtner, and Severin Sasso. "Use of Fibonacci Numbers in Lipidomics–Enumerating Various Classes of Fatty Acids." *Scientific Reports* 7 (January 2017): Article 39821.

Senghor, Bruno, Cheikh Sokhna, Raymond Ruimy, and Jean-Christophe Lagier. "Gut Microbiota Diversity According to Dietary Habits and Geographical Provenance." *Human Microbiome Journal* 7–8 (April 2018): 1–9.

Sengupta, Pallav. "Health Impacts of Yoga and Pranayama: A State-of-the-Art Review." *International Journal of Preventive Medicine* 3, no. 7 (July 2012): 444–58.

Sharma, Hari. "Ayurveda: Science of Life, Genetics, and Epigenetics." *Journal of Research in Ayurveda* 37, no. 2 (April–June 2016): 87–91.

Sharma, Hari, and Robert Keith Wallace. "Ayurveda and Epigenetics." *Medicina* 56, no. 12 (December 2020): Article 687.

Sharma, P. V., trans. "Vimanasthanum, Chapter 3." In *Charaka Samhita*. Delhi: Chaukhamba Orientalia, 1981.

Sharma, Parul, and Bhushan Sharma. "A Clinical Study to Assess the Impact of Lekhan Basti, Udvarthana, and Navak Guggulu in the Management of Obesity vis-à-vis Sthaulya." *IAMJ* 3, no. 2 (February 2015).

Sharma, Ram Karan, and Bhagwan Dash, eds. *Charaka Samhita of Agnivesa*. 3rd ed. Varanasi, India: Chowkhamba Sanskrit Series Office, 1998.

Sharma, Rohit, and Pradeep Kumar Prajapati. "Predictive, Preventive and Personalized Medicine: Leads from Ayurvedic Concept of Prakriti (Human Constitution)." *Current Pharmacology Reports* 6 (October 2020): 441–50.

Sharma, Tarkeshwar, Chetan Ram Meghwal, Monika Prajapat, Ashok Kumar Sharma. "Conceptual Study of Vata Dosha w.s.r. to Nervous System." *Journal of Ayurveda and Integrated Medical Sciences* 9, no. 2 (February 2024): 134–40.

Shastri, Kashinath, and G. Chaturvedi, eds. *Charaka Samhita*. Varanasi, India: Chaukhamba Bharti Academy, 2004.

Shastri, Kaviraj Ambikadatta, ed. *Sushruta Samhita Uttaratantra; Krimirogapratishedha Adhyaya: Chapter 54 verse 19,* with "Ayurveda Tattva Sandipika." Hindi commentary, Part-II. Reprint edition. Varanasi: Chaukhambha Sanskrit Sansthan, 2012.

Sheldon, William Herbert, S. S. Stevens, and W. B. Tucker. *The Varieties of Human Physique*. New York: Harper and Brothers, 1940.

Shukla, Babita, Sumedha Saxena, Shazia Usmani, and Poonam Kushwaha. "Phytochemistry and Pharmacological Studies of Plumbago Zeylanica L.: A Medicinal Plant Review." *Clinical Phytoscience* 7 (2021): Article 34.

Singh, R. H. *The Holistic Principles of Ayurvedic Medicine*. Delhi: Chaukhambha Sanskrit Pratishtan, 2003.

Siddiqui, Saliha, and Kalpana Patni. "A Review on Ayurvedic Concept of Krimi & Its Management." *International Journal of Research in Ayurveda and Pharmacy* 9, no. 5 (2018): 19–23.

Silvertooth, E. W. "Special Relativity." *Nature* 322, no. 6080 (1986): 590.

Simard, Suzanne W., David A. Perry, Melanie D. Jones, David D. Myrold, Daniel M. Durall, and Randy Molina. "Net Transfer of Carbon between Ectomycorrhizal Tree Species in the Field." *Nature* 388 (1997): 579–582.

Slika, Layal, and Digambara Patra. "Traditional Uses, Therapeutic Effects and Recent Advances of Curcumin: A Mini-Review." *Mini-Reviews in Medicinal Chemistry* 20, no. 12 (2020): 1072–82.

Smith, Leigh K., and Emily F. Wissel. "Microbes and the Mind: How Bacteria Shape Affect, Neurological Processes, Cognition, Social Relationships, Development, and Pathology." *Perspectives on Psychological Science* 14, no. 3 (2019): 397–418.

Sombra, Lorenna Rodrigues Silva, and Catherine Anastasopoulou. "Pharmacologic Therapy for Obesity." In *StatPearls* website. Treasure Island, FL: StatPearls Publishing, 2022.

Sonpipare, Manjusha, and Yogeshwar Pandey. "Deha-Prakruti and Its Importance in Daily Life." *World Journal of Pharmaceutical Research* 10, no. 2 (2021): 293–301.

Souza, Claudineia, Raquel Rocha, and Helma Pinchemel Cotrim. "Diet and Intestinal Bacterial Overgrowth: Is There Evidence?" *World Journal of Clinical Cases* 10, no. 15 (May 2022): 4713–16.

Spence, Charles. "The Tongue Map and the Spatial Modulation of Taste Perception." *Current Research in Food Science* (March 18, 2022): 598–610.

Spence, Charles, Katsunori Okajima, Adrian David Cheok, Olivia Petit, and Charles Michel. "Eating with Our Eyes: From Visual Hunger to Digital Satiation." *Brain and Cognition* 110 (December 2016): 53–63.

Srihagulang, Chanon, Jirapong Vongsfak, Tanat Vaniyapong, Nipon Chattipakorn, and Siriporn C. Chattipakorn. "Potential Roles of Vagus Nerve Stimulation on Traumatic Brain Injury: Evidence from In Vivo and Clinical Studies." *Experimental Neurology* 347 (January 2022): Article 113887.

Srivastava, Niraj, and Varsha Saxena. "Concepts of Prakriti (Human Constitution) and Its Association with Hematological Parameters, Body Mass Index (BMI), Blood Groups and Genotypes." *Journal of Natural Remedies* 19, no. 4 (October 2019): 162–68.

Srivastava, Shikha. *Current Traditional Medicine*. Bentham Science Publishers 10, no. 3 (2024): 75–83(9).

Stamp, Rebecca. "Average Person Will Try 126 Fad Diets in Their Lifetime, Poll Claims." *The Independent*, January 8, 2020.

Stinson, Lisa F., Mary C. Boyce, Matthew S. Payne, Jeffrey A. Keelan. "The Not-so-Sterile Womb: Evidence That the Human Fetus Is Exposed to Bacteria Prior to Birth." *Frontiers in Microbiology* 10 (June 4, 2019): 1124.

Su, Xueying, Ying Lyu, Weiyi Wang, Yanfei Zhang, Danhua Li, Suning Wei, Congkuo Du, Bin Geng, Carole Sztalryd, and Guoheng Xu. "Fascia Origin of Adipose Cells." *Stem Cells* 34, no. 5 (May 2016): 1407–19.

Suba, V. "Reverse Pharmacology: A Tool for Drug Discovery from Traditional Medicine." In *Evidence Based Validation of Traditional Medicines*, edited by Subhash C. Mandal, Raja Chakraborty, and Saikat Sen, Singapore: Springer, 2021.

Subrahmanya Sastri, V. V. *Tridosha Theory, Kottakkal Ayurveda Series 18*. Kerala, India: Kottakal, 2002.

Sultan, F., L. Eduardo Cardona-Sanclemente, D. Lagrange, C. Lutton, and S. Griglio. "Lipoprotein Lipase and Hepatic Lipase Activities in a Hypercholesterolaemic (RICO) Strain of Rat. Effect of Dietary Cholesterol." *Biochemical Journal* 266, no. 2 (March 1990): 349–53.

Sun, Ying, Peijun Ju, Ting Xue, Usman Ali, Donghong Cui, and Jinghong Chen. "Alteration of Faecal Microbiota Balance Related to Long-Term Deep Meditation." *General Psychiatry* 36 (January 2023): Article e100893.

Suśruta. *An English Translation of the Sushruta Samhita: Based on Original Sanskrit Text*. 2nd ed. Translated by Kaviraj Kunja Lal Bhishagratna. Varanasi, India: Chowkhamba Sanskrit Series Office, 1963.

Svoboda, Robert. *Prakruti: Your Ayurvedic Constitution*. Twin Lakes, WI: Lotus Press, 1988.

Swami, Viren, Samantha Hochstöger, Erik Kargl, and Stefan Stieger. "Hangry in the Field: An Experience Sampling Study on the Impact of Hunger on Anger, Irritability, and Affect." *PLoS ONE* 17, no. 7 (July 2022): Article e0269629.

Szmulewicz, Alejandro, Kerollos N. Wanis, Ashley Gripper, Federico Angriman, Jeff Hawel, Ahmad Elnahas, Nawar A. Alkhamesi, and Christopher M. Schlachta. "Mental Health Quality of Life after Bariatric Surgery: A Systematic Review and Meta-analysis of Randomized Clinical Trials." *Clinical Obesity* 9, no. 11 (November 2018): Article e12290.

Tengse, V. G., M. S. Baghel, S. N. Vyas, and J. R. Joshi. "A Survey on Etiopathological Correlation of Krimi (Intestinal Helminths) and Pandu (Anemia)." *Ayu* 32, no. 2 (2011): 165–170.

Thomas, Lorette W. "The Chemical Composition of Adipose Tissue of Man and Mice." *Quarterly Journal of Experimental Physiology and Cognate Medical Sciences* 47, no. 2 (April 1962): 179–88.

Törnwall, Outi, Karri Silventoinen, Jaakko Kaprio, and Hely Tuorila. "Why Do Some Like It Hot? Genetic and Environmental Contributions to the Pleasantness of Oral Pungency." *Physiology & Behavior* 107, no. 3 (October 2012): 381–89.

Tozzi, Paolo. "Does Fascia Hold Memories?" *Journal of Bodywork and Movement Therapies* 18, no. 2 (April 2014): 259–65.

Trappe, James M. "Frank and Mycorrhizae: The Challenge to Evolutionary and Ecologic Theory." *Mycorrhiza* 15 (2005): 277–81.

Travis, Frederick T., and Robert Keith Wallace. "Dosha Brain-Types: A Neural Model of Individual Differences." *Journal of Ayurveda and Integrative Medicine* 6, no. 4 (October–December 2015): 280–85.

Turányi, Csilla Zita, Katalin Zsuzsanna Rónai, Rezső Zoller, Orsolya Véber, Mária Eszter Czira, Ákos Újszászi, Gergely László et al. "Association between Lunar Phase and Sleep Characteristics." *Sleep Medicine* 15, no. 11 (November 2014): 1411–16.

Turnbaugh, Peter J., Ruth E. Ley, Micah Hamady, Claire M. Fraser-Liggett, Rob Knight, and Jeffrey I. Gordon. "The Human Microbiome Project." *Nature* 449 (October 2007): 804–10.

Ustun, Beyza, Nadja Reissland, Judith Covey, Benoist Schaal, and Jacqueline Blissett. "Flavor Sensing in Utero and Emerging Discriminative Behaviors in the Human Fetus." *Psychological Science* 33, no. 10 (September 2022): 1651–63.

Valiathan, M. S. *The Legacy of Sushruta*. Hyderabad, India: Orient Longman, 2007.

Valiathan, M. S. *Towards Ayurvedic Biology: A Decadal Vision Document*. N. p.: Indian Academy of Sciences, 2006.

Valk, Reimara, James Hammill, and Jonas Grip. "Saturated Fat: Villain and Bogeyman in the Development of Cardiovascular Disease?" *European Journal of Preventive Cardiology* 29, no. 18 (December 2022): 2312–21.

Vandana, K. S., and P. Sudhakar Reddy. "Survey to Assess Quality of Life in Obesity in Relation to Ashtadoshas of Ati-Sthoulya and Prakriti: A Cross-Sectional Study." *International Journal of Ayurvedic and Herbal Medicine* 10, no. 1 (January–February 2020): 3718–23.

van den Munckhof, I. C. L., A. Kurilshikov, R. ter Horst, N. P. Riksen, L. A. B. Joosten, A. Zhernakova, J. Fu, S. T. Keating, M. G. Netea, J. de Graaf, and J. H. W. Rutten. "Role of Gut Microbiota in Chronic Low-Grade Inflammation as

Potential Driver for Atherosclerotic Cardiovascular Disease: A Systematic Review of Human Studies." *Obesity Reviews* 19, no. 12 (December 2018): 1719–34.

Varambally, Shivarama, and B. N. Gangadhar. "Yoga and Traditional Healing Methods in Mental Health." In *Mental Health and Illness in the Rural World*, edited by Santosh Kumar Chaturvedi, 1–12. Singapore: Springer, 2020.

Vasudeva, Neeru, Neerja Yadav, and Surendra Kumar Sharma. "Natural Products: A Safest Approach for Obesity." *Chinese Journal of Integrative Medicine* 18 (2012): 473–80.

Vidal-Puig, Antonio. "Adipose Tissue Expandability, Lipotoxicity and the Metabolic Syndrome." *Endocrine Abstracts* 50, (2013).

Vinayaka, Venkatappa, and Patil Suchitra. "Effect of Udvarthana on Obesity." *The Journal of Alternative and Complementary Medicine* 20, no. 5 (May 2014): A148.

Virtue, Sam, and Antonio Vidal-Puig. "Adipose Tissue Expandability, Lipotoxicity and the Metabolic Syndrome—An Allostatic Perspective." *Biochimica et Biophysica Acta (BBA)—Molecular Basis of Disease* 1801, no. 3 (March 2010): 338–49.

Waehler, Reinhard. "Fatty Acids: Facts vs. Fiction." *International Journal for Vitamin and Nutrition Research* 93, no. 3 (June 2023).

Walker, William H. II, James C. Walton, A. Courtney DeVries, and Randy J. Nelson. "Circadian Rhythm Disruption and Mental Health." *Translational Psychiatry* 10 (January 2020): Article 28.

Wallis, Claudia. "Your Body Has a Clever Way to Detect How Much Water You Should Drink Every Day." *Scientific American*, September 2022, 25.

Walter, Jens, Inés Martínez, and Devin J. Rose. "Holobiont Nutrition: Considering the Role of the Gastrointestinal Microbiota in the Health Benefits of Whole Grains." *Gut Microbes* 4, no. 4 (July-August 2013): 340–46.

Wang, J. et al. "Effects of Mitochondrial Dynamics in the Pathophysiology of Obesity." *Frontiers in Bioscience (Landmark)* 27, no. 3 (2022): 107.

Wansink, Brian, and Audrey Wansink. "MyPlate, Half-Plate, and No Plate: How Visual Plate-Related Dietary Benchmarks Influence What Food People Serve." *Cureus* 14, no. 5 (May 2022): Article e25231.

Warraich, Haider. "It's Time to Rethink the Origins of Pain." *Scientific American*, September 2022.

Wekerle, Hartmut. "The Gut-Brain Connection: Triggering of Brain Autoimmune Disease by Commensal Gut Bacteria." *Rheumatology* 55 (2016): ii68–75.

Welch, Claudia. *Balance Your Hormones, Balance Your Life*. Philadelphia: Da Cap Press, 2011.

Wilding, John P. H., Rachel L. Batterham, Salvatore Calanna, Melanie Davies et al. "Once-Weekly Semaglutide in Adults with Overweight or Obesity." *The New England Journal of Medicine* 384, no. 11 (March 18, 2021): 989–1002.

Wilson, Annette S., Kathryn R. Koller, Matsepo C. Ramaboli, Lucky T. Nesengani, Soeren Ocvirk, Caixia Chen, Christie A. Flanagan et al. "Diet and the Human Gut Microbiome: An International Review." *Digestive Diseases and Sciences* 65 (2020): 723–40.

Wiseman, Nigel and Andy Ellis. *Fundamentals of Chinese Medicine.* Brookline, MA: Paradigm Publications, 1985.

Wittmann, Markus, Wolfgang Schreiber, Michael Landgrebe, and Göran Hajak. "Circadian Rhythms and Depression." *Fortschritte der Neurologie-Psychiatrie* 86, no. 5 (2018): 308–18.

Woldemariam, Kalekristos Yohannes, Juanli Yuan, Zhen Wan, Qinglin Yu, Yating Cao, Huijia Mao, Yingli Liu, Jing Wang, Hongyan Li, and Baoguo Sun. "Celiac Disease and Immunogenic Wheat Gluten Peptides and the Association of Gliadin Peptides with HLA DQ2 and HLA DQ8." *Food Reviews International* 38, no. 7 (2022): 1553–76.

World Health Organization. *Benchmarks for Training in Ayurveda.* Geneva: World Health Organization, 2010.

———. *Constitution of the World Health Organization.* New York: World Health Organization, 1948.

———. "Healthy Diet." World Health Organization website, October 23, 2018.

———. "Traditional, Complementary and Integrative Medicine," World Health Organization website, 2021.

———. *WHO Global Report on Traditional and Complementary Medicine 2019.* Geneva: World Health Organization, 2019.

Wozniak, Susan E., Laura L. Gee, Mitchell S. Wachtel, and Eldo E. Frezza. "Adipose Tissue: The New Endocrine Organ? A Review Article." *Digestive Diseases and Sciences* 54 (2009): 1847–56.

Xia, Peng-Fei, Xiong-Fei Pan, Chen Chen, Yi Wang, Yi Ye, and An Pan. "Dietary Intakes of Eggs and Cholesterol in Relation to All-Cause and Heart Disease Mortality: A Prospective Cohort Study." *Journal of the American Heart Association* 9, no. 10 (2020): Article e015743.

Xia, W., P. Veeragandham, Y. Cao et al. "Obesity Causes Mitochondrial Fragmentation and Dysfunction in White Adipocytes due to Rala Activation." *Nature Metabolism* 6 (2024), 273–89.

Yang, Felix T., and Kristin I. Stanford. "Batokines: Mediators of Inter-Tissue Communication (a Mini-Review)." *Current Obesity Reports* 11 (2022): 1–9.

Yarmohammadi, Fatemeh, Soghra Mehri, Nahid Najafi, Sanaz Salar Amoli, and Hossein Hosseinzadeh. "The Protective Effect of Azadirachta Indica (Neem) Against Metabolic Syndrome: A Review." *Iranian Journal of Basic Medical Sciences* 24, no. 3 (March 2021): 280–92.

Ye, Run Zhou, Gabriel Richard, Nicolas Gévry, André Tchernof, and André C. Carpentier. "Fat Cell Size: Measurement Methods, Pathophysiological Origins, and Relationships with Metabolic Dysregulations." *Endocrine Reviews* 43, no. 1 (February 2022): 35–60.

Yee, M. S. et al. "Impact of Microplastic and Nanoplastics on Human Health." *Nanomaterials* 11 (2021): 496.

Yeung, Anthony Y., and Prasanna Tadi. *Physiology, Obesity Neurohormonal Appetite And Satiety Control*. Treasure Island, FL: StatPearls, 2022.

Young, Allan H., Mario F. Juruena, Renske De Zwaef, and Koen Demyttenaere. "Vagus Nerve Stimulation as Adjunctive Therapy in Patients with Difficult-to-Treat Depression (RESTORE-LIFE): Study Protocol Design and Rationale of a Real-World Post-Market Study." *BMC Psychiatry* 20 (2020): Article 471.

Yu, Zimin, Jia-Jia Wang, Liang-Ying Liu, Zhanjun Li, and Eddy Y. Zeng, "Drinking Boiled Tap Water Reduces Human Intake of Nanoplastics and Microplastics," *Environmental Science & Technology Letters* 11, no. 3 (2024): 273–279.

Zare, Roghayeh, Fatemeh Heshmati, Hossein Fallahzadeh, and Azadeh Nadjarzadeh. "Effect of Cumin Powder on Body Composition and Lipid Profile in Overweight and Obese Women." *Complementary Therapies in Clinical Practice* 20, no. 4 (November 2014): 297–301.

Zhang, Shumin, Jingwen Zhao, Fei Xie, Hengxun He, Lee J. Johnston, Xiaofeng Dai, Chaodong Wu, and Xi Ma. "Dietary Fiber-Derived Short-Chain Fatty Acids: A Potential Therapeutic Target to Alleviate Obesity-Related Nonalcoholic Fatty Liver Disease." *Obesity Reviews* 22, no. 11 (November 2021): Article e13316.

Zhang, Yanfei, Xueying Su, Yingyue Dong, Tongsheng Chen, Yuanyuan Zhang, Bihan Wu, Hanxiao Li et al. "Cytological and Functional Characteristics of Fascia Adipocytes in Rats: A Unique Population of Adipocytes." *Biochimica et Biophysica Acta (BBA) - Molecular and Cell Biology of Lipids* 1865, no. 2 (February 2020): Article 158585.

Zhang, Youjie, Shun Tian, Dan Zou, Hengyan Zhang, and Chen-Wei Pan. "Screen Time and Health Issues in Chinese School-Aged Children and Adolescents: A Systematic Review and Meta-Analysis." *BMC Public Health* 22 (2022): Article 810.

Zinöcker, M. K., and I. A. Lindseth. "The Western Diet-Microbiome-Host Interaction and Its Role in Metabolic Disease." *Nutrients* 10, no. 3 (2018): 365.

INDEX